Health and Healing in the Middle Ages
Volume 1

Saints, Cure-Seekers and Miraculous Healing in Twelfth-Century England

Health and Healing in the Middle Ages

Series Editors
Linda Ehrsam Voigts (University of Missouri-Kansas City)
Peregrine Horden (All Souls College, Oxford)

The subject matter of this series is interpreted broadly, from studies of health or palaeopathology at one end of the spectrum to a medical humanities approach to the history of healing at the other. It welcomes both monographs and focussed edited collections written in English, covering any centuries or geographical areas to which the term 'medieval' can be productively applied.

Enquiries about the series may be sent to Peregrine Horden (peregrine.horden@all-souls.ox.ac.uk) and Linda Voigts (voightsl@umkc.edu). Book proposals should be supported by a one-page prospectus, a brief chapter outline, and a one-page curriculum vitae.

Saints, Cure-Seekers and Miraculous Healing in Twelfth-Century England

Ruth J. Salter

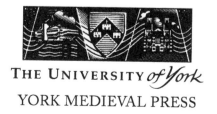

THE UNIVERSITY *of York*

YORK MEDIEVAL PRESS

First published 2021

A York Medieval Press publication
in association with The Boydell Press
an imprint of Boydell & Brewer Ltd
PO Box 9, Woodbridge, Suffolk IP12 3DF, UK
and of Boydell & Brewer Inc.
668 Mt Hope Avenue, Rochester, NY 14620–2731, USA
website: www.boydellandbrewer.com
and with the
Centre for Medieval Studies, University of York

ISBN 978 1 914049 00 2

A CIP record for this title is available
from the British Library

The publisher has no responsibility for the continued existence
or accuracy of URLs for external or third-party internet websites
referred to in this book, and does not guarantee that any content
on such websites is, or will remain, accurate or appropriate

This publication is printed on acid-free paper

To my family with my love

Contents

Illustrations

Map

Tables

Acknowledgements

This monograph was completed during the strange period that has been 2020–21, and I am incredibly grateful for the support I have received this year and throughout the research and writing of this book. This research could not have been achieved without the support of the Arts and Humanities Research Council to whom I am incredibly grateful. I also feel particularly thankful to Anne Lawrence-Mathers, Lindy Grant, Peregrine Horden and Helen Parish; all four are sources of inspiration and guidance. My thanks too to the editorial board at York Medieval Press and Boydell & Brewer for this opportunity and for the support you have all provided.

I was fortunate to undertake this research with the support of colleagues in the Department of History, the Graduate Centre for Medieval Studies, and the Centre for Health Humanities at Reading. My thanks too to colleagues and friends who are based at other universities across the UK and abroad. Your research has been inspiring and has provided me with much to think about, and you have been a source of support and friendship that I greatly cherish. I have been lucky to meet many people since I began my doctoral studies, whom I would now consider as friends. If I were to name everyone individually we would never get through the acknowledgements, but I hope you all know how much you mean to me. There are four people, however, who deserve particular recognition. So, my greatest thanks to Charlie Crouch, Harriet Mahood, Katie Phillips and Claire Trenery. You have been pillars of strength and patience and have always been there with supportive words (and caffeine) when I have needed you. Your unerring encouragement has been of the upmost importance to me during the past years. I am forever grateful that we met.

A source of continued support throughout has been my family and to them I offer my deepest gratitude. My parents, Delia and Frank, have always supported my curiosity and encouraged my love of history from an early age. I will always be grateful that you entertained my inquisitiveness and fostered my love of learning. To my sister, Claire, thank you for your support and your friendship (and your willingness to let me drag you around various medieval churches).

Abbreviations

Aimery Picaud, *Compostella*	Aimery Picaud, *The Pilgrim's Guide to Santiago de Compostela*, ed. and trans. W. Melczer (New York, 1993).
Bede, *De temporum ratione*	Bede, *The Reckoning of Time*, trans. F. Wallis, Translated Texts for Historians 29 (Liverpool, 1999).
Bede, *HE*	Bede, *Historia Ecclesiastica Gentis Anglorum*, ed. and trans. B. Colgrave and R. A. B. Mynors, OMT (Oxford, 1991).
Eadmer of Canterbury, *M. Dunstani*	Eadmer of Canterbury, *Miracula S. Dunstani*, in Eadmer of Canterbury, *Lives and Miracles of Saints Oda, Dunstan and Oswald*, ed. and trans. A. Turner and B. Muir, OMT (Oxford, 2006), pp. 160–211.
Geoffrey of Burton, *M. Moduenne*	Geoffrey of Burton, *Life and Miracles of St Modwenna*, ed. and trans. R. Bartlett, OMT (Oxford, 2002).
Gerald of Wales, *Itinerarium*	Gerald of Wales, *Itinerarium Kambriae et Descriptio Kambriae*, ed. J. F. Dimock, RS 6 (London, 1868); Gerald of Wales, *The Journey through Wales and The Description of Wales*, trans. L. Thorpe (London, 1978).
Kemp, 'The Hand of St James'	B. Kemp, 'The Miracles of the Hand of St James: Translated with an Introduction', *Berkshire Archaeological Journal* 65 (1970), 1–19.
Lanfranc, *Decreta*	Lanfranc, *Decreta Lanfranci Monachis Canturiensibus Transmissa*, in *The Monastic Constitutions of Lanfranc*, ed. and trans. D. Knowles and C. Brooke, OMT (Oxford, 2002), pp. 2–195.
L. Eliensis	*Liber Eliensis*, ed. E. Blake, Camden 3rd series 92 (London, 1962); *Liber Eliensis: A History of the Isle of Ely, from the Seventh Century to the Twelfth*, trans. J. Fairweather (Woodbridge, 2005).
L. Gilberti	*The Book of St Gilbert*, ed. and trans. R. Foreville and G. Keir, OMT (Oxford, 1987).
L. Henrici	*Leges Henrici Primi*, ed. and trans. L. Downer (Oxford, 1972).
M. Æbbe	*Vita et Miracula S. Æbbe Virginis*, in *Æbbe of Coldingham and Margaret of Scotland*, ed. and trans. R. Bartlett, OMT (Oxford, 2006), pp. 1–67.
M. Jacobi	*Miracula S. Jacobi*, Gloucester, Gloucester Cathedral Library MS 1, fols. 171va–175va.

M. Margarite	*Miracula S. Margarite Scotorum Regine*, in *Æbbe of Coldingham and Margaret of Scotland*, ed. and trans. R. Bartlett, OMT (Oxford, 2006), pp. 69–145.
M. Swithuni	*Miracula S. Swithuni*, in *The Anglo-Saxon Minsters of Winchester: The Cult of St Swithun*, ed. and trans. M. Lapidge, Winchester Studies 4.ii (Oxford, 2003), pp. 641–97.
ODNB	*Oxford Dictionary of National Biography* (Oxford, 2004), <https://www.oxforddnb.com/> [accessed 24 July 2020].
ODS	*The Oxford Dictionary of Saints*, ed. D. H. Farmer (Oxford, 1978).
OEH	*The Old English Herbarium*, in A. Van Ardsall, *Medieval Herbal Remedies: The Old English Herbarium and Anglo-Saxon Medicine* (New York, 2002), pp. 119–230.
OMT	Oxford Medieval Texts.
Reading Abbey Cartularies	*Reading Abbey Cartularies. British Library Manuscripts: Egerton 3031, Harley 1708 and Cotton Vespasian E xxv*, ed. B. Kemp, Camden 4th series 31, 33, 2 vols (London, 1986–87).
Reginald of Durham, *B. Cuthberti*	Reginald of Durham, *Libellus de Admirandis Beati Cuthberti Virtutibus quae novellis Patratæ sunt Temporibus*, ed. J. Raine, Surtees Society 1 (London, 1835).
Regularis Concordia	*Regularis Concordia: Anglicae Nationis Monachrum Sanctimonialiumque. The Monastic Agreement of the Monks and Nuns of the English Nations*, ed. and trans. T. Symons, Medieval Classics (London, 1953).
Regula S. Benedicti	*The Rule of St Benedict: In Latin with an English Translation*, ed. and trans. J. McCann (Tunbridge Wells, 1969).
RS	Rolls Series.
Thomas of Monmouth, *M. Willelmi*	Thomas of Monmouth, *The Life and Miracles of St William of Norwich*, ed. and trans. A. Jessop and M. R. James (Cambridge, 1896).
Thomas Walsingham, *C. Albani*	Thomas Walsingham, *Chronica Monasterii S. Albani: Gesta Abbatum Monasterii Sancti Albani*, ed. H. Riley, 3 vols, RS 28 (London, 1867).
VCH	Victoria County History.

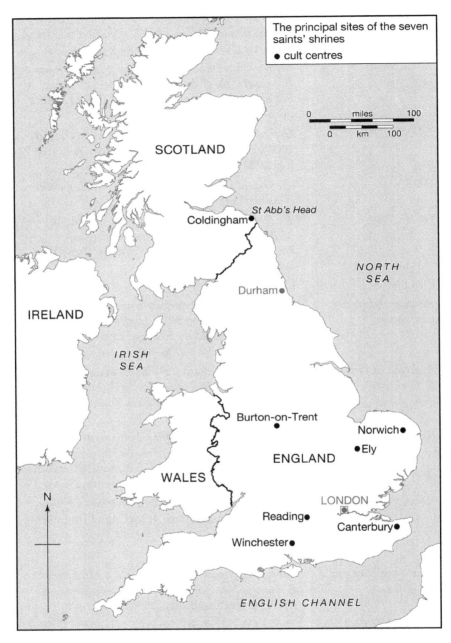

The principal sites of the seven saints' shrines

Introduction

The events at curative shrines are worthy of study because they provide a glimpse of the behaviour of medieval people at centres of popular religion and an indication of what sorts of people are involved. They illuminate many aspects of the beliefs of the Middle Ages in a way that other historical sources [. . .] cannot do.[1]

Ronald Finucane's statement, above, eloquently summarises a point at the heart of this current work. Hagiographies, and particularly the records of posthumous miracles (recorded in *miracula*), provide fascinating insight into lay religion and practices of belief.[2] The *miracula*, in their recording of the healing miracles that came about through saintly intercession, also reveal one aspect of the broad spectrum of medieval medical care that was available. Holy healing was a form of healthcare that stood alongside the various forms of worldly medical treatment. What sets miraculous healing apart, of course, is the divine source that was perceived to bring about cure. As Eamon Duffy commented, the saints were seen 'not primarily as exemplars or soul-friends, but as powerful helpers and healers in time of need', whether that was spiritual or, as is pertinent here, physical.[3] *Miracula*, albeit compiled by churchmen, provide unique insights into the practices and experiences of miraculous cure-seeking. These cure-seekers came to the saints with a variety of health complaints, but all with the faith that their petitions could bring about their desired healing.

---

[1]   R. C. Finucane, *Miracles and Pilgrims: Popular Beliefs in Medieval England* (London, 1995), p. 14.

[2]   I use 'lay' rather than 'popular' religion to denote everyday beliefs held by both laypeople and churchmen. For discussion regarding elite and 'popular' religion see: P. Brown, *The Cult of Saints: Its Rise and Function in Latin Christianity*, 2nd edn (Chicago, 2015); S. Yarrow, 'Narrative, Audience and the Negotiation of Community in Twelfth-Century English Miracle Collections', in *Elite and Popular Religion*, ed. K. Cooper and J. Gregory, Studies in Church History 42 (Woodbridge, 2006), pp. 65–77.

[3]   E. Duffy, *The Stripping of the Altars: Traditional Religion in England, c.1400–c.1580*, 2nd edn (New Haven, 2005), p. 178.

This book is an in-depth study of experiences of miraculous healing and the cure-seeking process through the lens of Latin miracle accounts produced in England during the twelfth century. It considers the practices involved in seeking and gaining miraculous healing (as portrayed in twelfth-century English hagiography) and analyses both the cure-seekers and their experiences of a cure. A central theme is the extent to which holy healing was perceived to exist within the broader medieval medical sphere. In short, how did cure-seekers experience the cure-seeking processes they underwent, and how was health-care presented within the hagiographical sources produced in England during this century?

The cults of saints are a recognised feature of the medieval Church. That there were individuals who were marked out for virtue and piety, and who continued to have an impact upon the temporal world posthumously, was taken as a given by both the Church and lay devotees.[4] Following the archetype of Christ in the Gospels, saints were understood to be capable of bringing about miraculous events, from saving ships from storms at sea to returning sight to the blind, and even reviving the recently deceased. Saints acted as guardians and patrons of religious communities which were the custodians of their shrines, but they also acted on behalf of those secular persons – regardless of age, gender, or social status – who had faith in their abilities. Some saints were martyrs, others confessors, and others still had questionable or tenuous claims to their sanctity.[5] Two elements were crucial: the faith placed in a saint by believers; and the ability of a saint, especially after death, to exert power across geographical and physical boundaries.[6] As a channel for God's power, a saint could intervene on behalf of God in the physical state of living humans. Often this took the form of providing miraculous healing, with the saint assuming the role of protective guardian and 'saintly physician'.

This book brings together studies of healthcare and pilgrimage to address questions relating to the ways that cure-seeking was understood, practised, and, importantly, experienced in twelfth-century England. Seven case-study *miracula*, detailed below, provide an in-depth insight into the cure-seeking process. The questions raised in the following chapters are deliberately focused on matter-of-fact issues, such as 'what complaints were the saints seen to be capable of curing?' Despite their apparent simplicity, questions about the basic practices and practicalities of miraculous cure-seeking often go unanswered.

---

4   R. Bartlett, *Why Can the Dead Do Such Great Things? Saints and Worshippers from the Martyrs to the Reformation* (Princeton, 2013), p. 37.

5   For further discussion of sanctity, its perception and definition, see A. Vauchez, *Sainthood in the Later Middle Ages*, trans. J. Birell (Cambridge, 1997), pp. 141–4.

6   Bartlett, *Why Can the Dead Do Such Great Things?*, p. 103.

Yet exploring these aspects is crucial to developing a greater understanding, and appreciation, of the processes involved in miraculous healing and of those who interacted with the saints and their representatives.

To achieve this, this book asks the following questions. Where did miracle cures fit within wider medical practices, and what knowledge did the monastic communities that housed the saints' shrines have of medicine? What ailments did saintly intercession cure, how were the afflictions described, and what does this reveal of the place of holy healing? Who were the cure-seeking pilgrims at the centre of these miracles, and what does their hagiographical presence suggest of wider practices of cure-seeking? Where did the cure-seekers come from? Was this a case of 'local cults for local people', or were the saints drawing in crowds from further afield? Practically speaking, how did the cure-seekers make their way to the shrines, what can be learnt of their travel experiences? And what could a cure-seeker expect on arriving at the shrine? Would they be welcomed by the monastic community or was their experience and engagement with these religious spaces limited? Combined, the answers to these questions reveal what was expected, accepted, and experienced of the process of seeking and securing a miraculous cure for bodily ill health.

The 'renaissance' of the long twelfth century has been recognised as a period of great change. This was a time in which papal control began to tighten over various aspects of the Church, including the process of canonisation.[7] This was also a point at which there was a cultural shift which saw the rise in the transmission and dissemination of translated Greek and Arabic works, and the development of the universities. In this century of change, the cults of the saints and their devotees, as recorded within the miracles, provide a point of entry into understanding practical processes and experiences of healing at a crucial point within English, and indeed Western, history. This period of English history is thus an important one for investigating miraculous healing.

Within this current work, the focus of these questions is on seven cults that were based within monastic, rather than secular, churches. The decision behind this was twofold. The first consideration was that the cults chosen, as discussed below, were established at a range of monastic institutions from across England and from great cathedral priories to small, more provincial, abbeys. Unifying these sites, despite their relative institutional independence, is the

---

[7] C. H. Haskins, *The Renaissance of the Twelfth Century* (Cambridge, MA, 1927), pp. 6–7. Also see C. Burnett, 'The Twelfth-Century Renaissance', in *The Cambridge History of Science. Volume 2: Medieval Science*, ed. D. C. Lindberg and M. H. Shank (Cambridge, 2013), pp. 365–84.

monastic emphasis on charity and hospitality, especially to the poor and pilgrims.[8] These ideals, considered in Chapter 6, had the potential for particularly
strong relationships to develop between the monastic community and local lay
cure-seekers who sought their, and their saints', aid. The second reason for this
focus was, admittedly, one of practicality. While there were secular cathedrals
in England, and while these institutions did champion the cults of their own
saints, this post-Conquest period was one in which monastic centres particularly thrived with revived interest in the cults of saints.[9] As noted, following
the Norman Conquest of 1066 there was a notable increase in hagiographical
production. With the arrival of new, Norman church leaders, the Benedictine
monasteries, in particular, were keen to celebrate their Anglo-Saxon saints
in the face of potential Norman scepticism.[10] As the post-Conquest period
settled into the twelfth century, a number of new and 'rediscovered' saints' cults
developed, further adding to the English cure-seeking scene. The 'vogue' for
bishop-saints, such as William of York (York Minster), emerged in the later
twelfth century and developed notably in the following centuries.[11]

The reinvigorated monastic interest at this time is also reflected in the pro-
liferation of hagiographic materials for such cults. Indeed, as Simon Yarrow
commented, the Benedictine monasteries dominated during this 'boom time'
of producing miracle collections following the Norman Conquest.[12] Secular
cults were not without twelfth-century mention. William of Malmesbury, for
instance, mentions Earconwald (London), Æthelbert (Hereford) and Chad
(Lichfield) in *Gesta Pontificum Anglorum* (*c.* 1125), alongside monastic saints
such as Cuthbert (Durham).[13] Arcoid's *Miracula S. Erkenwaldi Londoniensis
episcopi* (*c.* 1141) survives, abridged, in a later twelfth-century *Vitae Sanctorum*

[8]   *The Rule of St Benedict: In Latin with an English Translation* (hereafter *Regula
      S. Benedicti*), 36, ed. and trans. J. McCann (Tunbridge Wells, 1969), pp. 90–1.
[9]   P. Turner, 'Places of Worship in Britain and Ireland 1150–1350: An Introduction',
      in *Places of Worship in Britain and Ireland 1150–1350*, ed. P. S. Barnwell, Rewley
      House Studies in the Historic Environment 7 (Donington, 2018), pp. 1–9 (7–8).
      Also see: A. Clifton-Taylor, *The Cathedrals of England* (London, 1967), pp. 15–17;
      C. Daniell, *Atlas of Medieval Britain* (London, 2011), map 82, p. 92.
[10] S. Yarrow, *Saints and Their Communities: Miracle Stories in Twelfth-Century England*,
      Oxford Historical Monographs (Oxford, 2006), pp. 4–5.
[11] Turner, 'Places of Worship in Britain and Ireland 1150–1350', p. 8.
[12] Yarrow, 'Narrative, Audience and the Negotiation of Community', p. 68.
[13] William of Malmesbury, *Gesta Pontificum Anglorum* II.73.10–11, IV.170.1–2,
      IV.172.1, ed. R. M. Thomson and M. Winterbottom, 2 vols, OMT (Oxford, 2007)
      I, 226–9, 462–3, 464–5.

compilation.[14] However, the majority of hagiographical materials produced in Latin in England during the twelfth century relate to monastic cults, thus making these ideal for this current study of healing miracles. Future research, however, incorporating the surviving sources for the cults at secular cathedrals, would surely prove profitable.

Seven saints for whom hagiographies were compiled within twelfth-century England act as the central *miracula* for this current work.[15] These saints, and their associated cults, are spread geographically across England (from Winchester Cathedral Priory in the south to Coldingham Priory in the Scottish Borders), they come from a variety of monastic institutions (from smaller, rural monasteries to prominent, urban cathedral priories), and the dates of their hagiographies range across the century. Importantly, the case studies were selected specifically for the fact that they do not contain large volumes of cure-seekers and, as Chapter 4 reveals, these were cults primarily focused on localised care. In contrast to previous studies, such as those of Finucane, this one concentrates on a select, smaller group of miracle cures, allowing it to provide an attentive analysis of the cure-seeking pilgrims and their experiences. This localised focus also provides the opportunity to gain a familiarity with the individual cure-seekers and the cults they appealed to. What follows here is a brief introduction to each of the saints: Swithun, Dunstan, Æthelthryth, Modwenna, William of Norwich, Æbbe, and James the Greater (listed here in chronological order of their twelfth-century *miracula*'s production).

Three of the saints, Swithun, Dunstan, and Æthelthryth, had cults that were established prior to the twelfth century and for which their twelfth-century hagiographies were an addition to earlier productions of *vita* (life) and *miracula*.

A renowned saint, Swithun's (d. 863) cult at Winchester Cathedral Priory, and prior to the twelfth century Winchester Old Minster, was well-established.[16] Having spent his monastic career at Winchester, as bishop of the diocese for the last decade of his life, Swithun's connection to Winchester

[14] Cambridge, Corpus Christi College, MS 161, fols. 33r–45v; G. Whatley, '*Vita Erkenwaldi:* An Anglo-Norman's Life of an Anglo-Saxon Saint', *Manuscripta* 27 (1983), 67–81 (67); G. Whatley, 'Heathens and Saints: St Erkenwald in Its Legendary Context', *Speculum* 61 (1986), 330–63 (358 n. 85).

[15] I have used and cited published translations (where available) of the texts on which this book is based. On occasion, however, as indicated in the footnotes, to be more faithful to the Latin I have provided my own translation. Details of the published editions and translations for the seven *miracula* follow below.

[16] D. Knowles and R. N. Hadcock, *Medieval Religious Houses: England and Wales*, 2nd edn (London, 1971), p. 81; *A History of the County of Hampshire: Volume 2*, ed. H. A. Doubleday and W. Page, VCH (London, 1903), pp. 108–15.

was undisputed. Yet, despite being a highly regarded churchman, his fame comes from his posthumous miracle workings.[17] Following the arrival of Winchester's first post-Conquest bishop, Walkelin, work began on the Norman cathedral in 1079. The new church was consecrated in 1093, and Swithun's shrine was translated from the adjacent Old Minster into the new cathedral on his feast day, 15 July.[18] The production of Swithun's twelfth-century hagiography followed relatively quickly. The *Miracula S. Swithuni*, and accompanying *Vita S. Swithuni*, were produced by an unnamed Winchester monk at the beginning of the twelfth century.[19] *M. Swithuni*'s author built on a number of earlier editions of Swithun's hagiography, but the production of a new pair of hagiographies was clearly seen as necessary. The new *vita* and *miracula* marked the transition to the new cathedral and to a Norman-led community, while emphasising the longevity of Swithun's cult and the continued importance of Winchester as a pilgrimage location in the south of England.

Dunstan (d. 988) was also an Anglo-Saxon bishop and archbishop. Prior to Thomas Becket's murder (1170), he was Canterbury Cathedral's principal saint. Unlike Swithun, he is better remembered for his role in reforming the English Church than his posthumous career as miracle-giver.[20] While not a lone figure in the tenth-century reforms, Dunstan was influential in their implementation. Dunstan had risen quickly through the Church, holding several important positions, ultimately being appointed Archbishop of Canterbury Cathedral in 959. Following his death, Dunstan was rapidly added to liturgical calendars, achieving widespread veneration.[21] In the late eleventh century, however, his cult saw a series of setbacks. On 6 December 1067, a fire at Christ Church destroyed many of the priory buildings including the cathedral church. Following the fire, a temporary building was erected over the tomb of St Dunstan where the monastic community could say mass and perform their daily services. Dunstan continued to perform miracles in these tumultuous circumstances, as recorded in Eadmer of Canterbury's *Miracula S.*

---

[17] 'Swithun (Swithin) (d. 862)', in *The Oxford Dictionary of Saints* (hereafter *ODS*), ed. D. H. Farmer (Oxford, 1978), p. 365.

[18] J. Crook, *English Medieval Shrines*, Boydell Studies in Art and Architecture (Woodbridge, 2011), p. 125.

[19] *Miracula S. Swithuni* (hereafter *M. Swithuni*), in *The Anglo-Saxon Minsters of Winchester: The Cult of St Swithun*, ed. and trans. M. Lapidge, Winchester Studies 4.ii (Oxford, 2003), pp. 641–97; *Vita S. Swithuni Episcopi et Confessoris*, in *The Anglo-Saxon Minsters of Winchester: The Cult of St Swithun*, ed. and trans. M. Lapidge, Winchester Studies 4.ii (Oxford, 2003), pp. 611–39.

[20] 'Dunstan (909–88)', in *ODS*, pp. 111–13.

[21] Ibid., p. 113.

Dunstani, produced *c*. 1115.[22] Lanfranc's arrival to the archiepiscopate of Canterbury, in 1070, had seen the beginning of an extensive building project that resulted in Dunstan being translated to a new place of burial in the west of the church.[23] Under Anselm, Lanfranc's successor, and following the rebuilding, Dunstan was returned to a prominent position next to the high altar by the time Eadmer compiled *M. Dunstani*.[24]

Æthelthryth (d. 679) is one of the better-known female Anglo-Saxon saints. Her prominence at her cult centre in Ely certainly outshines the cathedral's three other Anglo-Saxon royal saints: her sisters, Seaxburh and Wihtburh; and her niece, Eormenhild. Æthelthryth was not initially destined for the Church and was married twice before becoming a nun.[25] According to the *Liber Eliensis*, Æthelthryth's first husband, Tondberht of Southern Gyrwe, gave her the Isle of Ely as a marriage-gift, and both husband and wife were devoted to chastity.[26] After Tondberht's death, Æthelthryth was married to Ecgfrith, son of King Oswiu of Northumbria. This marriage was decidedly less amicable, with Ecgfrith unwilling to accept his wife's chastity.

By the time Ecgfrith succeeded his father, in 670, Æthelthryth had gained the support of Wilfrid of Hexham, an influential figure in regional politics, who supported Æthelthryth's continued chastity.[27] Through Wilfrid's assistance, Æthelthryth was eventually granted leave to enter into a monastery, and she joined the double monastery at *Coludi urbs* under the abbacy of Æbbe,

---

[22] Eadmer of Canterbury, *Miracula S. Dunstani* (hereafter *M. Dunstani*) 14–15, in Eadmer of Canterbury, *Lives and Miracles of Saints Oda, Dunstan and Oswald*, ed. and trans. A. Turner and B. Muir, OMT (Oxford, 2006), pp. 160–211 (170–7).

[23] Ibid., pp. 176–9.

[24] Gervase of Canterbury, *Instructio nouiciorum* 'Of Terce and its psalms', in *The Monastic Constitutions of Lanfranc*, ed. and trans. D. Knowles and C. Brooke, OMT (Oxford, 2002), pp. 197–221 (212–13); J. Rubenstein, 'Liturgy against History: The Competing Visions of Lanfranc and Eadmer of Canterbury', *Speculum* 74 (1999), 279–309 (289–90).

[25] 'Etheldreda (Æthelthryth, Ediltrudis, Audrey) (d. 679)', in *ODS*, p. 138.

[26] *Liber Eliensis* (hereafter *L. Eliensis*) I.4, ed. E. Blake, Camden 3rd series 92 (London, 1962), pp. 14–15; *Liber Eliensis: A History of the Isle of Ely, from the Seventh Century to the Twelfth* (hereafter *L. Eliensis*) I.4, trans. J. Fairweather (Woodbridge, 2005), pp. 16–18. It should be noted that Blake's edition provides the Latin text for *L. Eliensis*, and Fairweather provides a modern translation. All further references to *L. Eliensis* include both texts unless the citation is specific to only one publication.

[27] Bede, *Historia Ecclesiastica Gentis Anglorum* (hereafter *HE*) IV.19, ed. and trans. B. Colgrave and R. A. B. Mynors, OMT (Oxford, 1991), pp. 392–3; *L. Eliensis* I.9, ed. Blake, pp. 23–5, trans. Fairweather, pp. 28–31.

Ecgfrith's aunt.[28] A year later, Æthelthryth departed and founded a monastery at Ely, where she was abbess for seven years before her death. Æthelthryth's sister, and successor, Seaxburh, later translated the sarcophagus into the church, marking the first time Æthelthryth's tomb was opened to reveal that her body lay incorrupt.[29] In 1106, Æthelthryth's relics, along with those of her sisters and niece, were translated into new shrines in the reconstructed choir. Æthelthryth was placed in a position of honour to the east of the high altar.[30] L. Eliensis, composed c. 1130–80, includes insights into the recent history of Ely that the author, an unknown Ely monk, seemingly experienced first-hand. The majority of L. Eliensis's chronicling can be found in the second of the three books, with books one and three constituting a vita and miracula for Æthelthryth.

Æthelthryth is one of three female saints in the case-study cults. The other two, Modwenna and Æbbe, were similarly Anglo-Saxon abbesses. However, unlike Æthelthryth, both saints appear to have been 'rediscovered' in the eleventh century, with their cults only becoming established in the twelfth century.

Modwenna's identity is somewhat obscure, yet by the twelfth century a connection had been made between Modwenna at Burton-on-Trent and St Moninne, founder of Killevy, Ireland (d. 571).[31] When and how this affiliation came about is unclear; however, Conchubranus's Vita S. Monenna (made at or for Burton's community in the early twelfth century), records that Monenna was rewarded with a grant of land in the Forest of Arden after curing the son of an English king.[32] Conchubranus recorded that Monenna was later buried on the island of Andressey, in the Trent, near Burton.[33] Modwenna, as recorded in Abbot Geoffrey of Burton's Vita et Miracula S. Moduenne Uirginis, was later translated into the abbey church, where her cult developed.[34]

---

[28] Bede, HE IV.19, ed. Colgrave and Mynors, pp. 392–3.

[29] Ibid.

[30] L. Eliensis II.144, ed. Blake, pp. 228–30, trans. Fairweather, pp. 275–8.

[31] R. Bartlett, 'Moninne (d. 517)', in Oxford Dictionary of National Biography (hereafter ODNB) (Oxford, 2004), <https://doi.org/10.1093/ref:odnb/18869> [accessed 24 June 2020].

[32] Conchubranus, Vita S. Monenna, in 'The Life of St Monenna by Conchubranus, Part I', I.14–15, ed. and trans. Ulster Society for Medieval Latin Studies, Seanchas Ardmhacha 9 (1979), 250–73 (268–73).

[33] Conchubranus, Vita S. Monenna, in 'The Life of St Monenna by Conchubranus. Part III', III.3, III.11, ed. and trans. Ulster Society for Medieval Latin Studies, Seanchas Ardmhacha 10 (1982), 426–54 (432–5, 444–7).

[34] Geoffrey of Burton, Life and Miracles of St Modwenna (hereafter M. Moduenne) 43, ed. and trans. R. Bartlett, OMT (Oxford, 2002), pp. 180–3.

This translation had occurred shortly after the foundation of Burton Abbey (*c.* 1004).[35] Abbot Geoffrey, who took over the abbacy in 1114, had previously been prior at Winchester Cathedral Priory.[36] Geoffrey, coming from an established cult centre, was keen to develop Modwenna's cult. To achieve this, he not only produced *M. Moduenne, c.* 1118–35, but also began a major building project and translated Modwenna's tomb to a more prestigious location.[37] *M. Moduenne* comprises a *vita* and *miracula* of unequal length. The *vita* was based upon Conchubranus's earlier hagiography, while the *miracula* recorded events that occurred after Burton's foundation, including a number of miracles that resulted from the rebuilding of Burton's abbey church.[38] The final miracle in *M. Moduenne*, that of a French penitent freed of his iron bonds and healed of the wounds they inflicted, was added to *M. Moduenne* by Prior Jordan shortly after the abbot's death, and is the only miracle in the collection not written by Geoffrey.[39]

Æbbe, previously mentioned regarding Æthelthryth's progression into the Church, founded her double monastery, *Coludi urbs,* in the late seventh century. Æbbe's monastery was situated overlooking the North Sea on Kirk Hill at St Abb's Head, Berwickshire, or at least this was the identified location in the high Middle Ages.[40] Æbbe's death (d. *c.* 683) had been followed by the divine destruction of her monastery following the improper behaviour of the inhabitants.[41] However, Æbbe herself was not named directly in the critique of the monastery, allowing her posthumous identity to remain untarnished by the downfall of *Coludi urbs.* Æbbe appears to have been forgotten about until the eleventh-century relic-collector Ælfred reportedly brought certain of her relics to Durham Cathedral Priory.[42] The most important development

---

[35] *A History of the County of Staffordshire: Volume 3,* ed. M. W. Greenslade and R. B. Pugh, VCH (London, 1970), pp. 199–213.

[36] Geoffrey of Burton, *M. Moduenne,* ed. Bartlett, p. xi.

[37] Ibid., pp. xi–xii, xxx.

[38] Ibid., 50, pp. 210–11.

[39] Ibid., 51, pp. 216–19. It should be noted that this last account is referred to here as '51', although it is presented unnumbered in Bartlett's edition of the hagiography.

[40] R. J. Salter, 'Memory, Myth, and Creating the Cult of St Æbbe of Coldingham', *Journal of Medieval Monastic Studies* 9 (2020), 31–49; R. J. Salter, 'Beyond the *Miracula*: Practices and Experiences of Lay Devotion at the Cult of St Æbbe, Coldingham', in *Northern Lights. New Directions in Late Medieval Insular Sanctity,* ed. C. Whitehead et al. (Turnhout, forthcoming).

[41] Bede, *HE* IV.25, ed. Colgrave and Mynors, pp. 420–7.

[42] Symeon of Durham, *Libellus de exordio atque procursu istius, hoc est Dunhelmensis ecclesie. Tract on the Origins and Progress of this the Church of Durham* III.7, ed. and trans. D. Rollason, OMT (Oxford, 2000), pp. 160–7.

in Æbbe's cult, however, proceeded from Durham's establishment of a daughter-house at Coldingham on land granted to them by Edgar of Scotland (d. 1107).[43] During the twelfth century, Æbbe's tomb was rediscovered at Kirk Hill, and the sarcophagus was translated to Coldingham Priory church. The specific date for this is not clear, but the anonymous *Vita et Miracula S. Æbbe Virginis*, compiled *c.* 1190–1200, described the translation in its third book.[44] The building of an oratory at Kirk Hill followed in 1188. A local layman, Henry, constructed the initial oratory, but the monks of Coldingham soon replaced this with a larger, more suitable structure.[45] The two-site location here is unusual, and is discussed further in Chapter 6.

The final two *miracula* that this book focuses on relate to two saints' cults which were new to the twelfth century: that of the young martyr William of Norwich (d. 1144), and that of St James the Greater whose cult developed at the twelfth-century foundation of Reading Abbey.

William had supposedly been murdered by Norwich's Jewish community.[46] His hagiography, *Vita et Passio S. Willelmi Martyris Norwicensis*, composed by Thomas of Monmouth, is the sole source for contemporary information about William's life and cult.[47] In 1140/41, aged eight or nine, William became an apprentice to a skinner in Norwich and, allegedly, became acquainted with the city's Jewish community.[48] On the Monday before Easter 1144, William and an unnamed messenger visited his mother to request her permission for

[43]   Salter, 'Memory, Myth, and Creating the Cult of St Æbbe', 36.
[44]   *Vita et Miracula S. Æbbe Virginis* (hereafter *M. Æbbe*) III, in *The Miracles of St Æbbe of Coldingham and St Margaret of Scotland*, ed. and trans. R. Bartlett, OMT (Oxford, 2006), pp. 1–67 (22–7).
[45]   *M. Æbbe* III, ed. and trans Bartlett, pp. 26–31.
[46]   For discussion of William and Norwich's Jewish community, see G. Bennett, 'William of Norwich and the Expulsion of the Jews', *Folklore* 116 (2005), 311–14; G. I. Langmuir, 'Thomas of Monmouth: Detector of Ritual Murder', *Speculum* 39 (1984), 820–46; V. D. Lipman, *The Jews of Medieval Norwich* (London, 1967); J. M. McCulloch, 'Jewish Ritual Murder: William of Norwich, Thomas of Monmouth, and the Early Dissemination of the Myth', *Speculum* 72 (1997), 698–740; C. Roth, *A History of the Jews in England*, 3rd edn (Oxford, 1964); M. Rubin, 'Making a Martyr: William of Norwich and the Jews', *History Today* 60 (2010), 48–54.
[47]   Thomas of Monmouth, *The Life and Miracles of St William of Norwich* (hereafter *M. Willelmi*), ed. and trans. A. Jessop and M. R. James (Cambridge, 1896). For a recent translation of this work see Thomas of Monmouth, *The Life and Passion of St William of Norwich*, trans. M. Rubin (London, 2014). This current work cites the 1896 edition of *M. Willelmi* as this contains the Latin text.
[48]   Thomas of Monmouth, *M. Willelmi* I.3, ed. Jessop and James, pp. 14–16.

William to join the kitchens of the archdeacon.[49] Supposedly, William was taken to the Jewry the following day, murdered on Maundy Thursday, and taken to Thorpe Wood, two miles east of Norwich, on Good Friday.[50] His body was found the next day and was buried in the wood on the Monday.[51] In the following week, William's uncle, the priest Godwin Sturt, accused the Jewish community of murder and, following a synod at which the Sheriff of Norwich protected the accused, the Jewish community were forced to retreat to Norwich castle.[52] On 24 April 1144, William was translated to the monks' cemetery at Norwich Cathedral resulting in the first miracles to be performed.[53] He was further translated four more times, as is further discussed in Chapter 6. Thomas of Monmouth, whose fervent interest in developing the cult is visible in *M. Willelmi*, was key to most of these translations. Thomas of Monmouth, who arrived in Norwich *c.* 1150, quickly adopted the role of William's shrine-keeper. He did this with seemingly little competition from the rest of the community. *M. Willelmi* was written in stages: the majority was compiled during the 1150s, shortly after Thomas's arrival, with additions in the 1170s; the final miracle was explicitly dated to 1172.[54]

The apostolic St James the Greater might have been one of the earliest saints, but Reading Abbey was a twelfth-century foundation.[55] Founded by Henry I in 1121, a year after the death of his only legitimate son in the White Ship Disaster, the abbey remained a focus of royal interest and patronage throughout its duration. Despite this prestige, Reading's cult did not gain major international renown; that honour was already held by Santiago de Compostela, Spain. The cult developed by Reading Abbey did not dispute the claims of Santiago regarding the location of James's body. What Reading possessed was 'the hand' of the saint, which had, apparently, been detached from James's body prior to his translation to Galicia.[56] The tradition of Reading's hand was that it had been in the possession of the German Emperors before being brought back to England by Matilda, daughter of Henry I,

---

[49] Ibid., I.4, pp. 16–19.

[50] Ibid., I.5–9, pp. 19–32.

[51] Ibid., I.10–15, pp. 32–42.

[52] Ibid., I.16, pp. 43–9.

[53] Ibid., I.17–19, pp. 49–55; Yarrow, *Saints and Their Communities*, p. 124.

[54] Thomas of Monmouth, *M. Willelmi* VII.19, ed. Jessop and James, p. 289.

[55] 'James the Great (d. 44)', in *ODS*, pp. 207–8.

[56] B. Taylor, 'The Hand of St James', *Berkshire Archaeological Journal* 75 (1994–97), 97–102 (97–8).

following the death of her first husband, Emperor Henry V.[57] The relic had come to the royal treasury of Germany following the death of Adalbert, bishop of Hamburg-Bremen, in 1072, who had, himself, received 'the arm' of St James from Vitalis, a bishop in Venice.[58] That this relic has been referred to as both 'arm' and 'hand' adds some validation to its apparent discovery in the ruins of Reading Abbey during building work in the eighteenth century. Now kept in St Peter's Catholic Church, Marlow, it includes the wrist bone and certain sinews which would have connected the wrist to the ulna and radius. That this hand was truly that of St James is highly unlikely, but there is a strong argument to be made for this being the relic belonging to Reading Abbey; a left hand is depicted in a seal of 1239, thus being comparable to the rediscovered mummified hand.[59] The miracle collection compiled at Reading in the later twelfth century survives only in one manuscript dating to the early thirteenth century which is now in Gloucester Cathedral's library.[60] When translating *Miracula S. Jacobi*, Brian Kemp referred to the survival of this *miracula* as 'a happy accident of fortune'.[61]

When using *miracula* it is important to recognise that, as with any source material, certain challenges must be identified. Further discussion follows in this introduction on my own approach to analysing the miracle accounts, but when discussing the case-study cults it is important to raise the issue of reading *miracula* as a source. Our twelfth-century *miracula* followed in a long tradition of recording posthumous miracles that dates back to the fifth century, with all such literature being inspired by Christ's miracles in the Gospels.[62] As Véronique Thouroude has noted, this was a 'highly conservative' form of literature in this manner, and Robert Bartlett commented on the 'stereotyped nature' of these short narratives.[63] Nevertheless, while *miracula* follow certain

---

[57] Ibid., 98.

[58] Ibid.

[59] Ibid., 100–1.

[60] *Miracula S. Jacobi* (hereafter *M. Jacobi*), in Gloucester, Gloucester Cathedral Library, MS 1, fols. 171va–175va.

[61] B. Kemp, '*The Miracles of the Hand of St James*: Translated with an Introduction', *Berkshire Archaeological Journal* 65 (1970), 1–19. Kemp's translation provides the modern English text for *M. Jacobi*, while the manuscript is used for the Latin (the transcription of which is my own). All references to *M. Jacobi* include references to both texts unless the citation is specific to only one publication.

[62] Bartlett, *Why Can the Dead Do Such Great Things?*, pp. 22–6.

[63] V. Thouroude, 'Sickness, Disability, and Miracle Cures: Hagiography in England, *c.*700–*c.*1200' (unpublished doctoral thesis, University of Oxford, 2015), p. 4; R. Bartlett, 'Medieval Miracle Accounts as Stories', *Irish Theological Quarterly* 82 (2017), 113–27 (114).

well-established structural and narrative conventions, the specific contents of the miracle accounts are diverse.[64] This is a genre with strong biblical and literary legacies, and these undoubtedly influenced twelfth-century writings and readings of *miracula*. That said, miracle accounts also include circumstantial details that reflect the contemporary world of their authors, and the cure-seekers whose experiences are represented in the reports. These circumstantial details are reflective of contemporary understandings of, and interactions with, the saints. To appeal to a contemporary audience these accounts needed to present plausible reflections of the experiences of cure-seekers, even if not all those who sought saintly aid were as successful in securing it as those recorded within these miracle collections.

These details, naturally, are of key interest to this current work yet we must recognise that here we are still faced with a refined record of the event. The details recorded are those details which were seen as worth recording for prosperity.[65] Hilary Powell, in her re-evaluation of the influence 'folklore' had on Anglo-Latin hagiographies, includes a thoughtful assessment of the genre and those who engaged with, and were represented within, these materials.[66] Powell argues that reading miracles requires taking a 'holistic approach' and recognising that these narratives are 'cultural products' reflective of their moment of creation.[67] *Miracula* are not historical texts but nor, despite being narrative, are they fictional; rather they are representative of both long-held patterns of Christian belief and contemporary world views. Acknowledging this makes it possible to use the details provided within the accounts to tease out the experiences of healing miracles. Attentive reading of these sources can prove rewarding, as is well reflected in the research produced in the last sixty years, with analysis of *miracula* resulting in productive, nuanced research into the cults of the saints and those who sought holy healing.

This current work sits within two distinct, although undoubtedly correlating, fields with medieval healthcare and medieval saints' cults brought together in this study on miraculous healing. Both areas of research have become prominent within medieval studies, with both often taking on a social or cultural focus. Within this introduction it would not be feasible to provide a full historiographical discourse on both elements, nor would it be fair to focus on one over the other. Consequently, what follows is a summary of both,

---

[64] Yarrow, 'Narrative, Audience and the Negotiation of Community', 69–71.

[65] Bartlett, *Why Can the Dead Do Such Great Things?*, p. 342.

[66] H. Powell, '"Once upon a time there was a saint...": Re-evaluating Folklore in Anglo-Latin Hagiography', *Folklore* 121 (2010), 171–89.

[67] Powell, '"Once upon a time there was a saint..."', 171, 185.

highlighting certain historians whose works have been of specific note to the development of this current text.

There have been more notable contributions to the growing field of medieval religion, saints' cults and pilgrimage than can possibly be given the full discussion they deserve within this introduction. Nevertheless, two overarching works on saints and their cults that cannot be overlooked due to their impressive weight in this field of studies are Duffy's pivotal *The Stripping of the Altars* (1992), and Bartlett's *Why Can the Dead Do Such Great Things?* (2013). Duffy's thoughtful and thorough work might focus on the closing medieval centuries, but its reflective study of the lay experience makes it a valuable resource. Focusing on lay devotion, Duffy's key argument was that this was a period in which devotion continued in the strong tradition of earlier centuries. Bartlett, who also edited the published *M. Æbbe* and *M. Moduenne*, has added greatly to the study of sanctity and the saints by producing an overview that begins with the early Christian martyr-saints and ends with the sixteenth-century Reformation. Bartlett has highlighted the importance of the saints and their relics throughout this *longue durée* and sheds light on the diverse range of saintly figures and their impact on the lives of their devotees. Both works add greatly to our contextual understanding of the developments in the cults of the saints, and the lay interaction with these cults. Both thus provide a sense of that important, broader framework in which to place the miracles and the cure-seeking pilgrims who sought out the saints' brand of healing. Within this work I follow in this focus on interaction (and primarily lay interaction) with the saints but move away from a broad approach to focus on a select group of smaller cults in order to get a sense of the local nuances of cure-seeking and miraculous cure.

The study of medieval hagiography, and especially posthumous miracles, gained increasing interest in later decades of the twentieth century. One of the first, and most notable, proponents of using these materials to consider social history and lay religion was the previously quoted Ronald Finucane. Finucane's *Miracles and Pilgrims* (1977) provided an impressive overview of saints' cults in England. Taking in more than 3,000 posthumous miracles, Finucane was also an early advocate for analysing miracles from a statistical perspective: a method which provides a picture of the trends and anomalies among collections. In 1997, Finucane applied the same method to *The Rescue of the Innocents*, his enquiry into the influence of miracles on children and family life.[68] Didier Lett's *L'Enfant des miracles* (1997) similarly proved the

---

[68]   R. Finucane, *The Rescue of the Innocents: Endangered Children in Medieval Miracles* (New York, 1997).

value of integrating statistical analysis, with Lett combining this with a study of children in relation to wider familial and societal dynamics and with an acknowledgement of the biblical traditions of such texts.[69] Statistical analysis was also used by Pierre-André Sigal and André Vauchez, who, respectively, produced studies of French saints and the canonisation process in the 1970s and 1980s.[70] Like Finucane, the studies produced by Sigal and Vauchez were broad, and brought together great numbers of miracle accounts, producing as a result fascinating overviews of the general trends of lay faith and the wider patterns of miraculous cure. As will become apparent in the following chapters, statistical analysis has also been adopted, albeit with a more focused and localised lens, within this current work.

Others have taken a more literary interest in the hagiographical texts. Benedicta Ward's *Miracles and the Medieval Mind* (1987), like Finucane's work before, presented the cults of saints within a more socially-focused context. Ward concluded that miracles provided 'a way to approach the ordinary day-to-day life of men and women in all kinds of situations and in all ranks of society'; in so doing she stressed the importance of these materials as a resource.[71] Literary analysis of hagiography has continued to prove an important method for engaging with the texts. In more recent years, Rachel Koopmans and Simon Yarrow have both shown this to be the case. Koopmans's *Wonderful to Relate* (2011) reflected on the late eleventh- and twelfth-century developments of the genre, and the move away from an oral tradition.[72] Yarrow's *Saints and Their Communities* (2006) provided a focused consideration of lay religion through a case-by-case study of six cults, two of which (William at Norwich, and James at Reading) also feature here.[73] Yarrow also lays out, in his introduction, the typical form of 'ritual healing', a pattern with which we will become familiar during this book.[74] This pattern begins with the recognising of the problem, followed by the identification of a shrine and the soliciting of the chosen saint, and engagement with the saint. The miraculous cure that follows is then witnessed, recorded, and recounted. Yarrow's attention to the social, and

---

[69] D. Lett, *L'Enfant des miracles: Enfances et familles au Moyen Âge (XIIe–XIIIe siècles)* (Paris, 1997).

[70] P.-A. Sigal, *L'Homme et le miracle dans la France médiévale (XIe–XIIe siècle)* (Paris, 1985); Vauchez, *Sainthood in the Later Middle Ages*.

[71] B. Ward, *Miracles and the Medieval Mind: Theory, Record and Event, 1000–1215* (Philadelphia, 1987), p. 214.

[72] R. Koopmans, *Wonderful to Relate: Miracle Stories and Miracle Collecting in High Medieval England,* The Middle Ages Series (Philadelphia, 2011).

[73] Yarrow, *Saints and Their Communities*.

[74] Ibid., pp. 18–19.

communal, aspects of the cults has been influential on the approach taken here, albeit the current work centres on the practices of miraculous cure-seeking.

In terms of the approach taken in this work, two historians in particular must be named here as both illustrate the benefits of analysing miracles in order to consider pilgrims and pilgrimage. Anne E. Bailey has addressed a broad range of topics relating to high-medieval cults and pilgrimages. Bailey's accessible and considered approach to the representation of female pilgrims, childhood and madness is notable within her publications.[75] Bailey's attention to detail in analysing the accounts relating to these individuals has brought attention to the journey to the shrine, a topic that I also find to be of great interest.[76] Powell, mentioned above, has also used miracle accounts to address aspects of pilgrimage and, importantly, miracles. Her study of parturient care has been beneficial in considering the miracles representing the dangers of childbirth.[77] Powell has also addressed the landscape of pilgrimage, both physically and spiritually (following in the biblical tradition), with her work on the landscape of Æbbe's cult being especially thought-provoking.[78] In taking into account the pilgrimages made to the shrines both Bailey and Powell have illustrated the importance of thinking about the journey too. This is evidently a vital part of the cure-seeking process and one which is given further attention in Chapter 5.

Following the cure-seekers in their process of searching for, and eventually securing, their desired healing, provides us with a route through which

---

[75] A. E. Bailey, 'Representations of English Women and Their Pilgrimages in Twelfth-Century Miracle Collections', *Assuming Gender* 3 (2013), 59–90; A. E. Bailey, 'Miracle Children: Medieval Hagiography and Childhood Imperfection', *Journal of Interdisciplinary History* 47 (2016), 267–85; A. E. Bailey, 'Miracles and Madness: Dispelling Demons in Twelfth-Century Hagiography', in *Demons and Illness: Theory and Practice from Antiquity to the Early Modern Period*, ed. S. Bhayro and C. Rider (Leiden, 2016), pp. 235–55.

[76] A. E. Bailey, 'Flights of Distance, Time and Fancy: Women Pilgrims and Their Journeys in Medieval Miracle Narratives', *Gender and History* 24 (2012), 292–309; A. E. Bailey, 'Women Pilgrims and Their Travelling Companions in Twelfth-Century England', *Viator* 46 (2015), 115–34.

[77] H. Powell, 'The "Miracle of Childbirth": The Portrayal of Parturient Women in Medieval Miracle Narratives', *Social History of Medicine* 25 (2012), 795–811.

[78] H. Powell, 'Pilgrimage, Performance and Miracle Cures in the Twelfth-Century *Miracula* of St Æbbe', in *Medicine, Healing and Performance*, ed. E. Gemi-Iordanou et al. (Oxford, 2014), pp. 71–85. Also see H. Powell, 'Following in the Footsteps of Christ: Text and Context in the *Vita S. Mildrethae*', *Medium Aevum* 82 (2013), 23–43; H. Powell, 'Saints, Pilgrimage and Landscape in Early Medieval Kent *c.* 800–1220', in *Early Medieval Kent, 800–1220*, ed. S. Sweetinburgh, Kent History Project 10 (Woodbridge, 2016), pp. 133–53.

to explore the practices and experiences of miraculous cure-seeking. As such, this sets the stage for the layout of this current work. Attention in the first chapter is on the place of miraculous cure within high-medieval medicine, with particular thought given to the medical knowledge of the monastic communities connected to the seven case-study cults. The second chapter then moves on to consider the ailments that the recorded cure-seekers brought to the shrine, the 'problem' as Yarrow refers to it.[79] This establishes the therapeutic angle, with the third chapter then developing a sense of who the cure-seekers were. Having developed this sense of who sought saintly aid, and the bodily complaints that caused them to seek holy healing, attention turns to the practicalities of the journey to the shrine itself; Chapter 4 considers the distances travelled by cure-seekers; and Chapter 5 addresses the practicalities of travelling on England's medieval roads. The final chapter brings us to the end of the cure-seeker's journey and to the shrines, to consider what was expected and experienced at the cult centre, and how accessible these spaces were. We leave our cure-seekers, therefore, at the point of their cure and the entering of their miracles into the records.

This book places the cure-seekers' experiences within the broader context of healthcare and medicine. Medieval medicine has been a growing area of historical interest since the mid-twentieth century.[80] Charles Talbot's *Medicine in Medieval England* (1967) must be acknowledged as being an important introduction that centred on close reading of primary materials.[81] While Talbot's limited citations are admittedly frustrating, this remains a useful overview of the medical landscape in medieval England. Medieval medicine has since received notable and increasing attention, with other important overviews including Edward Kealey's *Medieval Medicus* (1981), focused on Anglo-Norman medicine, and Nancy Siraisi's *Medieval and Early Renaissance Medicine* (1990), providing a valuable overview of the wider, European, sphere.[82] Research has also focused on specific manuscripts and their

[79] Yarrow, *Saints and Their Communities*, p. 18.

[80] For further discussion see P. Horden, 'Medieval Medicine', in *The Oxford Handbook of the History of Medicine*, ed. M. Jackson (Oxford, 2011), pp. 40–59 (43–5).

[81] C. Talbot, *Medicine in Medieval England*, Oldbourne History of Science Library (London, 1967); N. Siraisi, *Medieval and Early Renaissance Medicine: An Introduction to Knowledge and Practice* (Chicago, 1990).

[82] E. J. Kealey, *Medieval Medicus: A Social History of Anglo-Norman Medicine* (Baltimore, 1981); Siraisi, *Medieval and Early Renaissance Medicine*.

importance within contemporary contexts.[83] Thematic studies have included faith-healing, diseases, disability studies, the Black Death, and the emotions.[84]

The twelfth-century 'renaissance' is often championed as a turning point in Western medical learning.[85] The transmission of 'new' learned medicine added to previous monastic medical knowledge, including prognostic texts.[86] Research into high-medieval healthcare has also considered monastic charity and the development of hospitals.[87] Katherine Harvey's current work on episcopal interaction with medicine also promises to be illuminating.[88] Considering England's healthcare in relation to continental developments is imperative in ensuring that the broader context is also recognised. The networks which allowed for the transmission of learned medicine were of great importance in the arrival of new, scholastic medicine in high-medieval England. Monica H. Green has been a champion of such discussions in more recent years. Green, renowned for her work on women's medicine and medieval pandemics, has also helped to develop the discussion of the transmission of medical texts,

---

[83] *The Trotula: An English Translation of the Medieval Compendium of Women's Medicine*, ed. and trans. M. H. Green (Philadelphia, 2002); *The Alphabet of Galen: Pharmacy from Antiquity to the Middle Ages: A Critical Edition of the Latin Text with English Translation and Commentary*, ed. and trans. N. Everett (Toronto, 2012).

[84] For example: I. Metzler, *Disability in Medieval Europe: Thinking about Physical Impairment during the High Middle Ages, c. 1100–1400*, Routledge Studies in Medieval Religion and Culture 5 (London, 2006); L. Demaitre, *Medieval Medicine: The Art of Healing from Head to Toe*, Praeger Series on the Middle Ages (Santa Barbara, 2013); *Pandemic Disease in the Medieval World: Rethinking the Black Death*, ed. M. H. Green, The Medieval Globe 1 (Amsterdam, 2015); D. Bouquet and P. Nagy, *Medieval Sensibilities: A History of Emotions in the Middle Ages*, trans. R. Shaw (Cambridge, 2018); C. Trenery, *Madness, Medicine and Miracle in Twelfth-Century England* (Abingdon, 2019).

[85] Burnett, 'The Twelfth-Century Renaissance', pp. 365–84.

[86] F. S. Paxton, '*Signa mortifera*: Death and Prognostication in Early Medieval Monastic Medicine', *Bulletin of the History of Medicine* 67 (1993), 631–50 (633, 642–4).

[87] P. Horden, 'A Non-Natural Environment: Medicine without Doctors and the Medieval European Hospital', in *The Medieval Hospital and Medical Practice*, ed. B. S. Bowers, AVISTA Studies in the History of Medieval Technology, Science and Art 3 (Aldershot, 2007), pp. 133–46; P. Horden, *Hospitals and Healing from Antiquity to the Later Middle Ages*, Variorum Collected Studies (Aldershot, 2008), pp. 135–53; E. Brenner, *Leprosy and Charity in Medieval Rouen*, Royal Historical Society Studies in History, New Series (Woodbridge, 2015), pp. 38–57.

[88] For more on Harvey's current work, see 'Dr Katherine Harvey', Birkbeck, <http://www.bbk.ac.uk/history/our-staff/visiting-and-emeritus-staff/dr-katherine-harvey> [accessed 3 March 2019].

especially those created or translated in the environment of Salerno.[89] This has resulted in thoughtful consideration of the early arrival of such texts in England, an arrival that benefited from the Norman networks that reached across Europe.[90] Linda E. Voigts's research into medieval texts in England has similarly shed light on this topic, focusing on high to later medieval medicine and particularly the translation of these texts into the vernacular. Voigts and Michael R. McVaugh's study of phlebotomy texts and practices has been especially useful in considering a healthcare procedure also practised within the monastic communities.[91]

From the perspective of this current work, where healthcare and healing encompass more than the learned medicine studied within the developing high-medieval universities, the works of those who have considered the broadest remit of medieval medicine, and its social contexts, have been especially beneficial. One topic worthy of some attention is the medieval hospital, a quasi-monastic institution that attended as much to the soul as the body. Studies of these institutions have revealed how hospitals brought together both the temporal and spiritual, just as healing miracles can be seen to do. Peregrine Horden is among those who have considered healthcare and the hospital, and that these environments were not necessarily led by doctors.[92] Carole Rawcliffe has also researched hospitals, with particular interest in leper hospitals, as has Elma Brenner.[93] Rawcliffe's extensive study of healthcare in

---

[89] For examples, see: M. H. Green, 'Gendering the History of Women's Healthcare', *Gender and History* 20 (2008), 487–518; M. H. Green, *Making Women's Medicine Masculine: The Rise of Male Authority in Pre-Modern Gynaecology* (Oxford, 2008); *Pandemic Disease in the Medieval World*, ed. Green.

[90] M. H. Green, 'Salerno on the Thames: The Genesis of Anglo-Norman Medical Literature', in *Language and Culture in Medieval Britain: The French of England, c. 1100–c. 1500*, ed. J. Wogan-Browne et al. (York, 2009), pp. 220–32. Also see M. H. Green, 'The Re-Creation of Pantegni, Practica, Book VIII', in *Constantine the African and 'Ali ibn al-'Abbas al-Magusi: The 'Pantegni' and Related Texts*, ed. C. Burnett and D. Jacquart, Studies in Ancient Medicine 10 (Leiden, 1994), pp. 121–6; M. H. Green, 'Medical Books', in *The European Book in the Twelfth Century*, ed. E. Kwakkel and R. Thomson, Cambridge Studies in Medieval Literature 101 (Cambridge, 2018), pp. 277–92.

[91] L. E. Voigts and M. R. McVaugh, *A Latin Technical Phlebotomy and Its Middle English Translation*, Transactions of the American Philosophical Society 74.2 (Philadelphia, 1984).

[92] Horden, 'A Non-Natural Environment', pp. 133–46. Also see Horden, *Hospitals and Healing*.

[93] C. Rawcliffe, *The Hospitals of Medieval Norwich*, Studies in East Anglian History 2 (Norwich, 1995); C. Rawcliffe, *Leprosy in Medieval England* (Woodbridge, 2006); Brenner, *Leprosy and Charity*, pp. 19–37, 58–83.

medieval England has involved bringing to the fore the interplay between physical, bodily, healing, spiritual healing and charitable care, a dynamic which is also reflected in the saints' brand of therapy. Brenner, similarly, has reflected on the complexities of this care and the spiritual elements that it involved. Valuable overviews of this topic have also been provided by Nicholas Orme and Margaret Webster, and Sheila Sweetinburgh.[94] Sweetinburgh is noteworthy for approaching this from the perspective of the inter-relationships between hospitals, patrons and patients, and of achieving this through select case studies.[95] In a similar manner, I use case studies here to consider the saints, monastic communities and cure-seekers. Unsurprisingly, charity features frequently in discussion of all such institutions.[96] It is important to recognise the presence of these institutions in drawing a wider picture of the world which the cure-seekers inhabited, and their potential access to such institutions, even if mention of hospitals is rare within the *miracula*.

This religious aspect is naturally also reflected in studies of healthcare focused on the accounts of healing miracles, including those which fall within the context of disability studies. Disability studies have received increasing interest in the last two decades and, owing to the nature of many of the cure-seekers' complaints, these studies prove relevant here. Among those who have turned their attention to impairment, physical and mental, some are notable for their engagement with *miracula*. Irina Metzler, a prominent figure in disability studies, devoted a chapter to miracles in her informative work *Disability in Medieval Europe* (2006).[97] Metzler, rejecting a retrospective medical approach in favour of a social approach to disability, concluded that in considering the interaction between saint, shrine and sufferer she achieved 'a more fruitful approach [...] which placed greater emphasis on social and cultural factors than on medical ones alone'.[98] Others, such as Edward Wheatley, have since suggested further approaches to disability (Wheatley taking a religious approach to the study of blindness).[99] Yet a broad social approach can understandably prove beneficial in understanding miraculous healing and

---

[94] N. Orme and M. Webster, *The English Hospital, 1070–1570* (New Haven, 1995); S. Sweetinburgh, *The Role of the Hospital in Medieval England: Gift-Giving and the Spiritual Economy* (Dublin, 2004).

[95] Sweetinburgh, *The Role of the Hospital*, p. 14.

[96] Orme and Webster, *The English Hospital*, pp. 57–8.

[97] Metzler, *Disability in Medieval Europe*, pp. 126–85.

[98] Ibid., p. 185. For a more literary approach to the representation of the impaired within *miracula* see Thouroude, 'Sickness, Disability, and Miracle Cures'.

[99] E. Wheatley, *Stumbling Blocks before the Blind: Medieval Constructions of Disability*, Corporealities: Discourses of Disability (Ann Arbor, 2010), p. x.

those individuals who sought it, by taking into account the various, diverse elements which influenced contemporary views of saints and their cults, and contemporary understanding of affliction and cure. Awareness of the broader social context is important to ensure that the cure-seekers represented within the seven case studies are considered, as far as possible, within their contemporary environment.

Miracle accounts clearly hold value for those interested in medieval healthcare. Although, as discussed, we must approach these sources with a recognition of their literary nature, they provide important insight into the experiences of holy healing. The benefits of using *miracula* in this way have been well established, from the early analysis of Finucane and Sigal to more recent publications including Jenni Kuuliala's *Childhood Disability and Social Integration in the Middle Ages* (2016), and Claire Trenery's *Madness, Medicine and Miracle* (2019).[100] Kuuliala uses canonisation testimonies to explore attitudes to and lived experience of childhood impairment. Trenery, like Yarrow, takes a case-by-case approach to her work, but her focus is the definitions and diagnoses of conditions of the mind, including demonic possession and epilepsy. Importantly, Trenery highlights the limited extent of the 'medicalisation' of madness in miracle accounts. Similarly, in Chapter 2, this work looks at the language used to record the cure-seeker's afflictions and cures. What proves more revealing is the descriptions of how sufferers coped with, and sought remedy for, their various health complaints.

The historiographical discussion here has focused on some of the key publications that have influenced this book, with both miracles and medicine being given attention. One final researcher, Iona McCleery, must be mentioned here. McCleery's research has focused on medicine in medieval Iberia, and she has used miracle accounts for addressing this subject. However, it is her discussion of the representation of healthcare in the miracles, and the use of these materials by historians, which is of particular relevance here.[101] McCleery raised the issue of what 'medicine' means in relation to the study of saints' cults, noting that there have been two favoured methods for analysing healing miracles, the first being 'socio-statistical' (as used by Finucane and Sigal), the second

---

[100] J. Kuuliala, *Childhood Disability and Social Integration in the Middle Ages. Constructions of Impairments in Thirteenth- and Fourteenth-Century Canonization Processes*, Studies in the History of Daily Life 4 (Turnhout, 2016); Trenery, *Madness, Medicine and Miracle*.

[101] I. McCleery, "'Christ More Powerful Than Galen?' The Relationship between Medicine and Miracles', in *Contextualising Miracles in the Christian West, 1100–1500: New Historical Approaches*, ed. M. M. Mesley and L. E. Wilson, Medium Ævum Monographs 32 (Oxford, 2014), pp. 127–54.

cultural (an approach taken by Horden and Metzler).[102] The use of statistics, McCleery highlighted, 'is an essential start to any major study of saints' cults', but she cautions over the risk of 'reducing illness down to simplistic categories' or retrospectively diagnosing the recorded ailments.[103] In order to avoid such pitfalls I make no diagnostic judgements on the cures recorded, as further discussed below. The result of this is that some categories for statistical analysis must remain broader, as these must reflect the information within the miracles themselves, but that evaluation of the accounts does not stop at such an analysis. Like McCleery, I see this as a starting-point for further enquiry into the narratives and terminology of the accounts themselves. Statistics can provide us with an important overview, but it is within the account details that we find information of the experiences of cure-seeking and miraculous healing.

As noted above, this book progresses with the cure-seekers on their journey from ill health to the saints' shrines and their miraculous recovery. While the challenges of reading hagiography have been considered, attention is needed here to address how the miracles at the heart of this work are approached and analysed.

Like many of the above-mentioned works, the research presented here takes a social approach to the topic of miraculous healing and the practicalities and experiences that were connected to this. In so doing, the primary aim is to consider the cure-seekers who sought saintly assistance, but attention is also given to the monastic communities and their understandings of healthcare and healing. In reading *miracula*, it must be recognised that these reports come from a specific genre of writing that is not only a product of its time but also a reflection of wider, and older, Christian values, teachings and beliefs. At the heart of these accounts, though, are the reports of some of the many who petitioned the saints in the hopes of securing a remedy for their corporeal afflictions. This work takes the view that the accounts represent real, lived experiences of suffering and cure. That is not to say that miraculous remedy is taken as a given, but rather that we must understand that this is how these events were perceived in their own time. It is not the intention of this book to challenge this perception in order to find out 'what really happened'; rather, I work with the accounts to understand how holy healing was understood, practised and experienced. This allows for much more rewarding results in attempting to understand contemporaries' attitudes to health and healing.

As well as accepting the perceived miraculous nature of the cures, this work does not make any attempts to retrospectively diagnose the cure-seekers'

---

[102] Ibid., pp. 140–6.
[103] Ibid., p. 142.

complaints. In part, as will become clear in Chapter 2, this is because the level of detail and the language used within the *miracula* do not allow for in-depth diagnosis. As important, however, is recognising that understandings and terminology relating to ill health have changed over time. This is one area then where we might be slightly cautious of Finucane's approach to the miracles. Finucane attempted to rationalise the events of the accounts he ana-lysed, resorting, as McCleery has observed, 'to modern theories of remission, vitamin deficiency and psycho-somatic illness'.[104] This does not, of course, take away from the overall, pioneering, importance of Finucane's work, but there are recognised issues with retrospective diagnosis, especially when that diag-nosis is produced through modern science-based theories.[105] This current work does not rewrite the miracle accounts in terms provided by modern medical understanding; rather, it works to understand them, and the afflictions and impairments they record, within the context of medieval healing practices and the cure-seekers' experiences.

Although it is worth erring on the side of caution with regard to retro-spective diagnosis, and thus the rationalising of miracle cures, Finucane's foundational use of statistical analysis in the study of reported miracles is a method followed here, albeit on a smaller scale. While Finucane's work drew on thousands of miracles, I focus on a more select case-study group (just as Yarrow and Trenery have done). The seven *miracula*, detailed above, record 259 individuals whom I have termed 'cure-seekers'. All but two of these cure-seekers appear only once within the *miracula*, but *M. Willelmi* records two individuals who appear twice. The first, William, was sacrist of Norwich Cathedral Priory.[106] In both instances, his health complaint is the same and is seemingly connected to his increasing seniority. His second record within *M. Willelmi* sheds further light on his condition, but his suffering is consequently fatal (due to his reliance in the end on worldly medicines rather than faith in William).[107] Within the statistics, therefore, the two accounts relating to William the sacrist are counted as one and the same owing to these

[104] Ibid., p. 130.

[105] For further discussions of retrospective diagnosis see: J. Arrizabalaga, 'Problematis-ing Retrospective Diagnosis in the History of Disease', *Asclepio* 54 (2002), 51–70; A. Cunningham, 'Identifying Disease in the Past: Cutting the Gordian Knot', *As-clepio* 54 (2002), 13–34; J. Theilmann and F. Cate, 'A Plague of Plagues: The Prob-lem of Plague Diagnosis in Medieval England', *Journal of Interdisciplinary History* 37 (2007), 371–93.

[106] Thomas of Monmouth, *M. Willelmi* III.13, IV.9, ed. Jessop and James, pp. 145–7, 174–7.

[107] Ibid., IV.9, pp. 176–7.

circumstances, and to his ultimate passing. Alditha, first wife then widow of Toke, is another matter. Appearing twice in *M. Willelmi*, Alditha is first cured of her long-lasting illness, and later of deafness (associated with her increasing age).[108] As Alditha is clearly recorded as one and the same person, the number of cure-seekers stands as 259; however, in terms of interactions with the saints, her two separate cures mean that there are 260 instances of successful cure-seeking. This is a point worth noting in order to understand the statistical analysis relating to the individual cure-seekers (of which there are 259) and the analysis of separate occasions of successful cure (that being 260).

The research presented here, however, does not rely solely on statistical analysis. Rather, statistical methods are part of a multi-analytical approach alongside linguistic and textual analysis. Combining these methods provides for a multifaceted approach to the miracles to be adopted and thus best allows for the details of these fascinating insights into cure-seeking to be drawn out. In some instances, details are specifically given, while in others it is possible to tease out implicit details from close reading of the text. Where there is not enough available information to do the latter, care has been taken not to make such inferences, so as to best reflect the nature of the source material. Naturally, certain records of miraculous cure prove more revealing owing to their length and level of detail, and the result of this is that certain familiar names appear more frequently within this book. Among these are some of the accounts which I have found the most fascinating in my research, including that of the young girl Ysembela, who eventually secured miraculous cure through the merits of St James at Reading Abbey.[109] While such cure-seekers do stand out, the following chapters draw on the full range of cure-seekers recorded within the seven *miracula* to provide as rounded a picture as possible of the cure-seeking experiences that the hagiographers have recorded.

One final point to make here is about the use of terminology and what is meant by certain key terms. First, 'cure-seeker' is used to emphasise the motivation of these individuals' interactions with the saints and their cults. Quite early in my research I adopted this term to identify these individuals who desired the recovery of their physical health. While cure-seeking might be seen as a form of pilgrimage, the miracles rarely use the term *peregrini* to describe these individuals, and it is unlikely that many of them partook in officially sanctioned pilgrimage. Moreover, as Chapter 4 reveals, the great majority of cure-seekers were relative locals who sought out the assistance

---

[108] Ibid., III.14, V.23, pp. 147, 217–18. In the second account Toke is written as Thoche, but it is evident that the two are one and the same.

[109] *M. Jacobi*, fols. 174rb–va; Kemp, '*The Hand of St James*' XX, 14–16.

of the saint they saw as their neighbourhood patron. Can such individuals be considered as having made a pilgrimage to the cult centres? It is hard to believe that a resident of Canterbury, for instance, would have considered themselves as a pilgrim to Canterbury Cathedral. This is a point which others might wish to debate at greater length, but for the purpose of this work, and owing to the very specific reasons for engaging the saints, the choice here is to use 'cure-seeker' as the identifier of the miraculously healed individuals. I make no claim to be the only person to use the phrase 'cure-seeker(s)' but what is important here is the use of this term to specifically identify this group of cult devotees who sought, and successfully achieved, their miraculous cure.

The terms 'medicine' and 'healing' must also be addressed. Can miracles be considered a form of medicine? This is a question that needs consideration and one in which issues of terminology can prove most challenging. Medicine, and medical practice, tend to be associated with temporal, and often educated, methods of treatment. Miracle cures, in comparison, could be identified as a 'religious thaumaturgy' that sat within contemporary healthcare practices but beyond medical intervention.[110] Yet, the saints, following in the footsteps of Christ, might also be referred to as 'physicians'.[111] Augustine of Hippo, while not alone among the early Church Fathers in using such language, is notable for his frequent use of such terminology to promote the fact that Christianity was the 'remedy'.[112] The continued belief in *Christus medicus* (Christ the physician) is evident in religious writing throughout the medieval period.[113] Of course, Augustine played upon the concept of healing in relation to the health of the eternal soul (as opposed to the temporal body), and there is a distinction to be made between the two. *Miracula*, as Trenery observes, were not medical texts.[114] The term medicine, then, is used here to refer to worldly knowledge and practices, where curative knowledge was learnt either through

[110] I. Metzler, *A Social History of Disability in the Middle Ages: Cultural Considerations of Physical Impairment*, Routledge Studies in Cultural History 20 (London, 2013), p. 6.

[111] For example, *M. Swithuni* 6, ed. Lapidge, pp. 654–5.

[112] For example, Augustine of Hippo, *Enarratio in Psalmum* 118.9.2, in *Sancti Aurelii Augustini, Hipponensis Episcopi. Opera Omnia*, ed. J.-P. Migne, *Patrologiae cursus completus, series latina* 32–47, 12 vols (Paris, 1844–65), XXXVII (1865), col. 1523. For further discussion see R. Arbesmann, 'The Concept of "Christus Medicus" in St Augustine', *Traditio* 10 (1954), 1–54.

[113] J. Ziegler, *Medicine and Religion c. 1300: The Case of Arnau de Vilanova*, Oxford Historical Monographs (Oxford, 1998), p. 179.

[114] Trenery, *Madness, Medicine and Miracle*, p. 4.

practice or scholastic study (or both).[115] In referring to the miraculous cures produced through saintly assistance, the broader terms of 'healing' and 'cure' are employed to reflect this particular method that was both part of contemporary healthcare, and which also stood beyond the remits of earthly medicines. In a similar vein, this work is keen to recognise the difference between 'impairment' and 'disability' when discussing physically impaired individuals. As Metzler highlighted, impairment is corporeal but disability has strong socio-economic connotations that must be understood within its contemporary environment rather than retrospectively judged.[116]

*   *   *

In exploring experiences of miraculous healing at seven case-study shrines, I examine a very specific group of shrine visitors and an element of lay devotion for which there is still much to be revealed. In addressing health practices at shrines associated with healing in twelfth-century England, this book engages with the fields of medieval pilgrimage and saints' cults, and medieval medicine. By focusing on these areas, we can gain a detailed insight into cure-seeking pilgrims that will invite further development of the topic in the future.

---

[115] Horden, 'Medieval Medicine', pp. 40–2.
[116] Metzler, *Disability in Medieval Europe*, p. 157.

1

Miraculous Cures in Context:
Twelfth-Century Medicine and the Saints

Working one Sunday, a certain man suffered from divine vengeance while pulling up brambles.[1] His finger was pierced by a thorn which caused his hand and arm to swell. His life was despaired of and doctors gave him 'medicamenta' (medication) to reduce the inflammation, but this only increased the swelling.[2] Eventually, he was brought to the statue of Swithun at Sherborne where he was healed by the saintly bishop. Clarica, the wife of Gaufridus de Marc, came to William of Norwich's shrine having suffered for some years with kidney pain.[3] Prior to this she had 'multum expenderit' ('spent much') on doctors who had been unable to assist her. The moment her knees touched William's tomb, however, she found herself to be cured. These accounts are reflective of the attitude towards *medici* (doctors) found within the miracle accounts. The trope shows the biblical legacy within this genre of writing.[4] However, it is also indicative of the fact that cure-seekers had access to other avenues of medicinal, or at least therapeutic, aid than the miracles of the saints. Those with the means might look to *medici* although, as in the above cases, this could result in great expenditure or, reportedly, the worsening of symptoms. Others might turn to more simple medicines, including 'uires herbarum' ('the power of herbs').[5] Although the miracles portray these alternatives as less successful, and even resulting in greater suffering, these references also reveal the presence of other healthcare avenues and show that some cure-seekers may have looked to these channels before requesting saintly aid.

---

1   *M. Swithuni* 46, ed. Lapidge, pp. 680–3.
2   Ibid., pp. 682–3.
3   Thomas of Monmouth, *M. Willelmi* III.7, ed. Jessop and James, p. 132.
4   Mark 5.26; Luke 8.43. This book uses the Douay-Rheims Bible. See *Douay-Rheims Bible*, <http://www.drbo.org/> [accessed 10 October 2020].
5   *M. Æbbe* IV.8, ed. Bartlett, pp. 46–7.

Cure-seekers could look to various potential sources of healing, but miracle accounts portray the saint's aid, unsurprisingly, as superior to any earthly options. Nevertheless the twelfth century was a period of immense change in secular medical knowledge.[6] Monastic institutions, such as those that housed our seven case-study cults, were key in the initial transmission of this medical knowledge and showed increasing interest in collecting and producing medical texts, including the works of Constantine the African who had translated a number of important medical works into Latin resulting in their reintroduction into Western medicine.[7] Through the network of Norman territories, and between Norman churchmen, these materials found their way into English book collections from an early date, with strong links developing between England and Salerno.[8] This chapter opens with an overview of these developments before addressing what can be learned of the medical knowledge within the monasteries, as these were important centres for the collection and transmission of this knowledge. Addressing the monastic context provides an insight into the understanding of medicine and healthcare of monks within the monastic communities, including the hagiographers who compiled our seven case-study *miracula*. Care for the soul, which could be termed 'spiritual health', was also a major concern for contemporary churchmen who perceived a relationship between spiritual and physical well-being. These ideas were influenced by biblical models, and the emphasis placed on caring for the sick reflected the charity of Christ.[9] Considering what can be learned about healthcare within English monasteries during the twelfth century then, and especially at the seven case-study cult centres, is essential in placing healing miracles within their contemporary context.

The Medical Landscape

To place miracle healing and the medical knowledge developing in the English monasteries within its context it is important to provide a panorama of the

---

[6] For further discussion, see Talbot, *Medicine in Medieval England*, pp. 30–1, 42–5, 56–7; Siraisi, *Medieval and Early Renaissance Medicine*, pp. 13–16.

[7] V. L. Bullough, *Universities, Medicine and Science in the Medieval West*, Variorum Collected Studies 781 (Aldershot, 2004), p. 8.

[8] C. Burnett, *The Introduction of Arabic Learning into England*, Panizzi Lectures 1996 (London, 1997), pp. 220–32; Green, 'Salerno on the Thames', pp. 220–32; Green, 'Medical Books', pp. 277–92; E. Brenner, 'The Transmission of Medical Culture in the Norman Worlds, *c.* 1050–*c.* 1250', in *People, Texts and Artefacts: Cultural Transmissions in the Norman Worlds of the Eleventh and Twelfth Centuries*, ed. D. Bates, E. D'Angelo and E. van Houts, IHR Conference Series (London, 2017), pp. 47–64.

[9] Matthew 25.34–46.

wider medical landscape. Doing so is essential to understand the environment in which our cure-seekers turned to the saints for the health of their bodies. The long twelfth-century 'renaissance' is often seen as a turning point in Western medical knowledge due to the transmission and translations of 'new' medical works and the development of the study of medicine at the universities. Salerno and its environs were key among the locations that flourished during this period, with the work of Constantine the African translating many of the most important medical texts from Arabic into Latin at nearby Montecassino in the late eleventh century.[10] As Patricia Skinner has commented, there was a tradition of learned transmission in southern Italy prior to this point with the classical medical works that survived in Byzantine traditions being transmitted through Byzantine enclaves in Ravenna and the South.[11] Florence Eliza Glaze has shown that Salerno was renowned for medical and pharmacological expertise by the mid-eleventh century.[12] However, the high Middle Ages marked a point when the volume and interest in progressing learned medicine in the West notably increased. Salerno was an important early centre for these developments, and particularly well circulated were the Salernitan *Articella* texts.[13] Montpellier was also developing as a centre of medical learning at this point (although the foundation of the university would not occur until 1220).[14] John of Salisbury's *Metalogicon* (1159) provides the earliest known reference to the latter, noting that students were leaving behind their philosophical studies to study medicine at either Salerno or Montpellier.[15]

England, while geographically distanced from this Mediterranean medical boom, was in no way a backwater. Benefiting from the strong Norman connections to the Continent, the arrival of new medical works in England occurred notably early in the twelfth century. Indeed, the presence of 'Salernitan' Latin medical literature in England is greater than in many other places in Western

---

[10] E. Brenner, 'The Medical Role of Monasteries in the Latin West, *c.* 1050–1300', in *The Cambridge History of Medieval Monasticism in the Latin West. Volume 2: The High and Late Middle Ages*, ed. A. I. Beach and I. Cochelin (Cambridge, 2020), pp. 865–81 (877).

[11] P. Skinner, *Health and Medicine in Early Medieval Southern Italy*, The Medieval Mediterranean 11 (Leiden, 1997), p. 127.

[12] F. E. Glaze, 'Salerno's Lombard Prince: Johannes "Abbas de Curte" as Medical Practitioner', *Early Science and Medicine* 23 (2018), 177–216 (178).

[13] Green, 'Salerno on the Thames', p. 222.

[14] F.-O. Touati, 'How Is a University Born? Montpellier before Montpellier', *CIAN-Revista de Historia de las Universidades* 21 (2018), 41–78 (42–3).

[15] John of Salisbury, *Metalogicon* I.4, ed. J. B. Hall and K. S. B. Keats-Rohan, *Corpus Christianorum Continuatio Mediaevalis* 98 (Turnhout, 1991), p. 18.

Europe.[16] Importantly, the institutions in England (and Normandy) were not solely collecting texts created in southern Europe but, as Green highlights, appear to have been producing codices themselves.[17] Latin remained the primary language for such texts; however, some materials were also translated into Anglo-Norman from the late twelfth century onwards. These vernacular translations focused on the practical rather than the theoretical.[18] Tony Hunt's research has highlighted that the monastic *scriptoria* played an essential role in the early production of a wide range of Anglo-Norman works, with history and scientific texts produced alongside religious writings.[19] The use of the vernacular, and the focus on the practical, suggests a potential learned lay audience for these materials or even, as Green suggests, that they were used as 'self-help' texts.[20] Interestingly, the pragmatic focus within the Anglo-Norman works is reflective of pre-Conquest, Old English, medical texts such as Bald's *Leechbook* or Pseudo-Apuleius's *Herbarium*, which included medical knowledge derived from late antique continental sources but had also focused on the more hands-on application of such knowledge.[21]

But what do we know of English medical practitioners in this period? For later medieval centuries there is evidence of a range of practitioners, but it is more challenging to paint a comprehensive picture of the medical scene in England during the twelfth century. Clearly there were trained *medici* among whom were a number of notable monks. However, there would likely have been a wide variety of practitioners, many of whom learned their craft empirically and left few written records.[22] Interestingly, as further discussed in the following chapter, the miracle accounts refer to the *medici* (often negatively)

---

[16]   Green, 'Salerno on the Thames', p. 221.

[17]   Ibid. At least twenty-five per cent of the surviving medical manuscripts Green had studied indicate that they were produced in England or Normandy.

[18]   Ibid.

[19]   T. Hunt, 'The Anglo-Norman Book', in *The Cambridge History of the Book in Britain. Volume 2*, ed. N. J. Morgan and R. M. Thomson (Cambridge, 2008), pp. 367–80 (373). Also see T. Hunt, 'The Medical Recipes in MS. Royal 5 E. vi', *Notes and Queries* 33 (1986), 6–9.

[20]   Green, 'Salerno on the Thames', p. 229. Also see Rawcliffe, 'Medical Practice and Theory', in *A Social History of England, 900–1200*, ed. J. Crick and E. Van Houts (Cambridge, 2011), pp. 391–401 (391).

[21]   Siraisi, *Medieval and Early Renaissance Medicine*, p. 10; A. Van Ardsall, *Medieval Herbal Remedies: The Old English Herbarium and Anglo-Saxon Medicine* (New York, 2002), pp. 74–80. Also see L. E. Voigts, 'A New Look at a Manuscript Containing the Old English Translation of the *Herbarium Apulei*', *Manuscripta* 20 (1976), 40–60.

[22]   Rawcliffe, 'Medical Practice and Theory', p. 391.

but rarely mention other medical practices.[23] Of course, it might be questioned whether all those described as *medici* were fully trained in the learned, theoretical practices of medicine emerging at this point, or whether all cure-seekers would have had the means to consult these high-status practitioners. This seems unlikely on the grounds of cost for all but the wealthier cure-seekers. Nevertheless, it is evident that it was the *medici* whom the hagiographers saw as the alternative, or at least as the last possible earthly option before cure-seekers sought divine aid. Identifying the *medici* in this way was not new to the twelfth century but had a biblical precedent.[24] But how did learned medical theories, and spiritual concepts, of bodily health shape high-medieval understandings of the body, ill health and cure, including those of the cure-seekers and the monastic communities housing the cults?

The Theoretical Body

Humours and Complexions

Humoral theory – the concept that four humours (blood, black bile, yellow bile and phlegm) were produced and worked in balance within the body – is perhaps one of the longest-held theories to have governed medical understanding. With its roots in the Hippocratic Corpus (fifth century BCE), the practice of bloodletting to purge bad humours continued into the nineteenth century.[25] Humoral theory was central to medieval medical understanding and was interwoven with other four-way divisions that were observed in the natural world, including the elements, the seasons, and the ages of man.[26] Of particular importance, however, to humoral theory were the associated primary qualities or complexions. The complexions were two pairs of juxtaposing qualities (hot and cold, dry and wet) that were innate to all things, including the body. Each person had their own particular balance of these complexions, which were affected by both external influences (such as environment), and internal factors (for instance sex or age).[27] At its most elementary, ill health occurred when the complexions within an individual became unbalanced. To rectify this, the body would need to be purged of the excess, or have the excess counterbalanced by means of the application

---

[23] See below, pp. 73–4.

[24] Mark 5.25–34.

[25] Siraisi, *Medieval and Early Renaissance Medicine*, p. 97.

[26] J. A. Burrow, *The Ages of Man: A Study in Medieval Writing and Thought* (Oxford, 1986), p. 12.

[27] Siraisi, *Medieval and Early Renaissance Medicine*, p. 101.

of medicines that held the opposite qualities. The humours, and even more so the complexions, were thus of great importance to the basic principles that underpinned medieval medical theory.

To retain the correct balance for bodily health, it was important that the six non-naturals were also considered. The non-naturals, derived from Galenic medicine, covered a range of conditions that impacted upon health.[28] Of the non-naturals (air, exercise and rest, sleep and waking, food and drink, repletion and excretion, and the passions and emotions), diet was seen to be the most vital. This was due to the fact that food was required in order for the body to create the humours necessary for its maintenance.[29] In classical and medieval medical practice, therefore, diet played a key role in both maintaining and recovering health. That there was an awareness that poor dietary choices could impact on health is reflected in *M. Willelmi*. Gaufrid of Canterbury, having had three teeth removed, suffered a further complaint when his head became swollen after a meal of white peas, goose with garlic and new ale.[30] Gaufrid's choice of foods, Thomas of Monmouth noted, was 'contrarie diete' ('a contrary diet') to what he required.[31] *M. Willelmi* does not expand on why this meal was poorly chosen, but evidently there is a sense here of cause and effect. Furthermore, Thomas of Monmouth critiqued Gaufrid's actions as being gluttonous, drawing an association between his ensuing affliction and the sinfulness of his luxuriant dining choices.

Spiritual Health and the Body

Humoral and complexional theories accounted for one way in which health, ill health and recovery were understood in the high Middle Ages. However, it is also important to recognise another, and equally complex, concept of health that was based on a perceived connection between body and soul, sickness and sin. This intimate relation between the temporal body and immortal soul, Rawcliffe has noted, 'constitutes one of the most salient features of medieval medical practice'.[32] There was a concern that damage to the body or soul could

---

28   Ibid.

29   C. Rawcliffe, '"On the Threshold of Eternity": Care for the Sick in East Anglian Monasteries', in *East Anglia's History: Studies in Honour of Norman Scarfe*, ed. C. Harper-Bill, C. Rawcliffe and R. G. Wilson (Woodbridge, 2002), pp. 41–72 (58); Siraisi, *Medieval and Early Renaissance Medicine*, p. 106.

30   Thomas of Monmouth, *M. Willelmi* VII.19, ed. Jessop and James, pp. 289–94 (290). Also see below, pp. 72–3, 168–9.

31   Ibid. I have not followed Jessop and James's translation here in order to be closer to the Latin's meaning.

32   Rawcliffe, 'Medical Practice and Theory', p. 395.

affect the health of the other, and therefore caring for those who were suffering was seen as an important charitable act (and one that would also benefit
the souls of the altruistic). These spiritual concepts also had their roots in
antiquity, but rather than being influenced by classical medicine, these models
were biblical in their origins.

Christ's miracles, as recorded in the Gospels, presented him as *Christus
medicus* (Christ the physician) and this was reflected in the miracles performed
through later saintly intercession too. Christ's miracles illustrated the intercessory power of the divine over temporal bodies and emphasised the importance
of having faith in God. The Gospel story of the woman cured from 'profluvio
sanguinis' ('a flowing of the blood') after twelve years exemplifies this.[33] She
was cured immediately after having touched Christ's garment and, following
her cure, Christ said, 'Filia, fides tua te salvam fecit: vade in pace, et esto sana
a plaga tua' ('Daughter, thy faith hath made thee whole: go in peace, and be
thou whole of thy disease').[34] This woman is said to have first sought the help
of doctors, but to no avail and at great expense, thus reflecting the perceived
supremacy of God's divine will and the dominance of divine healing over
mundane treatments.[35] These characteristics were reflected in the medieval
miracula, with the saints' actions being *imitatio Christi* (an imitation of Christ)
and with earthly medicines being presented as less effective than divine remedy.
Faith and health were thus inextricably connected within medieval thought
and, as Duffy noted, such healing might also involve the wider community.[36]

The Old Testament also established similar connections between spiritual
and physical health, albeit with a more punitive nature than the Gospels. Here,
rather than the merciful Christ curing the faithful, God was depicted as the
defender of faith against blasphemers and doubters. Corporeal afflictions were
markers of sin, while confession was emphasised as an important process of
atonement.[37] Later hagiographical materials show the saints as vehicles of
divine punishment, as well as healing. Within the seven *miracula* focused upon
here, only *M. Swithuni* and *M. Æbbe* are without such accounts. Æthelthryth,
conversely, is recorded in *L. Eliensis* as having been particularly protective of
her shrine and her monastic community, with punishments meted out to both
the laity and to unworthy churchmen. Importantly, miracles of any nature

---

[33] Mark 5.25.
[34] Mark 5.30.
[35] Mark 5.26.
[36] Duffy, *The Stripping of the Altars*, pp. 188–90.
[37] Numbers 5.6–10.

stressed the omnipotence of God and divine ability to intervene in the lives of humans.[38]

Although this current work is focused on miraculous healing, it is important to acknowledge these punitive accounts. Such miracles, resulting in bodily harm, are indicative of wider, popular, understandings of the connection between impious behaviour and corporeal affliction. Drawing this connection between sinful conduct and divine punishment was a reflective process: both cause and effect had to have occurred for this to be recognised as heavenly intervention. Divine punishment was not necessarily permanent and could act as a corrective. When Ælfwine of Hopwas, a royal official, put his own eye out with his thumb – after delighting in causing harm to the monks of Burton – the action resulted in him learning from his mistake and amending his ways.[39]

Being able to identify with the suffering of Christ was another essential component in the connections drawn between physical and spiritual health.[40] Care for the health of the soul was believed to be of more importance than health of the body, and must have especially resonated within the Church. This is well illustrated in Bernard of Clairvaux's letter to the monks of St Anastasius, Italy, regarding their continuous issues with malaria. Bernard sympathises with the monastic community but stresses that 'sickness of the soul' is a greater fear than that of the body.[41] As such, Bernard argues, there were some merits in basic herbal remedies but seeking out specialised medicines provided by *medici* was contrary to the simplicity of religious life. The monks of St Anastasius, Bernard advises, should thus trust in humility and prayers to purge themselves of sin and ensure their spiritual health was maintained. What is key within Bernard's letter is that simple remedies, such as those that could be produced from the herbs grown within the monastery's own physic garden, were acceptable in extreme circumstances. However, Bernard, a strict Cistercian, did not consent to the purchase of specialised medicines or specialist care as this was not in keeping with Cistercian monastic life. The Benedictines, on the other hand, at whom Bernard's letter takes an

---

[38] For further discussion of medieval responses to biblical miracles, see Ward, *Miracles and the Medieval Mind*, pp. 20–4.

[39] Geoffrey of Burton, *M. Moduenne* 47, ed. Bartlett, pp. 190–3.

[40] C. Rawcliffe, 'Curing Bodies and Healing Souls: Pilgrimage and the Sick in Medieval East Anglia', in *Pilgrimage: The English Experience from Becket to Bunyan*, ed. C. Morris and P. Roberts (Cambridge, 2002), pp. 108–40 (123).

[41] Bernard of Clairvaux, *The Letters of St Bernard of Clairvaux* 388, ed. B. S. James (Stroud, 1998), pp. 458–9.

implicit and 'characteristic jibe', were more lenient in their allowance for medical treatment and medical practice.[42]

For some churchmen, like Bernard of Clairvaux, the recourse to more complex (and thus expensive) pharmacopeia was of grave concern. As a Cistercian, Bernard was especially troubled by what he perceived to be the lax attitude of the Benedictines towards the use of earthly medicines. Yet, as Horden has highlighted, even Cistercians were turning to these costly medicines in the twelfth century.[43] For Bernard, though, faith was to be put in God, and His will, and greater attention was to be placed on caring for the soul. These concerns were reflected by other high-medieval churchmen including Herbert of Losinga, bishop of Norwich. In a letter addressed to Norwich monk, Godfrey, Herbert cautioned the wayward monk over his frequent leave from the community.[44] Herbert critiqued Godfrey's constant requests to be permitted to bathe and have his blood let, two preventative and curative procedures that (as discussed below) were administered to monks. Herbert warned that bodily indulgences affected the health of Godfrey's soul, and the souls of those under his care.[45] Herbert's fears were focused on the liberties that Godfrey was taking with his monastic responsibilities, and his concern that the soul's health should be placed above that of the body is clear.

What must be remembered, however, is that those educated in scholastic medicine at this time would also have been churchmen. Indeed, there were a handful of great monk-physicians who balanced their monastic duties with their work as a *medicus*. Abbots Faricius of Abingdon and Baldwin of Bury St Edmunds are prime examples of this. Both men held important offices as monastic superiors of substantial communities. Both were also royal physicians. Baldwin's medical talents helped secure his abbacy, having impressed the monastic community when he attended to his predecessor, Abbot Leofstan.[46] Faricius likewise used his skill for the benefit of high-status patients including Henry I.[47] Faricius also attended Henry I's first wife, Matilda, during her pregnancies.[48] Faricius's and Baldwin's professional work benefited their

---

[42]   Rawcliffe, '"On the Threshold of Eternity"', p. 42.

[43]   P. Horden, 'Sickness and Healing', in *The Oxford Handbook of Christian Monasticism*, ed. B. M. Kaczynski (Oxford, 2020), pp. 403–17 (404).

[44]   *The Life, Letters and Sermons of Bishop Herbert de Losinga* 16, ed. E. M. Goulburn and H. Symonds, 2 vols (Oxford, 1878), I, 105–10.

[45]   Ibid., 109–10.

[46]   Rawcliffe, '"On the Threshold of Eternity"', p. 43.

[47]   P. Horden, 'Faricius (*d.* 1117), doctor and abbot of Abingdon', in *ODNB*, <https://doi.org/10.1093/ref:odnb/9157> [accessed 26 June 2020].

[48]   Ibid.

monasteries, with both men using their earnings to fund building schemes at their respective institutions.[49] However, Faricius also faced critique for his profession, especially his treatment of women, with the bishops of Lincoln and Salisbury raising concerns over his suitability to succeed Anselm at Canterbury.[50]

While some might have questioned monastic use and practice of medicine, it is clear that for many it was possible to justify the use of classical medical and natural philosophical theories, propounded by the great (pagan) thinkers, within the Christian world view. By taking the line of thought that God was the ultimate source of all endeavours, it was possible to argue that temporal medicine, and any successes that such treatments resulted in, were in themselves, ultimately, divinely willed. Reflecting on this, Rawcliffe commented that monk-physicians 'could legitimately claim both biblical and classical authority for their endeavours' by drawing on the exemplar of *Christus medicus* and classical writings.[51]

Monastic Medical Knowledge

The concept of *Christus medicus* would have been well known within the monasteries that housed our seven saints, and this message would have been embedded in the sermons but also the reading materials of the monks. *Lectio divina* (divine reading) was a compulsory element of daily life within the monastery. The monks would gather at least once a day for the *lectio divina* in the cloister, and reading in the dormitory following dinner was also permitted, especially in the summer.[52] The purpose of this reading time was clear, and biblical and spiritual texts were preferred. Concern was particularly taken that any novices should be provided with suitable material.[53] Senior members of the community had somewhat more say over their reading material come Lent, and those who held particular offices might borrow books which related more directly to their duties.[54] Those books not in use, or the reference books

---

[49] *A History of the County of Berkshire: Volume 2*, ed. P. H. Ditchfield and W. Page, VCH (London, 1907), pp. 51–62; Rawcliffe, "On the Threshold of Eternity"', p. 43.

[50] *Chronicon Monasterii de Abingdon*, ed. J. Stevenson, 2 vols, RS 2 (London, 1858), II, 287.

[51] Rawcliffe, "On the Threshold of Eternity"', p. 42.

[52] *Regula S. Benedicti* 48, ed. and trans. McCann, pp. 110–13; J. Kerr, *Life in the Medieval Cloister* (London, 2009), pp. 156–9.

[53] Kerr, *Life in the Medieval Cloister*, p. 181.

[54] Ibid., p. 182. Also see P. Meyvaert, 'The Medieval Monastic Claustrum', *Gesta* 12 (1973), 53–9 (54–5).

that were not lent out, were kept in *armaria* (cupboards) or libraries. Moreover, some monastic offices, which required particular skills and knowledge, might have had specific reference collections of their own which would have been kept separately, so that they were more accessible to that office. Medical works, unsurprisingly, would not have been likely materials for the *lectio divina*; nevertheless the twelfth-century monasteries were clearly interested in collecting these texts as surviving manuscripts and book lists reveal.

Monastic Book Collections

Developing a picture of the type and range of books available within monastic collections during the high medieval period is challenging and relies on the survival of either the manuscripts or detailed book lists, or both. Medical, and other scientific, material was being collected and produced at certain key monastic centres including St Augustine's Abbey, Canterbury; Bury St Edmunds Cathedral Priory; Durham Cathedral Priory; and Worcester Cathedral Priory. But definitive evidence of medical books elsewhere proves more elusive. Considering the importance of spiritual reading to monastic life it is no surprise that the great monasteries concentrated on liturgical and theological works. Indeed, the high medieval book catalogue from Cistercian Rievaulx Abbey, Yorkshire, reveals that only fifteen per cent of the abbey's collection consisted of works of history, philosophy, grammar, and medicine.[55] That spiritual and liturgical works were of such great importance is a given, so too is the fact that such items would be housed within the main library or book collection. These materials, therefore, were the ones most likely to be listed in any catalogues. As book lists tend to concentrate on these main collections, it does not mean a lack of medical manuscripts within the monastery, especially if such resources were kept elsewhere in smaller, specialised collections.

For the seven monasteries that act as case studies here, the survival of evidence of medical manuscripts is fragmentary. The abbeys of Burton and Reading both felt the full effect of the sixteenth-century Dissolution on their properties and holdings, with works being dispersed to other collections. The cathedral libraries survived somewhat better, with some maintaining more extensive records of their medieval holdings. Nevertheless, natural disasters have also impacted upon these resources; Norwich, for instance, suffered a devastating fire in 1272.[56] Canterbury was also affected by numerous fires and

[55] M. R. James, *A Descriptive Catalogue of the Manuscripts in the Library of Jesus College, Cambridge* (London, 1895), pp. 43–56; Kerr, *Life in the Medieval Cloister*, p. 182.

[56] *English Benedictine Libraries: The Shorter Catalogues*, ed. R. Sharpe et al., Corpus of British Medieval Library Catalogues 4 (London, 1996), pp. 288–99 (288).

was still recovering from the impact of the fire of 1067 in the early twelfth century, during Eadmer's production of *M. Dunstani*. This, and the arrival of the Norman archbishops (first Lanfranc, then Anselm), resulted in the restocking of the cathedral's book collection, albeit with an understandable focus on replenishing the liturgical collections.[57] As a major centre, Canterbury Cathedral Priory had strong connections with other important institutions, including Worcester and Durham. The results of these interactions are visible in Eadmer's works, which reveal intellectual exchanges between Eadmer, Symeon of Durham and John of Worcester; the latter, significantly, being a scholar to whom both historical and scientific works have been attributed.[58] One such work, partly written by John himself, contained astronomical works translated by Walcher, the prior of Great Malvern, from the Arabic, alongside works associated with Adelard of Bath and a treatise on the astrolabe.[59]

John of Worcester's work implies a high level of scientific knowledge, and interest, at Worcester in the early twelfth century. John's *Chronicon* is also noteworthy for its record of his meeting with Grimbald, Henry I's doctor. Grimbald provided John with details of his attendance on the king, and *Chronicon*'s account of this, at least partly in John's own handwriting, includes miniatures depicting Grimbald beside the king's bedside with the tools of his trade.[60] That healthcare and medical procedure were discussed by these great, learned figures is worthy of note, and the importance of such discourses for transmitting medical knowledge should not be overlooked. Worcester's continuing interest in acquiring medical texts from good sources is further reflected in its possession, by the thirteenth century, of two twelfth-century medical manuscripts.[61] These two manuscripts appear to have been produced in the ambience of Montpellier or one of the translation centres in Spain, suggesting that Worcester was keen to collect cutting-edge treatises and to maintain a high level of interest in scientific and medical knowledge.

[57]   R. Gameson, *The Earliest Books of Canterbury Cathedral: Manuscripts and Fragments to c.1200*, Canterbury Sources 4 (London, 2008), p. 23.

[58]   A. Lawrence-Mathers, 'John of Worcester and the Science of History', *Journal of Medieval History* 39 (2013), 1–20 (3); R. M. Thomson, *A Descriptive Catalogue of the Medieval Manuscripts in Worcester Cathedral Library* (Cambridge, 2001), p. xxiii; P. McGurk, 'Worcester, John of (*fl.* 1095–1140)', in *ODNB*, <https://doi.org/10.1093/ref:odnb/48309> [accessed 26 June 2020].

[59]   Oxford, Bodleian Library, Bodl. MS Auct. F.1.9, fol. 75v; Thomson, *A Descriptive Catalogue*, p. xxiii.

[60]   Oxford, Corpus Christi College, MS 157, fols. 382v–383r.

[61]   Worcester, Worcester Cathedral Library, MSS Q.40, Q.60; Thomson, *A Descriptive Catalogue*, pp. 142, 157.

Durham is a similarly noteworthy example of an important monastic institution that, during the twelfth century, was building a collection of medical
works. The twelfth-century catalogue is impressive, recording around 450
books in the priory's collection.[62] Durham, a wealthy and long-established
institution, owned a large number of pre-Conquest manuscripts, including
those inherited from the original community at Lindisfarne.[63] Of particular note, however, is a manuscript that contains *computus*, astronomy and
medical writings.[64] This manuscript's medical material included Isadore
of Seville's *Etymologies*, a list of medical remedies and charms, notes on the
four humours and their effects, and two folios of miniatures depicting cautery
points on the body.[65]

Durham also benefited from manuscript donations, including from *medicus*, Master Herbert.[66] Herbert donated several medical books to Durham
in the mid-twelfth century including herbals, a lapidary, and a number of
works that were part of the new medical corpus beginning to spread through
Europe.[67] New translations of classical medical texts, often with Arabic additions, together with the establishment of the European medical schools, led to
a wider range of medical and scientific knowledge being disseminated through
Western Europe and within the British Isles. Among Herbert's donations
were Dioscorides's *De Materia Medica*, and a collection of medical treatises
including Constantine's translations of Isaac Israeli ben Solomon's *Liber
Febrium* and Galen's *Microtegni*.[68] Few of the donations made by Master Herbert appear to have survived and it is not possible to tell whether the *Pantegni*
Herbert donated was a full copy. Green has argued that the *theorica* and books

[62] Durham, Durham Cathedral Library, MS B.iv.24. Also see A. Lawrence, 'The Artistic Influence of Durham Manuscripts', in *Anglo-Norman Durham, 1093–1193*,
ed. D. Rollason, M. Harvey and M. Prestwich (Woodbridge, 1998), pp. 451–70
(452).

[63] R. A. B. Mynors, *Durham Cathedral Manuscripts to the End of the Twelfth Century*
(Oxford, 1939), pp. 13–23.

[64] Durham, Durham Cathedral Library, MS Hunter 100; Mynors, *Durham Cathedral
Manuscripts*, p. 49.

[65] MS Hunter 100, fols. 85r–101v, 102r–118r, 119r–120r.

[66] *Catalogi Veteres Librorum Ecclesiæ Cathedralis Dunelm: Catalogues of the Library of
Durham Cathedral at Various Periods, from the Conquest to the Dissolution including
Catalogues of the Library of the Abbey of Hulne and the MSS. Preserved in the Library of Bishop Cosin, at Durham*, ed. B. Botfield, Surtees Society 7 (London, 1838),
pp. 7–8; Mynors, *Durham Cathedral Manuscripts*, pp. 46, 62.

[67] *Catalogi Veteres Librorum*, ed. Botfield, pp. 7–8.

[68] Cambridge, Jesus College, MS Q.D.2; Edinburgh, National Library of Scotland
Advocates MS 18.6.11, fols. 1r–81v, 85r–104r.

I, II and IX of the *practica* were in circulation together in the twelfth century, but that it was unusual for the two complete works to be in circulation prior to the late twelfth century owing to the rest of the *practica* being lost at sea.[69] Thus, it is likely that Durham's gifted copy was the *theorica*, possibly with the three books of the *practica* attached. The *Pantegni* aside, Herbert's donations include general works, such as the Hippocratic *Prognosis*, and more specialist resources, including 'Liber epidimiarum' and 'Liber stomachi s' constanter' [*sic*], specialising in epidemics and the stomach respectively.[70]

Bury St Edmunds also benefited from connections with medical practitioners, and importantly from the influence of their own monk-physician, Abbot Baldwin (d. 1097). Baldwin was physician to three kings of England: Edward the Confessor, William I, and William Rufus. He also treated his abbatial predecessor, Leofstan, which led to his succession as abbot.[71] Although there is no direct evidence of Baldwin having taught medicine at Bury, his medical legacy is notable in the medicalised terminology used in Archdeacon Herman's *Miracula S. Edmundi*, and in the surviving high-medieval medical texts attributed to Bury.[72] Debby Banham has commented that one of these

[69] Green, 'The Re-Creation of Pantegni, Practica, Book VIII', pp. 123–6; Glaze, 'Salerno's Lombard Prince', 190. There is no modern edition of Constantine's *Pantegni* but it survives in Renaissance print editions; for a complete edition see *Omnia opera Ysaac*, ed. A. Turinus, 2 vols (Lyons, 1515), via the *Bibliothèque Interuniversitaire de Santé*, <http://www.biusante.parisdescartes.fr/histoire/medica/resultats/index.php?cote=00122&do=livre> [accessed 10 September 2020]. Also see M. H. Green, '"But of the Practica of the Pantegni he translated only three books, for it had been destroyed by the water": The Puzzle of the Practica', *Constantinus Africanus*, 22 March 2018, <https://constantinusafricanus.com/2018/03/22/but-of-the-practica-of-the-pantegni-he-translated-only-three-books-for-it-had-been-destroyed-by-the-water-the-puzzle-of-the-practica/> [accessed 10 September 2020].

[70] *Catalogi Veteres Librorum*, ed. Botfield, pp. 7–8.

[71] A. F. Wareham, 'Baldwin (*d.* 1097)', in *ODNB*, <https://doi.org/10.1093/ref:odnb/1160> [accessed 14 July 2020].

[72] Herman the Archdeacon, *Miracula S. Edmundi*, in *Herman the Archdeacon and Goscelin of St Bertin*, ed. and trans. T. Licence, OMT (Oxford, 2014), pp. 1–125; Cambridge, Cambridge University Library MS li.6.5; Cambridge, Peterhouse College, MS 251; London, British Library MSS Royal 12. C. xxiv, Sloane 1621; London, Wellcome Library, MSS 801A, AMS/MF/5; Oxford, Bodleian MS Bodley 130. For further discussion, see: D. Banham, 'Medicine at Bury in the Time of Abbot Baldwin', in *Bury St Edmunds and the Norman Conquest*, ed. T. Licence (Woodbridge, 2014), pp. 226–46; M. Gullick, 'An Eleventh-Century Bury Medical Manuscript', in *Bury St Edmunds and the Norman Conquest*, ed. T. Licence (Woodbridge, 2014), pp. 190–225; V. Thouroude, 'Medicine after Baldwin: The evidence of BL, Royal 12. C. xxiv', in *Bury St Edmunds and the Norman Conquest*, ed. T. Licence (Woodbridge, 2014), pp. 247–57.

surviving manuscripts (Cambridge, Peterhouse College MS 251) is 'the near-est thing to a standard medical textbook in early medieval Europe', prior to the establishment of fixed curricula in the universities, although she remains uncertain about this manuscript's Bury provenance.[73]

What of the evidence for medical books at the seven cult centres focused upon here? Evidence of their collections is more obscure. Early twelfth-century Canterbury, as noted, was still in the process of renovation following the destruction of the greater part of the complex in 1067. From the surviving evidence of the books at Christ Church in the early twelfth century there is no indication that their collection included anything medical or overtly scientific. Nevertheless, Lanfranc and Eadmer, among others at Christ Church, were significant scholars with access to a mass of resources and connections to other major centres, as noted. In Canterbury, the archbishop could easily have had numerous books copied, or have brought in scholars and borrowed exemplars from elsewhere.[74]

Winchester proves similarly lacking in concrete evidence of a twelfth-century interest in medical works. However, as a long-established monastic institution, Winchester's Old Minster was a seat of learning from as early as the tenth century and, until the late twelfth century, was known for its production and patronage of quality books.[75] Thirty of the surviving works are pre-Conquest, suggesting an impressive early library.[76] Among these is one of the best-known Old English medical texts, Bald's *Leechbook*.[77] The *Leechbook* can be broadly connected to Winchester, but not directly to the Old Minster (and later, the Cathedral Priory). Nonetheless it does signal local interest in medicine and could indicate that the monastic community had related exemplars. The *Leechbook* was made with 'a conscious effort to trans-fer to Anglo-Saxon practice what one physician considered the most useful in native and Mediterranean medicine', with the compiler having brought together Greek, Roman, Byzantine and North African knowledge, indicating a high level of expertise.[78] Thus, the Old Minster monks could have had access to a compilation text that covered a range of health complaints and offered practical cures.

---

[73] Banham, 'Medicine at Bury', p. 277.

[74] Talbot, *Medicine in Medieval England*, p. 46.

[75] *English Benedictine Libraries*, ed. Sharpe, pp. 648–50.

[76] Ibid.

[77] London, British Library, MS Royal 12.D.xvii; N. R. Ker, *Medieval Libraries of Great Britain: A List of Surviving Books*, 2nd edn (London, 1964), p. 200.

[78] M. Cameron, *Anglo-Saxon Medicine*, Cambridge Studies in Anglo-Saxon England 7 (Cambridge, 2006), pp. 35, 42–5.

Approximately thirty years before the production of *L. Eliensis*, Ranulf Flambard made an inventory of Ely's possessions, including the priory's books.[79] This inventory, later copied into *L. Eliensis*, included 'xiiii textus magni vel parvi, auro et argento ornati' ('fourteen gospel books, large or small, ornamented with gold and silver') and 'ccc libri xiii minus; ex his xix missales sunt et viii lectionales et ii benedictionales, xxii psalteria et vii breviarii et ix antiphonarii et xii gradalia' ('[thirteen] short of 300 books; of these nineteen are missals, and eight lectionaries, and two benedictionals, twenty-two psalters and seven breviaries, and nine antiphonars and twelve graduals').[80] Flambard's attention was primarily on the more expensive books among Ely's collection. Yet, the inclusion of around 200 works, not counting *liturgica*, is impressive even if the late eleventh-century list of Ely's holdings does not specifically record any medical texts. This does not prove that the priory was devoid of any medical works as there is also no record of Ely holding a copy of *Regula S. Benedicti* (Benedict of Nursia's instructions for communal monastic living), and surely that was somewhat of an essential. Owing to the aforementioned fire of 1272, our other East Anglian monastery, Norwich Cathedral Priory, is sparse in terms of concrete evidence for its twelfth-century book collections.[81] The best evidence for Norwich's book collections is found in the late thirteenth- to early fourteenth-century obedientiaries' records.[82] The little that did survive the fire consisted of works 'kept elsewhere in the cloister', but there is a frustrating vagueness on what these items were.[83]

As a smaller institution, Burton Abbey, rather unsurprisingly, possessed fewer books than the great cathedral priories.[84] Fortunately, the late twelfth-century catalogue of these survives, highlighting that Burton had 'a modest but adequate collection of the Fathers and some other devotional reading, though it was not well supplied with *biblica*'.[85] Burton's book catalogue is doubtless characteristic of smaller monastic libraries in England, and makes no mentions of medical or scientific texts.[86] This confirms that medical texts, if owned, would have been considered as specialist materials that were unlikely to be part of the monastery's main collection. Coldingham

---

[79] *English Benedictine Libraries*, ed. Sharpe, pp. 127–31 (127).

[80] *L. Eliensis* II.139, ed. Blake, p. 224, trans. Fairweather, p. 269.

[81] *English Benedictine Libraries*, ed. Sharpe, pp. 288–99 (288).

[82] Ibid., pp. 288–9.

[83] Ibid., p. 289; Ker, *Medieval Libraries of Great Britain*, pp. 135–9.

[84] *English Benedictine Libraries*, ed. Sharpe, pp. 33–42.

[85] Ibid., p. 33.

[86] Ibid., p. 34.

Priory, equally small, though wealthy, paints a similar picture. Although, as a dependent daughter-house, the monks based at Coldingham were first and foremost monks of Durham. Though the extensive medical resources at the motherhouse were not instantly available to the Coldingham monks, these materials were potentially accessible to them.

Reading provides the most fortunate evidence for twelfth-century library holdings, with the library catalogue, like *M. Jacobi*, dating to the late twelfth century. Reading's catalogue, along with that of its daughter-house, Leominster, can be found within its cartulary.[87] Compiled in the early 1190s, with additions being made into the thirteenth century, the cartulary contains an inventory of the abbey's relics followed by a list of its books.[88] The catalogue begins with Bibles, then glossed books of the Bible, patristics, historical works, service books, and finally school texts.[89] Reading also owned a bestiary, bound alongside a copy of Petrus Alfonsi's *Dialogi contra Iudeos*.[90] Bestiaries, like herbals and lapidaries, contained medicalised notations regarding animals and their uses. More intriguingly, Reading's catalogue lists a work entitled '*Liber de physica, Passionarius scilicet, qui fuit abbatis Anscherii, in uno uolumine*'.[91] This could refer to Gariopontus's *Passionarius Galeni*, although several other medical works were also referred to as *passionarius*. This *passionarius* has not survived. Nevertheless its presence at Reading is interesting, especially as the catalogue entry suggests that it was acquired by Ansger, Reading's second abbot, who then gave it to the monks.[92] This indicates that Ansger had a personal interest in medicine, and that he wished to foster its introduction at Reading.

Writing Medicine

In addition to the collecting of medical books, it is worth drawing brief attention to the writing of medical texts within English monasteries in the twelfth century. The work of one English writer that is of importance is the *Anglicanus ortus* of Henry of Huntingdon (d. *c.* 1157), which consists of six

[87] London, British Library, MS Egerton 3031; *English Benedictine Libraries*, ed. Sharpe, pp. 419–61 (420); *Reading Abbey Cartularies. British Library Manuscripts: Egerton 3031, Harley 1708 and Cotton Vespasian E xxv*, 'Abbatial Acts and Abbey Documents 225–26', ed. B. Kemp, Camden 4th series 31, 33, 2 vols (London, 1986), I, 186; A. Coates, *English Medieval Books: The Reading Abbey Collections from Foundation to Dispersal*, Oxford Historical Monographs (Oxford, 1999), pp. 24–36.
[88] MS Egerton 3031, fols. 6v–8r, 8v–10v.
[89] Coates, *English Medieval Books*, p. 21.
[90] MS Egerton 3031, fol. 9v; Coates, *English Medieval Books*, p. 30.
[91] Coates, *English Medieval Books*, p. 33.
[92] Ibid.

books on medical herbs and spices, and two books on gemstones.[93] While primarily known for his production of *Historia Anglorum*, Henry of Hunting-don was a learned and well-read writer among whose poetic works *Anglicanus ortus* sits. This work is heavily influenced by other medical materials, most notably Constantine the African and Marbod of Rennes.[94] Importantly, however, Henry did not merely copy his exemplars but brought these materi-als together into a new poetic composition.[95] As Winston Black has argued, having rediscovered the sole surviving copy of *Anglicanus ortus*'s lapidary, *De gemmis preciosis*, the presence of Constantine's *Liber de gradibus* among Henry's sources is noteworthy for reflecting the early spread of Salernitan medicine through Europe and that English medical writers were part of the 'pan-European' adoption of Galenic theories that were resulting from the Salernitan translations at this time.[96]

A second Henry, Henry of Winchester (d. *c.* 1225), must also be recognised for his contribution to Anglo-Norman medical knowledge. The eleven-page, widely circulated, *Tractatus magistri enrici de egritudinibus fleubotomandis* ('Of Phlebotomie' in the later Middle English) has been attributed to Henry, who had been a medical master at Montpellier.[97] This treatise, as Voigts and McVaugh have noted, has little likeness to the earlier *Epistula de flebotomia* (which dates back to the ninth century), rather it frequently cites Constantine's *Megatechni* and *Viaticum*.[98] The Salernitan influence, but lack of reference to Galen or Avicenna's *Canon* – introduced to the Western medical schools in the second quarter of the thirteenth century – places production date of the treatise as *c.* 1150–1225.[99] Importantly, the treatise was compiled, like the vernacular texts, with practicality in mind. For this reason the tract is primarily structured around the diseases for which bleeding was to be undertaken, thus allowing the phlebotomist to easily confirm which vein was required.[100] The creation of such texts is important in establishing that medical information was not merely being collected and copied verbatim in English monasteries in

---

[93] Henry of Huntingdon, *Anglicanus Ortus: A Verse Herbal of the Twelfth Century*, ed. and trans. W. Black, Studies and Texts 180 (Oxford, 2012).

[94] W. Black, 'Henry of Huntingdon's Lapidary Rediscovered and His *Anglicanus ortus* Reassembled', *Medieval Studies* 68 (2006), 43–87 (46–7, 59, 64–7).

[95] Ibid., 64.

[96] Ibid., 66, 67 n. 57.

[97] Voigts and McVaugh, *A Latin Technical Phlebotomy*, pp. 1, 7.

[98] Ibid.

[99] Ibid., pp. 4, 7.

[100] Ibid., p. 9.

the twelfth century; some people were also using such texts as exemplars in the creation of their own additions to the Latin medical corpus.

'Old' and 'New' Medicine

Evidently, monasteries were not devoid of medical, or other scientific, works. Interest in these fields was often influenced by the presence of medically-minded individuals, such as Baldwin at Bury. However, with the increased dispersal of new medical texts, there was a chance for the monastic communities to broaden their understanding of health and healing. If the degree of change is to be understood, attention must first be given to the 'old' medical corpus.

Herbals, bestiaries, and lapidaries, as well as sources such as Isidore of Seville's *Etymologies* and Bede's *De temporum ratione*, shaped understandings of health and the human body. *De temporum ratione* contained a commentary on the 'Ages of Man', following the pattern of the classical Hippocratic Corpus's discussion of the same; this was important for conceptualising human life and the human body.[101] Herbals were important to the older corpus of medical works, especially the herbal of Pseudo-Apuleius, and the *Ex herbis feminis* attributed to Dioscorides. The latter survives in thirteen English manuscripts from the twelfth century or earlier.[102] Monastic interest in such texts was sanctioned by Cassiodorus, who compiled a small collection of Latin versions of Greek medical works at his influential monastery, Vivarium.[103] The tradition was further developed in Carolingian medical manuscripts, originating from houses which effected the Anglo-Saxon reform movement.[104]

The two herbals, Pseudo-Apuleius and *Ex herbis feminis*, are often found together, including in one of Bury's medical manuscripts.[105] The Bury herbal

---

[101] Hippocrates, Heracleitus, *Nature of Man. Regimen in Health. Humours. Aphorisms. Regimen 1–3. Dreams. Heracleitus: On the Universe*, trans. W. H. S. Jones, Loeb Classical Library 150 (Cambridge, MA, 1931), pp. xxxii–iv; Bede, *The Reckoning of Time* (hereafter *De temporum ratione*), trans. F. Wallis, Translated Texts for Historians 29 (Liverpool, 1999), pp. 100–1.

[102] J. M. Riddle, 'Pseudo-Dioscorides' *Ex herbis feminis* and Early Medieval Botany', *Journal of the History of Biology* 14 (1981), 43–81 (44). Additionally, see Van Ardsall, *Medieval Herbal Remedies*, p. 206 n. 234.

[103] Siraisi, *Medieval and Early Renaissance Medicine*, pp. 9–10.

[104] M. Frampton, *Embodiments of Will: Anatomical and Physiological Theories of Voluntary Animal Motion from Greek Antiquity to the Latin Middle Ages* (Saarbrücken, 2008), p. 297.

[105] MS Bodley 130. For other contemporary examples see London, British Library, MSS Harley 5294, Sloane 1975.

contains particularly detailed illustrations, including a stunning image of a bramble, or 'brimble' as the text calls it.[106] This image depicts the foliage, thorns and ripening blackberries of the plant, making identification easy. The presence of common plants within the herbals provided practical and accessible treatments. Brambles, for example, are notoriously free-growing in fields and hedges. The question remains as to whether monks would cultivate or be expected to collect such 'ingredients' themselves, or whether these would be purchased by the monastery from an external source, but it is clear that common and easily-accessible ingredients were key to simple medicines. The bramble commentary in the Bury herbal is an example of medical advice available within this widely distributed text. Capitalised words indicate the various medical uses for the plant, such as for 'AURIUM DOLOREM' ('pain in the ears'), 'PROFLUUIUM MULIERIS' ('the "flowing" of women'), and 'CARDIACOS' ('the heart').[107]

Another source of medicinal knowledge that might be found in a twelfth-century English monastery was the lapidaries.[108] Peter Kitson identified that the oldest (surviving) vernacular lapidary in Western Europe appears to have been produced in Canterbury in the mid-eleventh century.[109] A Hellenistic lapidary attributed to Damigeron was also known in Latin translation in Anglo-Saxon England.[110] According to Kitson, the Latin lapidary of Pseudo-Aristotle was translated in the twelfth century and came from Hebrew translations of an Arabic compilation.[111] By the thirteenth century, two early twelfth-century alphabetical editions of the Latin Damigeron belonged to Worcester Cathedral Priory and St Augustine's, Canterbury.[112]

Stones, like animals and plants, were thought to have therapeutic properties. As such, lapidaries were of interest to practising *medici*, including Master Herbert who donated his copy of *Liber de natura lapidum in uno volumine* to Durham.[113] Most often, though, lapidaries were to be found within other manuscripts, including bestiaries, as found in the *Aberdeen Bestiary* (produced

---

[106] MS Bodley 130, fol. 26r.

[107] Ibid.

[108] For further discussion of lapidaries see: P. Kitson, 'Lapidary Traditions in Anglo-Saxon England: Part 1, the Background; the Old English Lapidary', *Anglo-Saxon England* 7 (1978), 9–60; A. Lawrence-Mathers and C. Escobar-Vargas, *Magic and Medieval Society*, Seminar Studies in History (London, 2014), pp. 54–9.

[109] London, British Library, MS Cotton Tiberius A.iii; Kitson, 'Lapidary Traditions', 9.

[110] Kitson, 'Lapidary Traditions', 11–12, 17–19.

[111] Ibid., 12.

[112] Ibid., 13.

[113] *Catalogi Veteres Librorum*, ed. Botfield, pp. 7–8.

c. 1200).[114] Lapidaries focused on stones that were exotic or precious, such as rubies, pearls and crystals.[115] Unlike many of the plants within the herbals, these precious stones were expensive, luxury items and some of their perceived power might have come from their exotic origins and striking colours. The practical usage of luxury stones was, unsurprisingly, limited to a select few who had the money and means to obtain them. However the belief in the ability of precious stones to bring about a cure is well recorded, as can be seen in *M. Jacobi's* account of noblewoman Aquilina, who received gemstones from Henry II when she experienced a difficult labour.[116] *M. Jacobi* explained that these stones were 'parturientibus conferre credebantur transmisit' ('believed to bestow [help to] those in labour').[117]

Along with other medical texts, herbals, bestiaries and lapidaries would not form part of the *lectio divina* and were unlikely to have been accessible to the broader monastic community.[118] They were more likely to have been part of specialist collections under the care of the infirmarer or monastic superiors. That said, by the twelfth century, bishops were responsible for providing schools and masters to teach potential clerics, and the book collections of bishops, masters and wealthier clerics may have included highly illuminated encyclopaedias; some monks and monastic officials probably benefited from such education as well. Knowledge of humoral and complexional theories, and the 'Ages of Man' (in addition to some geographical knowledge, and awareness of the natural wonders of the world), was well established in twelfth-century monasteries. While specialist medical knowledge would have been largely confined to the sphere of the abbot's *familia* (household) and the specialist monastic officials who required it, a broader awareness of the body and health, and the natural world, would have been present within the wider monastery. Just as important, however, would have been the practical encounters with healthcare practices, ill health, and recovery experienced and witnessed.

Anglo-Norman Medical Texts

The materials discussed thus far were part of the growing collection of Latin medical texts that were being transmitted in England during this century.

---

[114] *Aberdeen Bestiary*, Aberdeen, Aberdeen University Library, MS 24, fols. 93v–103v.

[115] Ibid., fols. 100r–100v.

[116] *M. Jacobi*, fol. 174va-b; Kemp, '*The Hand of St James*' XXI, 16. It should be noted that Kemp translates this more simply as 'believed to help those in labour'; I have kept 'conferre' ('to bestow') in this translation.

[117] Ibid. Also see below, pp. 77–9.

[118] *Regula S. Benedicti* 48, ed. McCann, pp. 110–13; Kerr, *Life in the Medieval Cloister*, pp. 156–9, 178.

However it is also important to recognise the development of vernacular, Anglo-Norman, medical texts, which indicates a potentially broader readership. The production of Anglo-Norman medical materials, mentioned above, dates from the late twelfth century. They focus on the more practical rather than theoretical aspects of medicine. Hunt has produced a number of editions of surviving Anglo-Norman medical texts, based on surviving manuscripts from the thirteenth century onwards.[119] These materials not only illustrate England's connection to the Continent and especially to the Norman territories, including those in southern Italy, but also show that there was a broader, vernacular readership for these materials.[120]

Among the Anglo-Norman medical works, translated from their original Latin, that have been edited by Hunt are those found in a mid-thirteenth-century compendium.[121] From this manuscript, Roger Frugard's *Chirurgia* and Platearius's *Practica Brevis* were published in a single edition by Hunt.[122] A second volume contained four shorter medical texts, two of which – *De instructione medici* and a verse edition of the *Trotula* – also come from this manuscript.[123] The Anglo-Norman translations of *Chirurgia* and *Practica Brevis* both date from the twelfth century and are thus presumably reflective of a perceived contemporary need for such resources to be accessible in the vernacular. More challenging to ascertain is who the owners of these works were: evidence of medieval book collections best survives in relation to religious houses. Hunt argued that vernacular books within monastic institutions would have primarily arrived through donations, thus suggesting an initial lay audience.[124] Among a lay audience such medical materials would have been for a select readership including practitioners and, potentially, literate laypersons who used this resource for 'self-help'.[125] *De instructione medici* provides a good example of this, as it is concerned with setting out the process of visiting,

---

[119] *Anglo-Norman Medicine. Volume I: Roger Frugard's Chirurgia and The Practica Brevis of Platearius*, ed. T. Hunt (Cambridge, 1994); *Anglo-Norman Medicine. Volume II: Shorter Treatises*, ed. T. Hunt (Cambridge, 1997); *An Anglo-Norman Medical Compendium (Cambridge, Trinity College MS O.2.5 (1109))*, ed. T. Hunt, Anglo-Norman Text Society Plain Text Series 18 (Oxford, 2014); *An Anglo-Norman Medical Compendium (Oxford, Bodleian Library MS Bodley 761)*, ed. T. Hunt, Anglo-Norman Text Society Plain Text Series 19 (Oxford, 2017).

[120] Green, 'Salerno on the Thames', p. 229.

[121] Cambridge, Trinity College MS O.1.20.

[122] Hunt, *Anglo-Norman Medicine. Volume I*.

[123] Hunt, *Anglo-Norman Medicine. Volume II*, pp. 17–67, 68–128.

[124] Hunt, 'The Anglo-Norman Book', p. 380.

[125] Green, 'Salerno on the Thames', p. 229.

diagnosing, and healing the sick.[126] Green similarly sees a lay audience as being the key demographic for recipe collections and also suggests that these texts could have been produced for women.[127] Regardless of their ownership, these texts are an important indication of the growing interest in accessible learned medicine from the high into the late Middle Ages. Clearly there was a strong Salernitan tradition which lay behind much of this, one which was reflected in the medical works being collected and created by the twelfth-century monastic centres in which saints' cults, like the seven case studies here, were housed.

Monastic Care in the Community

It is vital to consider the practical healthcare delivered to the monks. Care for the sick was an important rule laid down in *Regula S. Benedicti* and it must be acknowledged that monks would also have experienced ill health and medical care.[128] These experiences would have contributed to monastic views of illness and healing. Those who were sick were given some respite from the usual monastic rules regarding duties and diet. Meat, theoretically 'off-the-menu' for healthy monks, was permitted for those who were sick or weak.[129] Diet, as noted, was key among the non-naturals, and meat was seen as a necessity for recovering monks, as was rest.[130] Many monks were highly aware of the dietary leniency sanctioned for medical reasons, leading to concern from churchmen, including Bernard of Clairvaux, that such leniencies might lead to false claims of ill health in order to enjoy this less rigorous regime.[131]

Bathing

The *Regula S. Benedicti* also permitted bathing for the sick; something which the healthy, and particularly the young, were rarely allowed.[132] As a method of evacuation and repletion, bathing was also an essential restorative practice for balancing the non-naturals.[133] However monastic attitudes to bathing

---

[126] Hunt, *Anglo-Norman Medicine. Volume II*, p. 19.

[127] Green, 'Salerno on the Thames', pp. 224, 227–8.

[128] *Regula S. Benedicti* 36, ed. McCann, pp. 90–1.

[129] Kerr, *Life in the Medieval Cloister*, pp. 48–9; Rawcliffe, "On the Threshold of Eternity"', pp. 41–72.

[130] Rawcliffe, "On the Threshold of Eternity"', p. 58.

[131] Bernard of Clairvaux, *Apologia* XIX.22–23, in *The 'Things of Greater Importance': Bernard of Clairvaux's Apologia and the Medieval Attitude toward Art*, ed. and trans. C. Rudolph (Philadelphia, 1990), pp. 232–87.

[132] *Regula S. Benedicti* 36, ed. McCann, pp. 90–1.

[133] Rawcliffe, "On the Threshold of Eternity"', p. 59.

were complex, as bathing for pleasure, rather than necessity, was seen as a self-indulgent luxury. Lanfranc thus limited healthy Canterbury monks to three baths a year, all of which preceded important festivals.[134]

Although bathing of the whole body was limited within the monastery, washing occurred daily. Monks were obliged to wash their hands before entering the refectory, a practice of both practical and symbolic cleansing.[135] The Maundy, carried out on a weekly basis, involved brothers washing each other's feet, and mirrored Christ's washing the feet of the disciples.[136] Washing therefore could offer cleansing on two levels – physical and spiritual – and this is again indicative of the intertwined nature of contemporary understanding regarding the health of the body and of the soul. That *Regula S. Benedicti* notes the importance of bathing, and specifically full-body immersion, as a treatment for the sick, is thus unsurprising. Conversely, immersion in icy water could be used to quell feelings of passion. Bernard of Clairvaux stood neck-deep in water to rid himself of lustful thoughts. St Cuthbert and Ailred of Rievaulx were likewise recorded as having submitted to this practice.[137] Later in his life, medicinal bathing (presumably using warmer water) also allowed Ailred of Rievaulx some relief from the discomfort of urinary stones. Ailred's biographer, Walter Daniel, stressed that this was by no means a luxury but an exhaustive process, and medical necessity. One occasion saw the abbot having to undergo forty successive baths.[138]

Bloodletting

Bloodletting, often noted for its frequent practice, was similarly deployed as both a preventative and curative process and, like bathing, had both physical

---

[134] Lanfranc, *Decreta Lanfranci Monachis Canturiensibus Transmissa* (hereafter *De-creta*) 7, in *The Monastic Constitutions of Lanfranc*, ed. and trans. D. Knowles and C. Brooke, OMT (Oxford, 2002), pp. 2–195 (14–17).

[135] Kerr, *Life in the Medieval Cloister*, pp. 22, 60.

[136] John 13.14–15.

[137] William of St Thierry et al., *Vita Prima Sancti Bernardi Claraevallis Abbatis: Liber Primus* I.6, ed. P. Verdeyen and C. Vande Veire, *Corpus Christianorum Continuatio Mediaevalis* 89B (Turnhout, 2011), p. 37; Bede, *Vita Sancti Cuthberti auctore Beda* 10, in *Two Lives of Saint Cuthbert: A Life by an Anonymous Monk of Lindisfarne and Bede's Prose Life*, trans. B. Colgrave (Cambridge, 1940), pp. 141–307 (188–91); Walter Daniel, *The Life of Ailred of Rievaulx by Walter Daniel* 16, trans. F. M. Pow-icke, Medieval Classics (London, 1950), p. 25.

[138] Walter Daniel, *The Life of Ailred of Rievaulx* 27, trans. Powicke, p. 34; Kerr, *Life in the Medieval Cloister*, pp. 60–1.

and spiritual connotations.[139] Yet, despite regular practice, bloodletting is discussed in neither the *Regula S. Benedicti* nor the tenth-century *Regularis Concordia*: an omission that suggests it was practised without formality.[140] Phlebotomy had roots in ancient medical theory and was a recognised method for correcting humoral imbalances. However, scholastic medical theory recognised that blood was not made up of solely one humour. These ideas first appeared in Islamic medicine in the ninth century in the work of Quṣṭā ibn Lūqā, although it is worth questioning how widespread these high-academic theories were among the working *medici* and barber-surgeons who had not undergone formal training.[141] Less scholarly *medici*, practising prior to the rise of academic medical education, might well have had a more simplistic understanding about the purpose and effect of bloodletting.

Monastic communities, however, as Voigts and McVaugh have shown, had access to texts on phlebotomy from the early ninth century onwards.[142] The *Epistula de Phlebotomia*, based on earlier Greco-Roman works, and found in numerous monastic libraries, emphasised the use of the three major veins of the arms for bloodletting and was 'probably a standard guide' to the procedure undertaken within monasteries.[143] With the development of medical learning in Salerno in the late eleventh and twelfth centuries these earlier treatises on phlebotomy were reworked in order to incorporate additional information including *descretio sanguinis* (explanations on how physicians could use the let blood to judge the patient's condition).[144] Such contemporary additions can be found in a later twelfth-century version of a phlebotomy tract believed to have been originally produced by Archimatteus, while Constantine the African's *Pantegni* added two further veins in the arm to the list of suitable veins for

[139] J. Burton, *Monastic and Religious Orders in Britain, 1000–1300*, Cambridge Medieval Textbooks (Cambridge, 1994), p. 146; J. G. Clark, *The Benedictines in the Middle Ages*, Monastic Orders (Woodbridge, 2011), p. 128; P. Fergusson, *Canterbury Cathedral Priory in the Age of Becket* (New Haven, 2011), pp. 21, 109, 167, 168 n. 7.1; Kerr, *Life in the Medieval Cloister*, pp. 73–4, 210; Siraisi, *Medieval and Early Renaissance Medicine*, p. 115.

[140] *Regularis Concordia: Anglicae Nationis Monachrum Sanctimonialiumque. The Monastic Agreement of the Monks and Nuns of the English Nations* (hereafter *Regularis Concordia*), ed. and trans. T. Symons, Medieval Classics (London, 1953), p. xxxix.

[141] E. Savage-Smith, 'Were the Four Humours Fundamental to Medieval Islamic Medical Practice?', in *The Body in Balance: Humoral Medicines in Practice*, ed. P. Horden and E. Hsu, Epistemologies of Healing 13 (New York, 2013), pp. 89–106 (96–8).

[142] Voigts and McVaugh, *A Latin Technical Phlebotomy*, p. 1.

[143] Ibid., p. 2.

[144] Ibid., p. 3.

phlebotomy.[145] Gerard of Cremona was similarly influential for translating Albucasis's *Chirurgia* which elaborated on bloodletting further still, identifying thirty suitable veins and detailing the techniques that were to be used to perform the procedure successfully, as has been beneficially summarised by Voigts and McVaugh.[146] Evidently, bloodletting came from a notable, learned tradition influenced by classical practices. For churchmen in particular, phlebotomy also had important spiritual connotations, as Rawcliffe explained: 'Christ had been phlebotomised on the Cross to purge the sins of the world, bloodletting offered the most immediate means of restoring a healthy balance and ridding the body of corruption.'[147]

There were inherent risks with phlebotomy, and bloodletting could not be undertaken without forethought and planning: certain days were inauspicious. Astrological knowledge and an awareness of important dates in the liturgical calendar prevented bloodletting from being performed on days that were dangerous or impractical, an issue already recognised in Anglo-Saxon monasteries.[148] Bede illustrates this in his recording of the disastrous bleeding of a nun at Watton.[149] So well-known were these dangerous days, or 'Egyptian Days', that they needed only to be marked by a 'D' within the calendar of one *c.* 1200 English psalter thought to have belonged to the Benedictine monastery at Amesbury.[150] Instructions for bloodletting were present in monasteries from an early date: St Gall's library contained a copy of *Epistula de phlebotomia* in the 800s.[151]

---

[145] Ibid., pp. 3–4.

[146] Ibid., pp. 5–6.

[147] Rawcliffe, '"On the Threshold of Eternity"', p. 64. Also see *Ancient Christian Writers 52: Cassiodorus: Volume 2: Explanation of the Psalms*, Psalm 57, trans. P. G. Walsh (New York, 1990), p. 50; Ziegler, *Medicine and Religion c. 1300*, pp. 182–3.

[148] Cameron, *Anglo-Saxon Medicine*, p. 163; *Prognostics. De observatione lunæ et quid cavendum sit. De somniorum eventu*, in *Leechdoms, Wortcunning and Starcraft of Early England. Being a Collection of Documents, for the most part never before printed, illustrating the History of Science in the Country before the Norman Conquest*, ed. and trans. O. Cockayne, 3 vols, RS 35 (London, 1866), III, 152–5.

[149] Bede, *HE* V.3, ed. Colgrave and Mynors, pp. 460–1.

[150] Imola, Biblioteca Comunale di Imola, MS 111, fol. 6v. Also see: 'Il Salterio inglese (MS 111)', Biblioteca Comunale di Imola, <http://www.bim.comune.imola.bo.it/content.php?current=8628#top> [accessed 27 June 2020]; *A History of the County of Wiltshire: Volume 3*, ed. R. B. Pugh and E. Crittall, VCH (London, 1956), pp. 242–59.

[151] G. B. Risse, *Mending Bodies, Saving Souls: A History of Hospitals* (Oxford, 1999), p. 104.

Bloodletting, like bathing, was a long-established aspect of monastic life by the twelfth century and a great deal of attention was paid to the care provided before and after bleeding, highlighting monastic awareness of the impacts the practice had on the body. Bishop John Kirkby of Ely was so badly bled in 1290 that he required Æthelthryth's intercession.[152] Recognition of the weakness that ensued from phlebotomy can be found in Lanfranc of Canterbury's *Decreta* which lists the days when bloodletting was to be avoided.[153] Lanfranc's primary concern was the involvement of the entire community at key ecclesiastical events, but there was obvious appreciation too that monks would be unable to cope with the rigours of feast days. Indeed, Terryl Kinder has suggested that up to four pints of blood might be let at a time.[154] If this were the case, it is no surprise that hours standing and singing in church would prove challenging.

Bedrest

Ill and bled monks were permitted time to recover but they did not necessarily spend this time within the infirmary. Lanfranc stated that following bloodletting brothers may stay away from choir for a day, or longer if necessary, but made no suggestion that this rest should occur outside the cloister.[155] Infirmaries, while an important part of the monastic complex, were not the first port of call for an ailing monk. Rather, the unwell individual, according to Lanfranc, was to confess his illness. The abbot would then permit the monk to treat himself as required and to stay away from conventual duties if necessary.[156] Presumably this involved resting in the dormitory and provided a lenience towards missing services as well as greater concession over diet. Indeed, the *Decreta* states that only when sickness increased, meaning the monk could not remain 'in conuentu' ('in the community'), should the abbot tell the infirmarer to take the afflicted brother in.[157] This implies that brothers suffering milder complaints remained within the cloister where the community at large would have witnessed their ill health and, if lucky, their recovery. Additionally, this suggests that monks were to judge their level of illness, at least up to the point where the abbot or infirmarer needed to intervene.

[152] Rawcliffe, 'Curing Bodies and Healing Souls', p. 114.
[153] Lanfranc, *Decreta* 95, ed. Knowles and Brooke, pp. 140–1.
[154] T. N. Kinder, *Cistercian Europe: Architecture of Contemplation* (Grand Rapids, 2002), p. 278.
[155] Lanfranc, *Decreta* 95, ed. Knowles and Brooke, pp. 140–1.
[156] Ibid., 111, pp. 176–7.
[157] Ibid.

Monastic infirmaries tended to be constructed east of the claustral buildings, set apart from the community but still accessible. Monastic superiors were expected to visit their infirm charges daily, offering them emotional and spiritual comfort. At Abingdon the cook made daily visits to the infirmary, where he 'quod appetent diligenter interrogabit' ('will diligently inquire what [the sick brothers] might desire').[158] That an attempt was made to treat each in-patient as an individual reveals an attentiveness that is important to recognise. However, not all who were in the infirmary were ill. The infirmarer himself was expected to reside there to care for the sick monks and make sure that a suitable level of monastic discipline was maintained, and he might also be joined by assistants.[159] More permanently, infirmaries housed older monks for whom age and its associated problems meant they were no longer able to fully partake in the rigorous day-to-day duties of monastic life. These long-term inmates benefited from the quieter pace and fuller diet of the infirmary.[160]

What was a serious enough illness to require a stay in the infirmary? Peter Peverell, a Norwich monk, suffered from a swelling on his right eye that caused him pain and made him into a 'horribile spectaculum' ('horrifying spectacle').[161] Despite his pain and facial disfigurement, Peter did not enter the infirmary. Rather, his cure occurred when William of Norwich visited Peter while he slept, presumably, in the dormitory.[162] Conversely, Thomas of Ely spent eight days in the infirmary while suffering from a fever.[163] Unusually, the course of Thomas's affliction is recorded first-hand, providing direct insight into his experience. *L. Eliensis* records that Thomas was 'miser' ('wretched') and 'anxius' ('anxious').[164] Thomas became increasingly languid, and his brothers became 'timidi de funere' ('fearful of death').[165] Thomas recovered following a vision in which Æthelthryth attended to him in his bed. On waking, Thomas found his condition had improved; he called the brothers to his bed and the community gave thanks to God and Æthelthryth.[166]

These accounts were recorded at different points in the twelfth century, and in two separate communities (whose superiors might have varying opinions on

---

[158] *Chronicon Monasterii de Abingdon*, ed. Stevenson, II, 391.

[159] Kerr, *Life in the Medieval Cloister*, p. 77.

[160] Ibid.

[161] Thomas of Monmouth, *M. Willelmi* V.20, ed. Jessop and James, p. 211.

[162] Ibid.

[163] *L. Eliensis* III.69, ed. Blake, pp. 312–14, trans. Fairweather, pp. 385–8.

[164] Ibid.

[165] Ibid.

[166] Ibid.

what qualified as infirmary-worthy afflictions), but the significant difference was that Thomas was expected to die and that the Ely community were preparing for this. Preparing for a good death was a serious matter. The *Regularis Concordia* and Lanfranc's *Decreta* both state that dying monks were expected to be within the infirmary at the time when last rites were to be performed.[167] Thomas's affliction was feared to be fatal, but while Peter's suffering was painful there was no suggestion it would lead to his death (although Peter himself wished for death because of it).[168]

Despite the differences in treatment, both accounts highlight the presence of other members of the monastic community. Peter's changing appearance and cure, and Thomas's prolonged presence in the infirmary, were both witnessed by their fellow brethren. Both men's experiences provided the wider monastic community with the opportunity to observe suffering up-close. Such first-hand encounters should not be underestimated. Practical experience and observance would have shaped monastic communities and their ideas of health, ill health, medicine, and cure. The poor health of one monk could impact upon all the members of the community, including the hagiographers. It is likely most, if not all, monks spent some time in the infirmary. They certainly would have known of, and visited, others who had.

Bathing, bloodletting, and bedrest allowed for a dissemination of humoral balance theories, and the importance of the non-naturals. Bathing and phlebotomy drew on spiritual connections too, making these practices multifaceted in their meaning. What does this imply about the way hagiographers would have perceived the cure-seekers whose miraculous cures they recorded? Although, theoretically, distanced from the world, monks were not distanced from poor health. They observed symptoms and suffering in themselves and were also taught the importance of caring for the sick, as Christ did. While guides such as the *Regula S. Benedicti* focused on caring within the community, monastic institutions also provided charity and compassion for suffering laity.[169] This charity took a number of forms, but, as with in-house care, the observances it led to would have impacted on the monks and their understanding of the body, health, ill health and healthcare.

---

[167] *Regularis Concordia* XII.65, ed. Symons, pp. 64–5; Lanfranc, *Decreta* 112, ed. Knowles and Brooke, pp. 178–9.

[168] Thomas of Monmouth, *M. Willelmi* V.20, ed. Jessop and James, p. 212.

[169] *Regula S. Benedicti* 36, ed. McCann, pp. 90–1.

Monastic Care for the Laity

Hospitals

Unlike monastic infirmaries, lay-focused *hospitia* (hospitals) could fall into a number of categories. Sethina Watson, in her recent study of the hospital, welfare and the law, referred to there being 'a dizzying array of charitable institutions' that could be termed 'hospitals'.[170] While there are various ways in which these welfare institutions could be identified, and categorised, Rawcliffe's three-way division of these institutions is perhaps the most useful from our current perspective, focusing on those places connected to monastic houses. Rawcliffe separates *hospitia* into those for lepers, those for short-term care, and those for long-term care.[171] Few miraculous cures involved healing leprosy, and hospitals for long-term inmates were, to an extent, forerunners of retirement homes. Within the hagiographies focused upon here, only one account, in *M. Swithuni*, refers to leprosy.[172] *M. Willelmi* also includes an account in which a woman had become so swollen that she appeared 'tanquam elephantino perculsa incommodo' ('as though affected with elephantiasis'); however this is a comparative description of her appearance rather than any claim of her being leprous.[173] This woman was healed from long-term sickness while she lay in the, now unidentifiable, hospital called 'Brichtiue'.[174] Regarding the cure-seekers, however, it is the short-term *hospitia* (often located on the boundaries of the monasteries) that are most relevant.

Certain obedientiary positions brought monks into closer contact with the laity than the majority of the claustral community. The almoner and guest-master chiefly fulfilled these outward-facing responsibilities, as did the porter (gate-keeper) when this position was filled by a monk, but much of the day-to-day work would have been undertaken by monastic servants or regular canons.[175]

---

[170] S. Watson, *On Hospitals: Welfare, Law, and Christianity in Western Europe, 400–1320*, Oxford Studies in Medieval European History (Oxford, 2020), p. 4.

[171] C. Rawcliffe, *Urban Bodies: Communal Health in Late Medieval English Towns and Cities* (Woodbridge, 2013), p. 317. Also see R. Gilchrist, *Contemplation and Action: The Other Monasticism* (London, 1995), p. 9.

[172] *M. Swithuni* 44, ed. Lapidge, pp. 680–1.

[173] Thomas of Monmouth, *M. Willelmi* III.15, ed. Jessop and James, pp. 148–9.

[174] Ibid., p. 148. For further discussion of Norwich's hospitals, see C. Rawcliffe, 'Sickness and Health', in *Medieval Norwich*, ed. C. Rawcliffe and R. Wilson (London, 2004), pp. 301–26.

[175] Burton, *Monastic and Religious Orders in Britain*, pp. 45, 49, 62, 172–3, 178–80, 251; J. Kerr, *Monastic Hospitality: The Benedictines in England, c. 1070–c. 1250*, Studies in the History of Medieval Religion 32 (Woodbridge, 2007), p. 65.

The almoner's duty to the sick and poor laity was the most pronounced, with Lanfranc instilling that he should 'ubi egri, et debiles iaceant, qui non habent unde se sustentare ualeant' ('take great pains to discover where may lie those sick and weakly persons who are without means of sustenance').[176] The *Decreta* also cautions that, if the almoner attends the sick himself, he must take with him two servants and any women there must leave, presumably to avoid gossip.[177] The almoner was to speak kindly, and comfort the sick individual and, if possible, obtain any requested items.[178] In the case of a sick woman, the almoner was to send his servants in his place and was never to enter the house.[179] Importantly, the *Decreta* stresses that the almoner always had to seek the permission of the monastic superior before acting; only then could he give alms.[180] Similar concerns are found in the decrees of the First Lateran Council (1123) which forbade abbots and monks from visiting the sick in their provisions of charity.[181] However the *Regula S. Benedicti* stated that the sick, like pilgrims, were to be treated charitably because it was in them that Christ was most visible.[182] This reflected biblical ideals of care and charity found in both the Old and New Testaments.[183] A fine balance thus had to be maintained between providing charity and safeguarding against secular distractions. Lateran I's decrees are reflective of this, and of the growing reforms that aimed to ensure the separation between the monastic brethren and the temporal world.[184]

This need to provide care at a distance was reflected in many monastic *hospitia*. Monasteries were the most prolific of hospital founders, but the running of these institutions was rarely carried out by the monastic brethren. Hospitals were often built at boundaries, either the boundary of the monastic

---

[176] Lanfranc, *Decreta* 91, ed. Knowles and Brooke, pp. 132–3.

[177] Ibid.

[178] Ibid.

[179] Ibid.

[180] Ibid.

[181] *Concilium Lateranense I* 16, in *Decrees of the Ecumenical Councils*, ed. and trans. N. Tanner, 2 vols (London, 1990), I, *Nicaea I – Lateran V*, 193.

[182] *Regula S. Benedicti* 53, ed. McCann, pp. 118–23.

[183] Deuteronomy 15.7–11; Matthew 25.36–7.

[184] For further discussion of twelfth-century monastic reform see: S. Williams, *The Gregorian Epoch: Reformations, Revolutions, Reaction?*, Problems in European Civilization (Boston, 1964); G. Constable, *The Reformation of the Twelfth Century*, Trevelyan Lectures 1985 (Cambridge, 1996).

and lay worlds or on the boundaries of the town or village itself.[185] In Bury St Edmunds five of the six hospitals were founded by the monastic community, or their abbots, and were thus dependent on the abbey. All were constructed outside the gates of Bury, and appear to have been staffed by external employees.[186] At Reading, St John's hospital, founded by Abbot Hugh II in 1190, was constructed next to the church of St Laurence and the main West Gate which led into the abbey. In his 1191 confirmation of the foundation, Hugh II granted free alms to St Laurence's for the care of thirteen lay poor, and promised a daily provision of food for another thirteen poor; this was also to be available to pilgrims.[187] St John's, as testified by the charter, was thus a hospital for the local poor, travelling poor, and pilgrims, reflecting the manifold nature of many such short-term *hospitia*.[188]

The administration of *hospitia* varied greatly. Augustinian canons oversaw certain foundations as they were less bound to a life of seclusion than other monastic orders. Elsewhere, and often in an Augustinian context, the laity took charge of the daily care, and elsewhere still it was lay-brothers, and occasionally lay-sisters, who were charged with this duty.[189] At Reading, St John's was attached to St Laurence's, and the priest of the church was to provide spiritual care to the hospital's inmates, in exchange for which he was granted the perpetual vicarage of the church and was to be provided with a horse when he was required to travel.[190] However, it was the responsibility of Reading's almoner, not the priest, to maintain the chapel and hospital and to provide oil for the lamps.[191] These responsibilities would not require the almoner, let alone any other member of Reading's community, to spend much time within St John's itself, but it does indicate that the almoner, in his administrative role,

---

[185] H. Mahood, 'The Liminality of Care: Caring for the Sick and Needy on the Boundaries of Monasteries', *The Maladies, Miracles and Medicine of the Middle Ages: Selected Papers from the Postgraduate and Early-Career Researcher Conference, March 2014. The Reading Medievalist: A Postgraduate Journal* 2 (2015), 50–70, <http://blogs. reading.ac.uk/trm/2015/04/01/proceedings-of-the-gcms-postgraduate-confer ence-2015-the-maladies-miracles-and-medicine-of-the-middle-ages/> [accessed 17 July 2020].

[186] *Charters of the Medieval Hospitals of Bury St Edmunds*, ed. C. Harper-Bill, Suffolk Charters 14 (Woodbridge, 1994), pp. 1–10; *A History of the County of Suffolk: Volume 2*, ed. W. Page, VCH (London, 1975), pp. 133–6.

[187] *Reading Abbey Cartularies*, 'Abbatial Acts and Abbey Documents 224', ed. Kemp, I, 185–6.

[188] Ibid.

[189] Mahood, 'The Liminality of Care', 51–2, 61–2.

[190] *Reading Abbey Cartularies*, 'Reading 848', ed. Kemp, II, 124–5.

[191] *A History of the County of Berkshire: Volume 2*, ed. Ditchfield and Page, 97–9.

was responsible for employing a guardian, or care-giver, for the hospital to attend to the inmates.

Importantly, these hospitals tended to the spiritual as well as palliative care of their charges. The level of medical care undertaken is less evident. The need to provide the laity with spiritual care was as important, if not more important, than care for the body, just as it was for the monks themselves, hence the provision of the priest of St Laurence's in Reading.[192] That care within such institutions was predominantly palliative and spiritual, rather than curative, is important to bear in mind. Horden has noted that the hospitals worked on a similar principle to the Church at large, exemplifying the 'subordination of the care of the body to the care of the soul [...] the earthly physician to *Christus medicus*'.[193] This attitude to the manner of care provided can be seen as paramount in all high-medieval *hospitia*.

In terms of considering the level of interaction between the hospitals and the monastic communities it is important to understand that many monks would have had little reason to engage with the lay poor and sick within these foundations. *Hospitia*, especially those for short-term care, were not medical as much as they were a combination of hospice and hostel, and the care they provided was for both the local laity and for pilgrims who required accommodation. For those seeking cure through petitioning the saints, though, it was the shrine and not the hospital that was the focus (as is further discussed in Chapter 6).[194] Nevertheless, it is worth considering that cure-seekers, successful or not, provided monastic communities with further opportunities to observe suffering and recovery. In addition to learned medicine, and spiritual understanding of the body and soul, these observations would have shaped the ways in which monks saw, understood, and interpreted ideas about the body and health. That miraculous healing was a performance of divine intervention would have also strengthened the perceived connection between physical health and divine cure.

*   *   *

This chapter has emphasised that, while access to specialist medical texts was rare for the majority of monks, the monastic communities of the twelfth-century cloisters were not unaware of the issues of health and healing. Their

---

[192] Kerr, *Monastic Hospitality*, pp. 121–61.
[193] Horden, 'A Non-Natural Environment', p. 141.
[194] See below, pp. 178–80.

knowledge almost certainly came more from their experiences of the practical side of medicine than from 'book learning'. However, regular experience of phlebotomy and ritual bathing would have functioned as a reminder of the concepts of, and connections between, both physical and spiritual health. This was further reflected in the ways that monasteries treated their afflicted brethren and approached the charitable care they provided for the laity. *Hospitia* were not solely spaces for the ill, they were also locations where the local poor and pilgrims could find charity and respite. The monks themselves were unlikely to take part in the day-to-day care provided within the *hospitia*; but any monk might be required to assist the almoner, the infirmarer, or act as porter, during their monastic career. These responsibilities would bring that brother into closer contact with those who sought monastic charity.

This chapter has deliberately focused on the monastic understanding of medicine and healthcare practices not only because these were the institutions primarily involved in the earlier transmission of medical knowledge, but also because it was within these monastic communities that miraculous healing tended to occur. Furthermore, it was the monastic hagiographers who committed to writing the wondrous cures brought about through saintly intercession. In terms of considering whether the *miracula* indicate medical awareness, therefore, it is to the knowledge present within the monasteries that we must turn. Many monks, however, would have also been influenced by the witnessing of ill health, as, no doubt, would many laypeople. There would have been broader understandings that certain simple remedies could ease discomfort and provide remedial benefits. Beyond the monasteries and their written records, however, this evidence is more elusive and the *miracula* are thus advantageous for the references they provide in this regard.

In their recording of miraculous healing, hagiographers were keen to highlight how initial recourse to earthly medicine and practitioners failed where divine therapy succeeded. While the miracles accounts are dismissive of these other avenues of healthcare, their very mention within the reports highlights that cure-seekers had a range of curative options available to them (so long as they had the means to afford treatment). Particularly depicted as the alternative to saintly remedy, however, were the *medici*, many of whom must have benefited from the increased medical knowledge that was being transmitted across the Continent from centres such as Salerno and Montpellier. In promoting the importance of holy healing, and emphasising its superiority to earthly medicine, hagiographers thus sought to record the important details of the healing miracles, ensuring, at the least, that the nature of the cure-seekers' afflictions was accurately recorded. In many instances, however, the *miracula* provide further details that can assist in establishing an understanding of the afflictions suffered and the healthcare experiences of those who ultimately secured their cure through holy healing. It is to this topic, to the recording of the miracle cures, that the next chapter turns.

2

Holy Healing:
An Analysis of the Ailments

Our cure-seekers shared one common goal: the desire to secure the saints' intercession to bring about miraculous healing. The afflictions that these cure-seekers were relieved of are therefore central to the narratives recorded within the *miracula*, and to this current study. The accounts of holy healing that were documented in the miracle accounts must, of course, be recognised as only a literary representation of healing experiences. Nevertheless, they have the potential to indicate wider patterns of miraculous cure-seeking, providing an insight into the range and variety of complaints that were brought to the saints' shrines.

The previous chapter established that monks, hagiographers included, would have had some understanding of health and healing but little reason to consult the medical literature available within their monasteries, unless their obedientiary responsibilities required it. That the period under discussion here also sat on the cusp of the wide dissemination of the translated classical medical corpus into the monasteries, and that cure-seekers had other avenues of healthcare available to them, makes the study of the twelfth-century accounts of miraculous healing all the more valuable. As well as providing an insight into how ill health and impairment were experienced, the language of the miracles can also be analysed to consider evidence of medical knowledge on the part of their compilers. Here it is worth exploring whether the hagiographers, and the cure-seekers who experienced these afflictions, demonstrate any medical awareness.

The reports of miraculous healing, and their representation of the afflictions brought by cure-seekers to these seven shrines, are central to this chapter, and here the use of statistical analysis is advantageous. Analysis of health concerns recorded in miracle accounts has been a feature of hagiographical studies since Finucane's foundational *Miracles and Pilgrims* and continues to prove a useful method for revealing the range and patterns of curative miracles. As noted in the introduction, a key difference here from many previous studies is the intentional focus on a select, small group of *miracula* and the cure-seekers represented within these works. This focus allows this chapter to tease out the details from these accounts and to provide comprehensive discussion of some of the more notable cases that are included in the *miracula*. This results in a more 'up close and personal' approach than can be achieved with the great overview studies. A focused approach proved fruitful in Eleanora Gordon's study of medieval children, including their afflictions, which concentrated on five posthumous *miracula*, and in Metzler's study of impairment in eight hagiographies.[1] The analysis here brings together elements of these previous studies by focusing on select cults but not on a singular category of cure-seeker or health complaint.

Prior to engaging with the analysis into the complaints miraculously cured, the categories used to produce this analysis must be addressed. To avoid retrospective diagnosis the following study purposefully keeps the categories of affliction it uses as broad groupings. Finucane demonstrated that the broad grouping of miracles by the similarities in reported symptoms proved the most efficient method and the one that best reflected the hagiographical records.[2] Metzler further supported this by stressing that there are disparities between medieval and modern uses of medical terms.[3] To offer further guidance, however, a number of these broader categories include further commentary to highlight the types of accounts that they cover (these details are provided within parentheses).

The Cures in Question

The Ailments in the Hagiographies

Following in the footsteps of Christ's miracles, and those of the early saints, certain cures feature prominently within the seven case studies. The most commonly occurring complaints recorded in these miracle accounts were paralysis, illnesses, and eye afflictions (chiefly blindness). Of the 260 reports of miraculous healing, these three categories represent more than half of all the complaints recorded (Table 2.1). Within this there appears to be an indication of a possible shift in 'popular' afflictions during the twelfth century. *M. Swithuni* and *M. Dunstani*, compiled in the first twenty years of the century, record greater numbers of eye afflictions, yet in later hagiographies, *M. Willelmi*

---

[1] E. C. Gordon, 'Child Health in the Middle Ages as Seen in the Miracles of Five English Saints, A.D. 1150–1220', *Bulletin of the History of Medicine* 60 (1986), 502–22 (507–20); Metzler, *Disability in Medieval Europe*, pp. 131–3.

[2] Finucane, *Miracles and Pilgrims*, p. 103.

[3] Metzler, *Disability in Medieval Europe*, p. 127.

and *M. Jacobi*, reports of illness become more notable. However, we should be wary of taking these changing patterns as clear proof of the saintly specialisms and must ask whether differences between the miracle compilers could have also impacted on the type, and frequency, of healing miracles represented in these materials. In the case of Norwich, a growing urban settlement, it is not surprising that illnesses could have spread rapidly through the city. Reading, likewise, while not on the same city scale as Norwich, was a developing town in the twelfth century and might have faced similar issues. Indeed, *M. Jacobi* refers to a plague that swept through Reading and resulted in fatalities among both the lay and monastic communities of the town.[4] Rawcliffe, in *Urban Bodies*, highlighted that health was particularly impacted during periods of population growth when overcrowding and food shortages placed additional strain on the health of urban communities.[5]

Table 2.1. Afflictions recorded within the seven *miracula*

	M. Swithuni	*M. Dunstani*	*L. Eliensis*	*M. Moduenne*	*M. Willelmi*	*M. Æbbe*	*M. Jacobi*	**Total**
Blindness and other eye afflictions	18	8	4	1	3	8	2	44
Blood complaints	0	0	0	0	2	0	0	2
Bodily paralysis (partial or full paralysis, humps, curvature of the spine or knees, etc.)	16	6	5	2	13	11	7	60
Combinations of sensory affliction and paralysis (blindness/deafness/muteness and partial/full paralysis)	1	1	0	0	2	1	0	5
Combinations of sensory afflictions and illness	0	0	0	1	0	0	0	1
Combinations of sensory afflictions and swelling	0	0	0	1	0	0	0	1
Complaints relating to bodily pain (internal, with no reference to sickness or paralysis)	0	0	0	0	5	0	1	6

---

4   *M. Jacobi*, fol. 172ra; Kemp, 'The Hand of St James' IV, 7–8.
5   Rawcliffe, *Urban Bodies*, p. 62.

	M. Swithuni	M. Dunstani	L. Eliensis	M. Moduenne	M. Willelmi	M. Æbbe	M. Jacobi	Total
Complaints relating to the mouth (toothache, ulcers, etc.)	0	0	2	0	3	0	0	5
Deafness and other ear afflictions	1	1	0	0	1	0	0	3
Difficult labour	0	0	0	0	1	0	1	2
Eye and speech impediments (blindness and muteness)	0	0	0	0	1	0	0	1
Ear and speech impediments (deafness and muteness)	1	0	0	0	0	1	0	2
Eye, ear and speech impediments (blindness, deafness and muteness)	0	0	0	0	1	1	0	2
Illness (unspecific but including sickness, fever, etc.)	2	3	5	1	26	1	8	46
Injuries (accidents, incidents, animal bites/stings/attacks resulting in bodily damage)	2	0	3	5	2	1	1	14
Insomnia	0	0	0	0	1	0	0	1
Leprosy	1	0	0	0	0	0	0	1
Lower body complaints (dysentery, piles)	0	0	0	0	2	0	0	2
Mental health complaints (madness, possession, epilepsy, etc.)	3	2	2	0	11	3	0	21
Muteness and other speech impediments	2	0	3	0	1	6	1	13
Tumours, swellings and growths (including cancer, gout, dropsy)	2	0	2	1	9	9	2	25
Unexplained weakness/ feebleness (no obvious reference to illness or paralysis)	0	0	0	0	0	0	1	1
Wounds caused by penitential bonds/irons	1	0	0	1	0	0	0	2

The one complaint to remain consistently present across all seven *miracula* was cases of paralysis. These complaints could take various forms, with impairment being partial or affecting the entire body. The lack or loss of sight, and the lack or loss of mobility, had the potential to severely impact the life of the individual. Metzler has argued that while physical impairment might not have prevented some from economic activity, this was not the same as social tolerance.[6] That some saw the physically impaired as a burden is further reflected by Metzler in her examination of the thirteenth-century *Summa pastoralis* that stressed almshouses were not to be used to support those with physical impairment, despite attempts by families and neighbours to place such individuals in these institutions' care.[7] While physical impairment might result in socio-economic disability for a sufferer, illnesses could prove fatal and there is a clear sense of urgency in the majority of accounts that record ill cure-seekers, many of whom are described as being close to death.[8] The resulting challenges faced by the paralysed and blind, and the dangers presented by illness, would have greatly impacted upon cure-seekers, thus their continuous presence within miracle stories is understandable.

Two smaller, but nevertheless important, categories of affliction were those of tumours (including swellings, and other growths), and mental health complaints (madness, demonic possession, and epilepsy); combined, these account for almost a fifth of the miracles. The former were more numerous in the later texts, while the latter remain relatively constant. This suggests increasing contemporary attention to the physical health of the body as Christ's miracles provide few exemplary precedents of miraculously healing swellings. Various forms of tumorous swelling and growths have been dealt with collectively here, in keeping with medieval medical understandings of these conditions. As Luke Demaitre has noted, a range of apostemes (unnatural swellings of the skin, often containing fluid) were often treated as one and the same.[9] This is perhaps best summed up in Guy de Chauliac's *Magna chirurgia* produced in the mid-fourteenth century: 'the aposteme, tumour, swelling, thickening, ridge, bump, and growth are names which mean pretty much the same thing'.[10] Following the argument proposed by Finucane, afflictions that affected the mind or brain have been categorised here under the heading of 'mental health

[6]   Metzler, *Disability in Medieval Europe*, p. 26.
[7]   Metzler, *A Social History of Disability*, p. 174.
[8]   For example, see: *M. Dunstani* 26, ed. Turner and Muir, pp. 206–7; *L. Eliensis* III.59, ed. Blake, p. 306, trans. Fairweather, p. 375.
[9]   Demaitre, *Medieval Medicine*, p. 79.
[10] Guy de Chauliac, *Magna chirurgia* (1363), cited in Demaitre, *Medieval Medicine*, p. 79.

complaints' owing to the similarity in the experiences and consequences of these afflictions.[11] It should be noted though that Trenery, in her thorough analysis of madness, has convincingly shown that afflictions of the mind and of the brain were beginning to be identified more specifically by the later twelfth century, even if the experiences of such sufferers continued to be similar.[12]

The presence of accounts relating to injuries is also striking. *M. Moduenne* features heavily within this category, accounting for almost half of the total number of incidents. Many of these can be found within the one compilatory account and relate to incidents caused by the building work on Burton's church roof, highlighting the dangers which were involved with such projects. Builders are recorded as having fallen from the roof scaffolds, while a mother and her son were saved from potential injury when the church's bell fell on them.[13] Julie Kerr, addressing accidents within the monasteries, highlighted how construction posed risks to those within the buildings.[14] Other accidental incidents within the miracle accounts include references to manual labour including agricultural work. One unfortunate youth fell asleep while watching his flock and 'dumque aperto sterteret ore, subito in ipsum coluber introiuit' ('as he lay snoring with open mouth, a viper suddenly crept in').[15] It is not in itself surprising that accidental injuries occurred with some frequency. However, the range of varying injuries and accidents that appear in the hagiographies offer valuable insight into the limitations of twelfth-century medical practitioners. Injuries were taken very seriously, and saintly intervention was an important recourse. One of the most interesting of these accounts is found in *L. Eliensis*. A seemingly mundane accident became life-threatening for a man punished for dishonouring Æthelthryth.[16] The unnamed man had been instructed by his parish priest to observe the abbess's feast, but when he failed to do so, divine vengeance struck. He fell headlong into a hedge and 'in quam subito irruens sude acutissima infra vertebras transfixus est' ('colliding with this [hedge] at high speed, he was pierced between the ribs by a very sharp stake').[17] He extracted himself from the hedge, but was still impaled with

[11] Finucane, *Miracles and Pilgrims*, p. 107.
[12] Trenery, *Madness, Medicine and Miracle*, pp. 86–99.
[13] Geoffrey of Burton, *M. Moduenne* 50, ed. Bartlett, pp. 210–13.
[14] J. Kerr, 'Health and Safety in the Medieval Monasteries of Britain', *History* 93 (2008), 3–19 (7).
[15] Thomas of Monmouth, *M. Willelmi* V.3, ed. Jessop and James, pp. 189–91.
[16] *L. Eliensis* III.58, ed. Blake, pp. 305–6, trans. Fairweather, pp. 373–4.
[17] *Ibid.*, p. 374. Fairweather translated 'vertebras' as 'ribs' as he fell headlong into the hedge; a more accurate translation of *vertebras* would be 'joint'. Considering the context, the same translation has been given here.

part of the wooden stake and 'dolor in dies et supraducta cicatrice ceperat iam introrsus putrescere' ('his pain increased for days, though the scar had closed over, he began to putrefy internally').[18] Physicians were unable to help, and in fact caused further harm, and the man spent a year in pain before successfully seeking Æthelthryth's aid (and forgiveness).

One health matter notable for its rarity among these miracles is parturient concerns: there are only two references made to childbirth. Bothilda, wife of Girard, found her difficult labour eased by William of Norwich, and then gave birth to her son.[19] Aquilina, wife of Gilbert Basset and daughter of Reginald of Courtenay, was saved from a life-threatening labour that resulted in a stillborn child.[20] Childbirth, understandably, involved risks and complications so the scarcity of references within these accounts is intriguing. However, these seven *miracula* are not alone in this scarcity, nor was this specific to England, although Powell has noted that there was a shift in twelfth-century hagiographical patterns that resulted in later *miracula* being more likely to include occasional references to miracles of parturition.[21] Importantly, however, the lack of these 'gynocentric' accounts appears to be the result of the hagiographical trends on the part of the male, monastic authors rather than women's requirement for aid in childbirth.[22] In addition to hagiographical editorial choices, the practicalities of childbirth must be considered. First, women would have predominantly given birth within the home, and the majority of accounts, as discussed in Chapter 6, relate to healings that occurred within the cult centres.[23] Related to this is the importance of recognising time, or the lack thereof, with difficult labour. Unlike so many of the other ailments recorded, which have a much less pressing time schedule, a difficult labour required a quick resolution. Even after the birth there was, for some time, a great risk to both mother and newborn from dangers such as fever, bleeding and infection.[24] Further still, childbirth had (and still has) its own universal patron saint in the guise of St Margaret of Antioch and she would likely have been the first choice for expectant mothers.[25] One final point to consider is

---

[18] *L. Eliensis* III.58, ed. Blake, pp. 305–6, trans. Fairweather, p. 374.

[19] Thomas of Monmouth, *M. Willelmi* II.6, ed. Jessop and James, pp. 78–9.

[20] *M. Jacobi*, fol. 174va–b; Kemp, 'The Hand of St James' XXI, 16.

[21] Powell, 'The "Miracle of Childbirth"', 795–6, 799, 800–1.

[22] Ibid., 811.

[23] N. Orme, *Medieval Children* (New Haven, 2001), pp. 16–18.

[24] Ibid., pp. 13–21.

[25] 'Margaret of Antioch (Marina of Antioch)', in *ODS*, pp. 260–1.

whether monastic authors would either have known much about labour or have felt particularly comfortable writing on this topic.[26] The lack of parturient cure-seekers does not indicate that women did not call upon the saints in such times of need. It is known that there were portable relics and aids lent by churches to women in labour, and this will be further addressed below.

Gender and Affliction

Naturally, childbirth would have only been an issue for female cure-seekers. With that in mind it is worth questioning whether there was a noticeable difference in the representation of other cures sought depending on the gender of the cure-seeker. When separated by gender, it is evident that eye complaints, illnesses, and paralyses are relatively evenly represented (Tables 2.2–2.3). However, there is a difference in the frequency with which each of these three afflictions are recorded. For men paralysis remains the most frequent, yet for women accounts of blindness and other eye afflictions slightly predominate. There is also a greater diversity in the miraculous cures provided to male cure-seekers across the board.

Table 2.2. Afflictions suffered by male cure-seekers
within the seven *miracula*

	M. Swithuni	M. Dunstani	L. Eliensis	M. Moduenne	M. Willelmi	M. Æbbe	M. Jacobi	Total
Blindness and other eye afflictions	11	2	0	1	1	2	2	19
Bodily paralysis (partial or full paralysis, humps, curvature of the spine or knees, etc.)	13	5	3	1	6	6	3	37
Combinations of sensory afflictions and paralysis (blindness and/or deafness and/ or muteness and partial/full paralysis)	1	1	0	0	1	0	0	3

[26] Powell, 'The "Miracle of Childbirth"', 795–811.

Table 2.2. (*Continued*)

	M. Swithuni	*M. Dunstani*	*L. Eliensis*	*M. Moduenne*	*M. Willelmi*	*M. Æbbe*	*M. Jacobi*	**Total**
Complaints relating to bodily pain (internal organs or limbs, or both, but with no reference to sickness or paralysis)	0	0	0	0	2	0	0	2
Complaints relating to the mouth (toothache, ulcers, etc.)	0	0	2	0	3	0	0	5
Deafness and other ear afflictions	1	0	0	0	0	0	0	1
Eye and speech impediments (blindness and muteness)	0	0	0	0	1	0	0	1
Ear and speech impediments (deafness and muteness)	1	0	0	0	1	0	0	2
Illness (unspecific but including sickness, fever, etc.)	0	2	5	1	15	1	5	29
Injuries (accidents, incidents, animal bites/stings/attacks or other unfortunate events resulting in bodily damage)	1	0	1	4	2	1	1	10
Insomnia	0	0	0	0	1	0	0	1
Leprosy	1	0	0	0	0	0	0	1
Lower body complaints (dysentery, piles)	0	0	0	0	2	0	0	2
Mental health complaints (madness, possession, epilepsy, etc.)	2	2	2	0	8	0	0	14
Muteness and other speech impediments	1	0	3	0	1	2	1	8
Tumours, swellings and growths (including cancer, gout, dropsy)	2	0	2	1	3	5	1	14
Unexplained weakness/feebleness (no obvious reference to illness or paralysis)	0	0	0	0	0	0	1	1
Wounds caused by penitential bonds/irons	1	0	0	1	0	0	0	2

Table 2.3. Afflictions suffered by female cure-seekers within the seven *miracula*

	M. Swithuni	M. Dunstani	L. Eliensis	M. Moduenne	M. Willelmi	M. Æbbe	M. Jacobi	Total
Blindness and other eye afflictions	7	6	4	0	2	6	0	25
Blood complaints	0	0	0	0	2	0	0	2
Bodily paralysis (partial or full paralysis, humps, curvature of the spine or knees, etc.)	3	1	2	1	7	5	4	23
Combinations of sensory afflictions and paralysis (blindness and/or deafness and/or muteness and partial/full paralysis)	0	0	0	0	1	1	0	2
Combinations of sensory afflictions and illness	0	0	0	1	0	0	0	1
Combinations of sensory afflictions and swelling	0	0	0	1	0	0	0	1
Complaints relating to bodily pain (internal organs or limbs, or both, but with no reference to sickness or paralysis)	0	0	0	0	3	0	1	4
Deafness and other ear afflictions	0	1	0	0	1	0	0	2
Difficult labour	0	0	0	0	1	0	1	2
Eye, ear and speech impediments (blindness, deafness and muteness)	0	0	0	0	1	1	0	2
Illness (unspecific but including sickness, fever, etc.)	2	1	0	0	11	0	3	17
Injuries (accidents, incidents, animal bites/stings/attacks or other unfortunate events resulting in bodily damage)	1	0	2	1	0	0	0	4
Mental health complaints (madness, possession, epilepsy, etc.)	1	0	0	0	3	3	0	7
Muteness and other speech impediments	1	0	0	0	0	4	0	5
Tumours, swellings and growths (including cancer, gout, dropsy)	0	0	0	0	6	4	1	11

Analysing the health complaints by gender also identifies that all five references to oral complaints (toothache and mouth ulcers) relate to male sufferers. Surely, there would have been little difference in diet, or dietary requirement, that meant women had significantly superior oral health. Further investigation highlights a significant finding: four of the six men were members of monastic communities.[27] This could indicate that there were significant differences between monastic and lay diets, with the monastic diet being wider-ranging and richer than that of the majority of the laity.[28] Although monks were not supposed to have rich diets, this was not the reality, as Bernard of Clairvaux's *Apologia* reveals.[29] But why should such accounts not feature more prominently among the laity? The statistics suggest that this was a complaint that the laity rarely sought miraculous healing for, especially as the solution to toothache might be found by removing the tooth. In fact, even physicians were unlikely to see cases of toothache, as observed by Giovanni Michele Savonarola two centuries later. Savonarola revealed that patients only sought physicians when their pain was intense and after they had tried other remedies, commenting this was 'something that is considered to have become a barber's affair and is treated mostly by vulgar entrepreneurs on street corners'.[30]

Trusting in the abilities of barber-surgeons was not without risk. *M. Willelmi* offers proof that extraction was a standard treatment for severe toothache, and that saintly intervention was only perceived as necessary when complications ensued. Gaufrid of Canterbury had three teeth extracted, but then over-indulged by eating 'pisas, ac pinguissimum cum allio anserem' ('peas, and the fattest goose with garlic') and drinking 'ceruisiam nouellam' ('new ale').[31]

[27] *L. Eliensis* III.36, III.130, ed. Blake, pp. 274–6, 379, trans. Fairweather, pp. 332–5, 469; Thomas of Monmouth, *M. Willelmi* III.5, ed. Jessop and James, p. 129. In comparison, see Thomas of Monmouth, *M. Willelmi* III.4, VII.19, ed. Jessop and James, pp. 128, 258–60.

[28] For further discussion see: D. Banham, *Food and Drink in Anglo-Saxon England* (Stroud, 2004); A. Hagen, *Anglo-Saxon Food and Drink* (Little Downham, 2010); P. Patrick, *The 'Obese Medieval Monk': A Multidisciplinary Study of a Stereotype*, BAR British Series 590 (Oxford, 2014); C. M. Woolgar, 'Meat and Dairy Products in Late Medieval England', in *Food in Medieval England: Diet and Nutrition*, ed. C. M. Woolgar, D. Serjeantson and T. Waldron, Medieval History and Archaeology (Oxford, 2006), pp. 88–101 (97–9).

[29] Bernard of Clairvaux, *Apologia* XIX.22–3, ed. Rudolph, pp. 232–87.

[30] Giovanni Michele Savonarola, *Practica medicinae: sive de egritudinibus* (Venice, 1497), as cited in Demaitre, *Medieval Medicine*, p. 193.

[31] Thomas of Monmouth, *M. Willelmi* VII.19, ed. Jessop and James, pp. 289–94. This translation slightly differs from that of Jessop and James as 'pinguissimum' is a superlative.

These foods were not suitable for his needs and resulted in pain and swelling.[32] The swelling was so severe that Gaufrid's friends 'ori eius palustrem quo respiraret inmittunt calamum, ne interclusa spirandi uia spiritum suffocaret' ('inserted a reed into his mouth to enable him to breathe, lest he should be suffocated by the choking of the passages').[33] While the extraction is not taken as the direct cause for Gaufrid's suffering, his health was clearly impacted by the procedure, and Thomas of Monmouth implies that his diet should have been altered to be more fitting for his recovery. Whether or not Gaufrid was provided with any advice on 'after-care' is not recorded in *M. Willelmi*, but this account does illustrate the severe consequences that could result from a simple medical procedure.

Where miracles do make references to medicine and medical practitioners, the attitude taken is categorically critical. *Medici* were frequently recorded as having been unable to help, charging extortionate fees, often increasing the patient's suffering, or even adding further discomforts to their original complaint. Of course, when earthly medicines did succeed, the patient would not have had a reason to seek saintly assistance. Evidence such as the low number of accounts of toothache implies that, for some complaints at least, other options would be tried before troubling a saint, and that these might provide satisfactory relief. It was those afflictions beyond the skills of temporal medicine, such as paralysis, blindness, or a potentially fatal sickness, that miraculous healing alone was able to remedy.

Saintly Remedy

Medicine in the Miracles

The presence of other healing practices, and other healers, within the hagiographic sources (as noted in the previous chapter) is the first issue that requires attention here.[34] Alternative methods of cure, such as herbal remedies, appear infrequently within these seven *miracula*. References to physicians, however, are made in a number of accounts.[35] Nevertheless, these references are not

---

[32] Ibid., p. 290.

[33] Ibid.

[34] See above, pp. 30–31.

[35] *M. Swithuni* 9, 13, 22, 29, 37, 46, ed. Lapidge, pp. 654–5, 658–9, 664–5, 668–89, 674–5, 680–3; *L. Eliensis* I.44, III.36, III.58, ed. Blake, pp. 58, 274–6, 305–6, trans. Fairweather, pp. 78, 332–5, 373–4; Thomas of Monmouth, *M. Willelmi* III.7, IV.9, V.5, V.6, V.18, V.19, VI.12, VI.13, VI.16, VII.6, ed. Jessop and James, pp. 132, 174–7, 192–4, 209–11, 244–50, 253–4, 266–7; *M. Jacobi*, fols. 172vb, 173va–b, 174va–175ra; Kemp, '*The Hand of St James*' IX, XVII, XXI, XXII, 10, 13, 16.

evenly spread throughout the sources, and *M. Dunstani*, *M. Moduenne* and *M. Æbbe* make no direct mention of medical practitioners. Of the cases where physicians are recorded it is interesting to note that the Latin term used is *medicus*. There is only one instance in these accounts where the term *physicus* (physician) is used, and that account relates to Æthelthryth's fatal punishment of Ralph Fitz Olaf rather than a curative miracle.[36] As noted, when medical practitioners are referred to it is in critical terms. Frequent among this critique are complaints of their fees and ineffectiveness. More seriously still, some treatments are recorded as having caused greater suffering for the patient. For cure-seekers like Clarica and the man pierced by a thorn (referred to in Chapter 1), the ineffective and costly treatments offered by *medici* resulted in seeking out saintly aid as an alternative.[37] Of course, the miracles tend to present the saints as the final, successful, route of cure. *M. Willelmi*, however, does record that when William, the sacrist of Norwich, suffered from a return of his affliction, he turned back to doctors and their medicines, having received an earlier remedy from William the boy-martyr. But, having previously vowed that he would not use earthly medicines again, he died three days later.[38] Thomas of Monmouth records this as evidence of the superiority of saintly healing and the importance of keeping one's vows to the saints.

Abbot Osbert of Notley, likewise, found his condition growing worse following the application of ointments. Osbert suffered from an eye complaint, but with the 'colliriis usus medicaminaque plurima' ('ointments and several medicines') he took, Osbert experienced 'intensior cruciatur sentiebatur acutior' ('more intense pain and more acute torment').[39] While the medicines and topical applications Osbert tried only made matters worse it is interesting to note that this was a man of the Church who initially resorted to a range of temporal medicines. The Latin used here, *colliria*, specifically referred to eye-salves, thus implying a recognised treatment. It should be noted that *M. Jacobi* makes no mention of Osbert having lost his sight, or having suffered from any swelling or discharge, merely that his eyes became painful, especially when exposed to high levels of light.[40] In the '*Liber de Oculis*' of Constantine's *Pantegni* the ingredients listed in remedies for eye complaints include eggs and

---

[36] *L. Eliensis* III.138, ed. Blake, p. 386, trans. Fairweather, p. 477.

[37] Thomas of Monmouth, *M. Willelmi* III.7, ed. Jessop and James, p. 132; *M. Swithuni* 46, ed. Lapidge, pp. 680–1. Also see above, p. 27.

[38] Thomas of Monmouth, *M. Willelmi* IV.9, ed. Jessop and James, pp. 174–7.

[39] *M. Jacobi*, fol. 174ra; Kemp, '*The Hand of St James*' XIX, 14.

[40] Ibid.

rose oil.[41] In particular the comments concerning the cure of a 'petia' ('attack') on the eyes match the terminology of Osbert's story:

> Petia curatur sanguine columbino oculis instilato deinde cum albumine oui oleo quasi roseo lauentur: et collyrium quod dicitur diarodon: in modu[m] piperis valet in augmento doloris ophthalmie.

> (Attacks are cured by dropping doves' blood into the eyes then they should be washed with the albumin of an egg and oil like that made from roses: [whilst] the eye-salve called *diarodon*, like pepper, serves [only] to worsen the ophthalmic problem.)[42]

That a seemingly commonly known salve is criticised here is not without precedent in the *Pantegni*. Why *diarodon* should cause a peppery sensation is unclear, but this side effect was clearly a concern. Constantine's preferred salve was relatively simple and is made of only three components all of which appear to have been applied in their natural state. These 'new' remedies did not differ much from the 'older' medicines, and were predominantly based on natural products, and were, potentially, quite simple in their production and application. 'New' medicine was not, necessarily, a more advanced medicine in practice, and the classical heritage that acted as a foundation for medieval medical theories is evident (as Chapter 1 discussed). *The Old English Herbarium* – a collection of medicinal, herbal, recipes translated *c.* 1000 into Old English from Pseudo-Apuleius's *Herbarium* – makes multiple references to cures for eye complaints, many of which rely on accessible plants.[43] The majority of the recipes in the *OEH* refer only to the plant under whose name they are listed, but there are instances in which the recipe is more complex and the plant in question acts as the primary ingredient. The eye-salve Osbert applied might have been one of these more complex medicines. Common centaury (*Centaurium umbellatum*) was to be mixed with honey to restore sharper vision.[44] Combining the roots of greater celandine (*Chelidonium maius*) with honey, aged wine, and pepper provided a treatment that could be used for a variety of ocular complaints.[45]

The above ingredients might have created relatively mild *colliria*, nevertheless the ingredients might still have acted as an irritant to the eyes if wrongly

---

[41]   *Liber de Oculis* 17, 30, in *Omnia opera Yssac*, fols. 172r–178r (177v–178r).

[42]   Ibid., fol. 178r.

[43]   *The Old English Herbarium* (hereafter *OEH*), in Van Ardsall, *Medieval Herbal Remedies*, pp. 119–230.

[44]   Ibid., 36, p. 166.

[45]   Ibid., 75.1, p. 181.

made, or incorrectly applied. It cannot be overlooked that the recipe based around greater celandine also included pepper among its ingredients. *OEH* additionally noted that pounded rue could be used for eye pain and swelling. Rue could have adverse effects. In the poetic *Anglicanus ortus*, introduced in the previous chapter, Henry of Huntingdon states that rue has 'vim desiccantem, uim fertur habere calentem' ('a drying power and a heating power').[46] That rue was widely recognised for its abilities to remedy eye complaints is further supported by its inclusion within Hildegard of Bingen's *Physica*.[47] Indeed, rue is still used in herbal remedies, although it has been acknowledged as causing burn-like symptoms on the skin when exposed to sunlight.[48] This final point is interesting considering Osbert's suffering intensified when he was exposed to light; perhaps at least one of his *colliria* included rue.

Rue aside, Hildegard included several other remedies for irritated or painful eyes in *Physica*. Among these recipes' ingredients are: ginger-infused wine; goose bile mixed with wine; and an unguent of figs cooked in water with bear fat and butter.[49] All three were given with instructions that they were to be rubbed around the eyes. Hildegard's *Physica*, although unlikely to have been available in twelfth-century England, does highlight that there was a broader, European, knowledge of various types of herbal remedies, influenced by similar understandings of the body. Whether any of these worked is another matter. Neither details of the *colliria* used by Osbert, nor information regarding who prescribed or produced them, were recorded in *M. Jacobi*. That *M. Jacobi* does not include a reference to physicians within this account could, however, indicate that Osbert had consulted medical books and experts in his own abbey, rather than utilising external expertise.

One other account worthy of brief attention regarding its reference to herbal remedies is the account of a young boy cured of a tumour, which had prevented him from sleeping for fifteen days, recorded in *M. Æbbe*.[50] Before Æbbe healed the boy, his parents had 'apponebant ipsi medicamenta et funiculis circumligabant sed apposita' ('treated him with medicines tied onto him with cords').[51] However, these remedies repeatedly fell off, leading

---

[46] Henry of Huntingdon, *Anglicanus Ortus* I.10, ed. Black, pp. 96–7. Also see below, pp. 43–4.

[47] *Hildegard von Bingen's Physica: The Complete English Translation of Her Classical Work on Health and Healing*, trans. P. Throop (Rochester, 1998), p. 38.

[48] S. Arias-Santiago et al., 'Phytophotodermatitis Due to *Ruta graveolens* Prescribed for Fibromyalgia', *Rheumatology* 48 (2009), 1401.

[49] *Hildegard von Bingen's Physica*, pp. 17–19, 115–16, 184.

[50] *M. Æbbe* IV.8, ed. Bartlett, pp. 46–7.

[51] Ibid.

M. Æbbe's hagiographer to explain that this was a heaven-sent message to the boy's parents to teach them that he could not be cured by herbal remedies, and instead required divine aid.[52] No mention is made of what the herbal remedies involved, but notably there is no mention either of medical professionals, rather it was the parents who were active in providing this remedy. While ultimately unsuccessful, the account indicates a level of awareness of the healing properties of plants beyond learned medicine and medical texts.

Non-Herbal Remedies

It can be assumed that the majority of pre-miracle attempts at cure were based on herbal treatments. However, as noted in Chapter 1, these were not the only natural materials seen to have therapeutic properties. One account stands out within these miracles for the cure-seeker's (unsuccessful) use of another method of cure: the application of stones. This is the previously mentioned account of Aquilina's difficult labour, recorded within *M. Jacobi*. Aquilina, a noblewoman, had already consulted physicians, but they had been unable to assist. Henry II then sent Aquilina 'gemmas lapidesque preciores quotquot habuit' ('as many gems and precious stones as he had').[53] Which specific stones Henry II sent to Aquilina is unclear, but evidently these were valuable items. However, *The Aberdeen Bestiary's* lapidary (produced *c.* 1200) recommended several stones for complaints connected with pregnancy, labour, and childbirth. Carnelian, hematite, and jasper were believed to restrain the flow of blood.[54] Crystal was said to restore the ability to lactate.[55] Eaglestone and penantes were beneficial to pregnant women and women during childbirth.[56]

Both *The Aberdeen Bestiary* and Hildegard's *Physica* refer to jasper's abilities to restrain the flow of blood, and to protect infants after birth.[57] *Physica* also attributes suitable properties to sard.[58] *The Aberdeen Bestiary*, conversely, comments that sard was the 'vilissima gemmarum' ('the most common of precious stones').[59] Notably *Physica* states that sard was not to be used on its own but in combination with healing words to help alleviate the discomforts of

---

[52] Ibid.
[53] *M. Jacobi*, fol. 174vb; Kemp, '*The Hand of St James*' XXI, 16.
[54] *The Aberdeen Bestiary*, fols. 100v, 102v, 103r.
[55] Ibid., fol. 100v.
[56] Ibid., fols. 103r, 103v.
[57] *Hildegard von Bingen's Physica*, pp. 146–7.
[58] *The Aberdeen Bestiary*, fol. 100v; *Hildegard von Bingen's Physica*, p. 144: Orme, *Medieval Children*, p. 16.
[59] *The Aberdeen Bestiary*, fol. 102r.

labour.[60] According to Hildegard, using the stone alongside words and a belt channelled the power of sard. This combination of physical *materia medica* and healing words is common throughout medieval healing, as Louise Bishop has noted.[61] Placing trust in the powers of external objects and spiritual words might have assisted in alleviating the anxiety of parturient women, and might also have relieved some of the sense of personal responsibility for a successful birth.[62] Certainly, curative objects with Christian significance were widely used during medieval childbirth. One example of this was the practice, already in place in Canterbury in the early twelfth century, of lending St Anselm's belt to women in labour.[63] Eadmer comments in his *Vita S. Anselmi* that the sick, but particularly parturient women, would borrow this belt in times of need, and this might explain why *M. Dunstani* is without accounts of this nature.[64] In early sixteenth-century Burton-on-Trent, Modwenna's staff was similarly lent to pregnant women; however this appears to be a later addition to the cult, following the building of a new shrine in the early fifteenth century, and no mention of the staff is found within *M. Moduenne*.[65]

The use of physical, tangible, objects like saints' belts, and Henry II's precious stones, reveals a striking point: that there was a belief in, and requirement for, external sources of comfort and assistance in times of anxiety and danger. In Aquilina's case this danger was a genuine medical concern. She had been in labour for some days prior to Henry II sending her these precious stones; it was then another four days before she drank the water of St James, and only then was she able to expel her stillborn baby.[66] The description of her condition during these four days is graphic and emphasises the seriousness of her condition. *M. Jacobi* records that: 'enim sepultum uidebatur mortuum in moriente, corpus in corpore, funus in funere, genitum in genitrice' ('it really

---

[60] *Hildegard von Bingen's Physica*, p. 144.

[61] L. M. Bishop, *Words, Stones and Herbs: The Healing Word in Medieval and Early Modern England* (Syracuse, 2007), pp. 93–4.

[62] Orme, *Medieval Children*, p. 16.

[63] Ibid.; Powell, 'The "Miracle of Childbirth"', 798.

[64] Eadmer of Canterbury, *Life of St Anselm: Archbishop of Canterbury, by Eadmer*, ed. and trans. R. Southern, OMT (Oxford, 1972), p. 165. Also see Powell, 'The "Miracle of Childbirth"', 798, 801.

[65] *Letters and Papers, Foreign and Domestic, Henry VIII, Volume 13 Part 2, August–December 1538*, 256, ed. J. Gairdner (London, 1893), p. 101. See also: *A History of the County of Staffordshire: Volume 9, Burton-on-Trent*, ed. N. J. Tringham, VCH (London, 2003), p. 108; Orme, *Medieval Children*, p. 16.

[66] *M. Jacobi*, fol. 174vb; Kemp, 'The Hand of St James' XXI, 16.

looked like a dead body buried in a dying body, a corpse within a corpse, a child within its mother').[67]

The level of observation of Aquilina's plight appears surprising. As mentioned previously, childbirth would not be considered a natural area of expertise for monks. The description of what occurred, it must be assumed, came from the report made by Aquilina when she came to Reading following her recovery, and having waited for her period of purification to elapse.[68] The account impresses on the audience the level of danger that Aquilina faced prior to securing James's aid. Neither the briefly mentioned physicians, nor the king's gemstones, were able to bring about any relief, thus divine healing succeeded where temporal treatments failed, bringing Aquilina back almost from the dead. The hagiographer's provision of these details, however, does not necessarily confirm his personal interest in medicine.

The Language of Affliction

Describing Ill Health

A complete analysis of the language used to record all the conditions described in the miracle stories, and comparison of the terminologies, would constitute a worthwhile but separate project. As a preliminary study, this chapter, using select *miracula* from the seven case studies, considers three categories of health conditions cured through miraculous means: eye complaints, forms of paralysis, and tumours (including swellings and growths). All three afflictions might have caused the cure-seeker long-term suffering that could have resulted in disability, leaving the individual to depend on others for assistance. In cases of paralysis and swellings, it was also possible that sufferers would find themselves physically altered by their impairment. The paralysed might find their mobility restricted. A young boy, brought by his mother to Swithun's tomb, was 'debilitatis incommodo a natiuitate correptum' ('crippled from birth by an unfortunate debility') and 'digitis in manum conuersis et pene ad ulteriora traductis, utraque manus miserabiliter clausa' ('the fingers on each hand curled and almost twisted outwards [...] with each hand wretchedly closed up').[69] Severe swellings, as Gaufrid of Canterbury's aforementioned case highlights, could result in disfigurement and lead to related, secondary issues.[70]

---

[67] Ibid.
[68] Ibid.
[69] *M. Swithuni* 5, ed. Lapidge, pp. 652–3.
[70] Thomas of Monmouth, *M. Willelmi* VII.19, ed. Jessop and James, p. 290.

Eye complaints could be impairments in themselves, or could be the result of other underlying issues, including vitamin deficiency.[71] Within the records of healing miracles simple language is used to identify these complaints, with 'ceca' ('blind') appearing most frequently in *M. Swithuni* and *M. Æbbe* (Table 2.4). The only variations in this can be found when the hagiographers used phrases that played on the connection between light and sight, and blindness and darkness or night. The evidence from these two hagiographies regarding the prominence of blindness among eye complaints is reflective of the other five case-study materials too, all of which favour this simple language to describe these complaints. One account worth attention, however, is Geoffrey of Burton's report of Raven, a blind beggar from nearby Tutbury. Raven 'per accidentiam egritudinum oculorum lumen amiserat et, multo tempore iam transacto, cecitate ingruente, uidere aliquid omnimodo non ualebat' ('had lost his eyesight through an illness that had befallen him and as time passed his blindness increased until he could not see at all').[72] Here, Raven evidently identified the cause of his impairment, and reported this on receipt of his miraculous healing. Nevertheless, the terminology within the account differs little from that in *M. Swithuni* and *M. Æbbe*. Such terms may not reveal 'medicalised' language, but the details of these accounts do indicate whether blindness was congenital or occurred later in life.

Accounts of paralysis provide similar insight into when the impairment occurred, and the language here also tends to be more varied. Words such as *contractus* (contracted), *distortio* (distorted) and *paraliticus* (paralysed) appear frequently. Little in this language indicates any specialised medical training on the part of the hagiographers or, for that matter, the cure-seekers. However, it does imply attention to detail in terms of observing the manner in which the paralysis presented itself, as can be seen in the above account of the young boy with hands that were 'conuersis' ('twisted outwards').[73] Accounts such as this, where paralysis affected only part of the body, offer further details regarding the limb, or limbs, affected. These accounts also reveal how partial paralysis impacted on the cure-seeker. A young mute and paralysed man was described by Eadmer of Canterbury as having been unable to look upwards owing to his severely 'incuruis scapulis' ('curved shoulder blades').[74] The *miracula* might not be overtly medicalised, but Metzler has argued that discussion of

---

[71]   C. Rawcliffe, 'Health and Disease', in *A Social History of England, 900–1200*, ed. J. Crick and E. Van Houts (Cambridge, 2011), pp. 66–75 (72).

[72]   Geoffrey of Burton, *M. Moduenne* 45, ed. Bartlett, pp. 186–7. Also see below, pp. 166–7.

[73]   *M. Swithuni* 5, ed. Lapidge, pp. 652–3.

[74]   Eadmer of Canterbury, *M. Dunstani* 5, ed. Turner and Muir, pp. 162–5.

impairments, deemed difficult or impossible to cure, rarely features within medical writings.[75] This makes the inclusion of these cases in *miracula* all the more valuable for the insight they provide into the lived experiences of impaired individuals.

Table 2.4. Terminology used in the initial reference to eye
afflictions in *M. Swithuni* and *M. Æbbe*

		Latin	**English**
M. Swithuni	4	*ceca*	blind
	6	*cecitatis*	blindness
	9	*cecitatem*	blindness
	15	*cecatus*	blinded
	16	*cecitatis*	blindness
	18	*cecus*	blind
	19	*cecitas*	blindness
	20	*ceca*	blind
	22	*noctis tenebras*	shadows of the night
	29	*cectitatem*	blindness
	30	*cecus*	blind
	37	*luce priuatus*	deprived of light
	47	*cecum*	blind
	55	*amissioni oculi unius*	one eye removed
M. Æbbe	IV. 2	*cecitatem*	blindness
	IV. 15	*ceca*	blind
	IV. 19	*cecutierat*	had been very blind
	IV. 21	*apertis oculis nichil uidebat*	saw nothing [even] with her eyes open
	IV. 26	*tenebras oculorum incurrit*	incurred a darkness of the eyes
	IV. 27	*cecus*	blind
	IV. 28	*uisu priuata*	deprived of vision
	IV. 29	*unius oculi lumen*	[loss of] light of one eye

[75]   Metzler, *Disability in Medieval Europe*, p. 139.

Although more infrequent in their recording within the miracle accounts, tumours, swellings and growths provide a category of complaints that are varied in their description. Within the seven *miracula* there are twenty-five relevant accounts, and only *M. Dunstani* is without such a reference. Thus, it is worth considering them all here (Table 2.5). Despite the seemingly differing natures of these accounts (at least from a modern perspective) all these complaints share one important common feature: all of them resulted in some form of swelling to, or just under, the skin. Swellings can be found in *miracula* from across the twelfth century, but these cases appear in greater numbers in the later twelfth-century texts. It is, therefore, possible to consider the language used and whether there are any significant changes in the manner in which these details are recorded across the century. Do the *miracula* become more technical in their terminology as new medical knowledge, such as the translations of Constantine the African, begins to be dispersed more widely?

The most frequently used terms are *tumor* (tumour or swelling) and *inflatus* (inflated or swollen). These terms are frequently used alongside details of where on the body the swelling has occurred or how it appears, such as the cure-seeker with an 'inflacione uentris' ('inflation of the stomach') recorded in *M. Æbbe*, or John (a young monk of Ely) who suffered with a 'pessimo ulcere' ('harmful ulcer').[76] References to dropsy use the specific term *ydropicus*, which indicates the recognition of dropsy, or at least dropsical symptoms, as a particular affliction within the context of swelling. Gout and gout-like symptoms are, similarly, specified by the terms *gutta* and *podagra*. What is striking here is the use of two different terms for the affliction. It is worth considering the account of a cleric named Goscelin, who was punished rather than cured by Æthelthryth, for why this might be the case. *L. Eliensis* states that Goscelin was suddenly afflicted by pain in the feet 'quem medici *podagra* Grece nuncupant' ('which physicians call, in Greek, *podagra*').[77] *Podagra* affected the foot and came to be synonymous with gout.[78] It was considered to be a more technical term for gout, as used by physicians, and – coming from a Greek tradition – implies a potential difference between medical and common terminologies for gout and, possibly, specialised knowledge on the part of *L. Eliensis*'s compiler. Such medical terminology is rarely evident, appearing in only one other account in the seven *miracula*, so the appearance of this Greek term in *L. Eliensis* suggests specialist reading by the author.[79]

---

[76] *M. Æbbe* IV.22, ed. Bartlett, pp. 56–7; *L. Eliensis* III.130, ed. Blake, p. 379, trans. Fairweather, p. 469. Also see below, p. 140.

[77] *L. Eliensis* III.92, ed. Blake, p. 340, trans. Fairweather, p. 417.

[78] Demaitre, *Medieval Medicine*, p. 323.

[79] *M. Swithuni* 13, ed. Lapidge, pp. 658–9.

Table 2.5. Terminology and phrasing used to describe tumours, swellings and growths

		Latin	**English**
M. Swithuni	13	*tumore podagrico*	the swelling of gout
	46	*tumore turgescere*	began to bulge with a swelling
L. Eliensis	III.30	*ydropis morbo inflatum*	swollen by the disease of dropsy
	III.35	*morbum quem vulgo fellone nuncupant*	a disease commonly called felon
	III.92	*podagra*	gout
	III.92	*tumescere*	began to swell
	III.138	*pessimo ulcere*	a severe ulcer
M. Moduenne	50	*uerruca*	a wart
M. Willelmi	III.22	*gutta*	gout
	III.26	*ýdropicus*	dropsy
	III.32	*egrotauerat inflatura*	had been sick with an inflation
	V.20	*tumor*	a swelling
	V.22	*tumentia*	becoming swollen
	VI.13	*tumorem*	a swelling
	VI.14	*guttumosa*	goitre
	VI.16	*tumore*	a swelling
	VII.6	*cancrum*	cancer
M. Æbbe	IV. 6	*gutte tumor*	swollen [with] gout
	IV. 8	*tumor noxius*	[a] harmful tumour
	IV. 16	*inflata tumuerat*	had been inflated with [a] tumour
	IV. 22	*inflacione*	an inflation
	IV. 23	*consimili*	a similar [affliction]
	IV. 24	*inflatum*	an inflation
	IV. 30	*inflacione tumuerat*	had been swollen with an inflation
	IV. 32	*inflacio*	a swelling
	IV. 39	*distensus*	distended
M. Jacobi	2	*morbo tumescan ydropico.*	swollen with the disease of dropsy
	9	*tumorem*	a swelling

Although these miracle accounts do not contain high levels of medicalised language, that does not mean there was a lack of awareness of potential medical procedures and processes the cure-seekers might undertake, as Thomas of Monmouth's recording of Gaufrid's dental procedure highlights.[80] It is also worth contemplating an unusual reference to self-burning that is recorded in *M. Æbbe*, and considering this alongside an account of failed cautery recorded within Reginald of Durham's *Libellus de Admirandis Beati Cuthberti Virtutibus quae novellis Patratæ sunt Temporibus*.[81] These two accounts, while not identical, suggest that there might have been a wider belief, beyond learned medicine, in the benefits of applying heated implements to an affliction. Within *M. Æbbe* it is evident that this is a case of self-inflicted burning. The unnamed man, who came from the Edinburgh area, suffered from a paralysis that 'a planta pedis usque ad uerticem graue dolorum accidens perfudit et a sui status rectitudine ad beluinam usque similitudinem inclinauit' ('affected him from the soles of his feet to the top of his head and twisted him from his upright position into the likeness of a beast'), and he required a staff to aid his mobility.[82] *M. Æbbe* records that:

> Ad sui uero corporis redempcionem ferro simul et igne frequenter adhibito renes cicatricibus repleuerat sibique sentiens non adesse medicine carnalis auxilium, inspirante Deo confugit ad diuinum.

> (He frequently applied fire and iron to cure his body, so that he had covered his sides with scars, and feeling that no help would come from earthly medicine, he was inspired by God to take refuge in divine medicine.)[83]

What is not made clear within *M. Æbbe* is whether this self-burning was undertaken on the instigation of a *medicus*, or whether this reflects a more general belief in the potential benefits of such a procedure. Either way, it appears that this was done in the hope it would cure the affliction. Nevertheless, it is worth questioning the choice of the term 'redempcionem' here and whether that could indicate an attempted ransoming or redemption and thus suggest the act of burning in itself was a punitive action undertaken to secure divine aid. As *M. Æbbe* does not include any further details here to indicate the perceived need for redemption, though, the answer remains elusive and it could

---

[80] Thomas of Monmouth, *M. Willelmi* VII.19, ed. Jessop and James, pp. 289–94.

[81] *M. Æbbe* IV.5, ed. Bartlett, pp. 36–9; Reginald of Durham, *Libellus de Admirandis Beati Cuthberti Virtutibus quae novellis Patratæ sunt Temporibus* (hereafter *B. Cuthberti*) 119, ed. J. Raine, Surtees Society 1 (London, 1835), pp. 264–5.

[82] *M. Æbbe* IV.5, ed. Bartlett, pp. 36–7.

[83] Ibid.

be that 'redempcionem' is used here only to imply he was willing to undergo this practice of burning in order to bring about his cure (thus ransoming his skin for the sake of his recovery).

The account from *M. Æbbe* might, on its own, be dismissed as an unusual one-off, however it becomes more intriguing when read in conjunction with the work of another, contemporary, Durham monk. Reginald of Durham's *B. Cuthberti* can be dated to the third quarter of the twelfth century. Victoria Tudor stated that 'tangles of words and the characteristic use of gerunds' are features in Reginald's writing.[84] Despite these difficulties Reginald's reference to the practice of *cauterio* (cautery) is clear and detailed.[85] In this account the unnamed wife of John Vicecomes is cured of an affliction that affected her bowels.[86] John had suffered a similar complaint and had already secured St Cuthbert's curative assistance.[87] John's wife suffered from a 'yliaca' ('colicky') ailment that no physician had been able to cure.[88] As part of her treatment she underwent a form of cautery procedure:

> Unde et ipsa acrius circa ipsa ylia cauteriata, et in ipsis exustionum cicatricibus, setis equinis tripliciter intortis et deintro impositis, gravissime diutius est afflicta. Credidit enim se hiis medicinae doloribus infirmitatis diutinae posse miserias delenire, et dolorem doloris aculeo diminuendo confodere.

> (Indeed, she was sharply cauterised around the groin itself, and then these fiery wounds were made very much worse by the further insertion of triple-twisted horsehairs, which caused her suffering for a long time. For she [had] believed that, with such pains as medicine, she could eradicate the miseries of her long-drawn-out illness.)[89]

The result of this treatment was the exacerbation of her suffering from both the wounds caused by the cautery and further irritation caused to her intestines and groin. The resulting incontinence, detailed in Reginald's reporting of

---

[84]   V. Tudor, 'Reginald of Durham and St Godric of Finchale: A Study of a Twelfth-Century Hagiographer and His Major Subject' (unpublished doctoral thesis, University of Reading, 1979), pp. 91, 98.

[85]   *Cauterio, -are, -avi, -atus* indicates a practice of burning (or branding), but in the context of this miracle this is a purposeful, medical practice akin to cauterising, therefore the latter is used here in translating the account.

[86]   Reginald of Durham, *B. Cuthberti* 118, ed. Raine, p. 263 n. 1.

[87]   Ibid., pp. 263–4.

[88]   Ibid., 119, pp. 264–5.

[89]   Ibid. My gratitude to Anne Lawrence for her assistance with the translation of this particular piece of Latin.

her suffering and cure, meant that she had to change her underclothes three times a day. Her fluctuating temperature meant that sometimes she could wear little more than a 'camisiam' ('nightgown'), but then would quickly find herself becoming too cold and could not be warmed.[90] That *medici* and medicines were unable to cure her suffering, and in fact only made it worse, fits within the common hagiographical trope. What is unusual is this detailed reference to a specific procedure.

Durham Cathedral's awareness of cautery was referred to in the previous chapter, with regard to one of the surviving manuscripts within the cathedral's collections and its miniatures depicting the cautery points.[91] These diagrams include the positioning of cautery points in the lower intestinal area, and it might be that John's wife experienced cautery in similar places. Who performed this cauterising procedure is not recorded in *B. Cuthberti*, possibly it was one of the *medici* who attended her. Importantly, unlike *M. Æbbe*, she is referred to as having been 'cauteriata' ('cauterised'), and as experiencing 'medicinae doloribus' ('the pains of the medicine'), suggesting the presence of learned practitioners.[92] The reference made to the triple-twisted horsehair as part of her ineffective treatment might imply some attempt to close the wound, and thus a further surgical procedure. Whether these details were part of the sufferer's report or a result of Reginald's knowledge of cautery practice is unclear. What is interesting is that two accounts with references to burning treatments should be included in hagiographies connected to an institution with known cautery instructions.

The use of cautery reflects the contemporary reliance upon the theories of the four humours. Simply put, the woman was suffering from colicky symptoms which would have appeared cold and wet, so the remedy needed to counteract this was something hot and dry. Siraisi notes that it was often the patients not the doctors who 'wanted the cure by contraries to be rigidly followed'.[93] Both cautery and phlebotomy were frequently prescribed for complexional, internal, complaints owing to the fact that through their application they were believed to rebalance the body. Importantly, cautery became more widespread in the West following the translation of Albucasis's surgical manual into Latin during the twelfth century.[94] This was advanced medicine and suggests that

---

[90] Ibid.
[91] MS Hunter 100, fols. 119v–120r. Also see above, p. 39.
[92] Reginald of Durham, *B. Cuthberti* 119, ed. Raine, pp. 264–5; *M. Æbbe* IV.5, ed. Bartlett, pp. 36–9.
[93] Siraisi, *Medieval and Early Renaissance Medicine*, p. 117.
[94] Ibid., pp. 137, 161–2.

sufferers were prepared to try new and very painful medical procedures. The use of burning in *M. Æbbe*, however, suggests a more simplistic practice, and it is significant that this appears to have been self-inflicted.[95] Perhaps a medicalised reason cannot be provided for this self-burning, but taken together, these two accounts indicate that the communities of Durham and its dependent daughter-house at Coldingham were perfectly aware of the application of heat as a medical procedure.

A similar awareness, and use of, medicalised terminology was identified by Koopmans in William of Canterbury's *Miracula Sancti Thomae Cantuariensis* (produced in the 1170s).[96] However, and relevant to the above accounts too, Koopmans argues that the use of medical terminology cannot be taken as a guarantee of scholastic medical learning and comprehension.[97] Trenery's study of the epilepsy accounts in William's *Miracula Sancti Thomae Cantuariensis* further supports this argument. While William initially divided *epilensia* (epilepsy) into three categories, these differentiations are not used consistently within these miracle accounts.[98] Louise Wilson's analysis of the miracles of St Edmund of Abingdon (d. 1240), compiled in the late thirteenth century, has highlighted a similar awareness of medicine and medical theory, and nature, which indicates the increasing access within the monasteries to books of medicine and natural philosophy.[99] These references underline the fact that many monks would have had an awareness of medical practices, but it does not prove that they would have had a comprehensive understanding of learned medicine. It must be remembered that most hagiographers were not medical experts and *miracula* were not intended to be read as medical case studies. Thus, it is rare for accounts of miraculous healing to include scholastic medical commentaries, such as a discussion of humoral or complexional imbalance. The miracle accounts, however, provide important insight into the lived conditions and experiences of those who suffered from a range of illnesses and impairments, an insight that the contemporary medical texts cannot match.

---

[95] *M. Æbbe* IV.5, ed. Bartlett, pp. 36–7.

[96] William of Canterbury, *Miracula Sancti Thomae Cantuariensis*, in *Materials for the History of Thomas Becket, Archbishop of Canterbury*, ed. J. C. Robertson, 7 vols (London, 1875), I (1875), 137–546.

[97] Koopmans, *Wonderful to Relate*, pp. 183–4.

[98] Trenery, *Madness, Medicine and Miracle*, pp. 90–3.

[99] L. E. Wilson, 'Conceptions of the Miraculous: Natural Philosophy and Medical Knowledge in the Thirteenth-Century *Miracula* of St Edmund of Abingdon', in *Contextualising Miracles in the Christian West, 1100–1500: New Historical Approaches*, ed. M. M. Mesley and L. E. Wilson, Medium Ævum Monographs 32 (Oxford, 2014), pp. 99–125 (117–19).

Miracles and Healthcare

As established within this and the previous chapter, cure-seekers potentially had a range of healthcare options open to them, even if the miracles do not paint these other avenues in a positive light. With this in mind, one final point to consider in this chapter is how the cure-seekers perceived miraculous healing and where they situated it within the broader spectrum of healthcare on offer. Cure-seekers clearly recognised that the saints were a source of remedial care, if not medical intervention. The restoration of bodily health features heavily in the tradition of miracles, going back to the Gospels themselves. Many of those touched by Christ's miracle working were cured of bodily afflictions, and this same pattern, as noted, was replicated in the later posthumous *miracula* produced for the saints. Unlike physicians and barber-surgeons, miraculous healing was an option that did not come with an extortionate price tag or with the risk of exacerbating symptoms and suffering.

In discussing disease and treatment, Siraisi placed prayer, pilgrimage and visits to shrines amongst the wide range of 'self-help' practised by patients, noting that medical practitioners did not monopolise medical treatment.[100] That there was no single, or even dominant course of healthcare is important to remember, and the miracles prove that many cure-seekers tried multiple methods before the saints interceded. Of course, not all of those who sought healing miracles would have been successful; the *miracula* naturally only recorded cases where the saints succeeded. Yet Paul Hayward has suggested that, even when the saints did not intercede, pilgrims would have been provided with some consolation at having undergone the 'curative ritual' of appealing to the saints.[101] Rituals were also an important part of the preparation and application of temporal medicines; healing words, as noted above, often accompanied herbal and lapidarial treatments. The powers inherent in these natural objects were, in the eyes of medieval practitioners, God-given.[102] What set the saints apart was their close connection to God and their ability to bridge the celestial and temporal worlds in a way that other health providers could not, and the fact that their method of health-giving did not require the sufferer to take medicines or undergo invasive treatments.

It is of the utmost importance to avoid retrospective and anachronistic judgements when considering medieval concepts of health and ill health. As was seen in the previous chapter, when setting the context for miraculous

---

[100] Siraisi, *Medieval and Early Renaissance Medicine*, p. 137.

[101] P. A. Hayward, 'Saints and Cults', in *A Social History of England, 900–1200*, ed. J. Crick and E. Van Houts (Cambridge, 2011), pp. 309–20 (310).

[102] Rawcliffe, 'Medical Practice and Theory', p. 394.

cures, the idea of physical health was intrinsically linked to spiritual well-being.[103] Thus, there can be no simple separation between the spiritual and the corporeal. Saints were more than just healthcare providers; rather they were protectors of their communities and devotees. Nevertheless, healing miracles feature heavily in the *miracula* and, while the remedies provided by the saints were not medicinal, it is clear that their therapeutic abilities did place them within the gamut of healthcare available.

*   *   *

Miracula offer a valuable lens through which insight into the understandings and experience of ill health and impairment can be attained. It is also possible to place miraculous healing within the broader remit of medieval healthcare and to consider the extent of medical awareness in the twelfth century. While this chapter reveals that there are trends throughout the *miracula*, it also becomes evident that the miracle reports were not carbon copies of each other. At the heart of these accounts are the experiences of individuals who put their faith in the saints to recover their physical health. What also emerges is that hagiographical terminology for affliction tended to be relatively simplistic. Yet, there were also instances of more advanced knowledge. The term *podagra* in *L. Eliensis*, and the recognition of its Greek origins, indicated some medical awareness on behalf of *L. Eliensis*'s compiler. Likewise references to medicines and medical procedures, like the cautery documented in Reginald of Durham's *B. Cuthberti*, emphasised an awareness of other curative practices. Indeed, in instances of toothache, the sources imply that barber-surgeons were likely to be the first recourse for many sufferers. The saints were only to be turned to if further complications arose, as in Gaufrid of Canterbury's experience.

   That medicine should be given negative treatment in miracle accounts was to be expected. What is striking is that this indicates an etiquette and under-lying process in which the cure-seekers were likely to approach the saints only after they had exhausted other, earthly, healing options. Where this poten-tially differs is in the cases that required immediate attention, such as with an illness that brought the cure-seeker close to death. Attempting to find cures using temporal remedies first suggests that the cure-seekers did not wish to appear presumptuous or demanding of the saint. That an ill-advised attempt to find a cure had already been pursued might also heighten the sympathy felt towards the afflicted by their saintly intercessor. Such a process, curing the

---

[103] See above, pp. 32–6.

seemingly incurable, certainly heightened the miraculous nature of the saints' intercession.

For those who suffered from either insurmountable impairments or complaints that required rapid resolution, such as difficult childbirth, the saints and their brand of medical assistance offered a solution that earthly medical practitioners were unlikely to equal. It is easy to understand why the *miracula* include so many accounts of blindness and paralysis, two seemingly incurable conditions. It was a great triumph for a saint to produce miraculous cures for such ailments as this followed the precedent laid down by Christ in the Gospels. Yet the account of self-burning in *M. Æbbe* should not be forgotten as this suggests that some with paralysis did investigate other remedial avenues before turning their attention to holy healing.

For the hagiographers as well as the cure-seekers, miraculous healing was more than just an alternative treatment within the available forms of help for medical problems. Saints provided cures for those who had been let down by medical practitioners, herbal treatments or invasive surgery. The biblical precedent must be recognised, but there is evidence here too that hagiographers were keen to reflect and represent the experiences of cure-seekers who sought out the saints' assistance. Consequently, no two accounts are the same, and many provide tantalising details of the individual's personal experiences of affliction and eventual miraculous recovery. This by no means meant that monastic hagiographers ignored or rejected other forms of care for the sick and suffering. What emerges from their accounts is a much more complex model of the relationship between the medical, the spiritual and the miraculous.

3

The Great and the Good: Identifying the Cure-Seekers within the Miracles

H aving established the healthcare context, our journey towards miraculous cure begins by identifying the individuals at the heart of these selected miracles. While the primary aim of posthumous hagiography was to document, promote and celebrate the miraculous events themselves – as signs of divine intervention in the temporal world – accounts of holy healing required cure-seekers. As such, the individuals were central to the miracle stories and their encounters with the miraculous further our understanding of medieval cure-seeking.

The cure-seekers have unsurprisingly become the focus of many studies of medieval miracles, beginning with Finucane's *Miracles and Pilgrims* which identified a general trend for wide social interaction with the shrines, but with a greater number of lower-status men recorded with accidental injuries.[1] Sigal, similarly, highlighted that over ninety per cent of cure-seekers cured of blindness were 'd'origine populaire' ('of popular origin').[2] As Yarrow has demonstrated, though, statistics are not the only method for analysing these individuals; anecdotal comments can provide a wealth of information.[3] Using these methods together, as is done here, allows for the development of a rounded picture of these cure-seekers which considers them both as individuals and as representative of wider contemporary practices. This also offers a valuable method for comparative analysis between hagiographical collections. Within this chapter the focus is on identifying who these individuals were. The following chapter will consider the distances between the cure-seekers and the site of the cult.

Categorising the Cure-Seekers

Before analysing the cure-seekers within these seven sets of *miracula*, some consideration is needed of how the individuals in question have been

---

[1]   Finucane, *Miracles and Pilgrims*, p. 151.
[2]   Sigal, *L'Homme et le miracle*, p. 231.
[3]   Yarrow, *Saints and Their Communities*, p. 114.

categorised by age, gender and social status; and of the nature of the hagiographic materials. Throughout this book statistical analysis is based on what can be drawn from the twelfth-century accounts selected. In this chapter, where the details of the reports do not provide enough guidance to make a decisive categorisation, the cure-seeker has been categorised as 'unclear'. This ensures that the cure-seekers are represented as they have been recorded and remembered within the miracles, for example with regard to details about their social status. It is also for this reason that the social categories employed here have been kept broad, to reflect the hagiographical data.

It is additionally important to acknowledge the fact that the *miracula* are edited collections of selected miracles reported at the shrines. When considering the proportional representation of the cure-seekers within these texts, for example the balance of male to female cure-seekers, or laypeople to religious men, we must bear in mind the author's likely intention in compiling these collections. The purpose of the *miracula* was to champion the saints and their intercessory abilities. That is not to say that these accounts are inevitably unrepresentative of those who sought the saints' aid, but that caution must be exercised in making statements about what the *miracula* reveal of cult practices more broadly. There would have been many more individuals whose experiences did not make it into these collections, not least because they did not receive a cure. Nevertheless, the miracle records of successful petitions by cure-seekers shed a light on experiences of holy healing and represent a level of social engagement with our seven saints.

A Notable Lay Presence

Immediately evident in analysing the miracle accounts is the predominance of the laity within the records of successful cure-seeking (Table 3.1). Lay devotees feature heavily in all seven case studies. In fact, in both *M. Moduenne* and *M. Æbbe* the laity are the sole demographic represented. Within the remaining *miracula*, there are a small number of references to cure-seeking religious men (monks and clerics), who are discussed below. In total, though, the laity account for an impressive ninety-two per cent of the cure-seekers recorded within these materials. The importance of the saints to the laity, and the laity to the success and longevity of a saint's cult, has long been recognised, and this 'mutual relationship', as Bartlett describes it, was no different for our seven cults.[4] Within this broad category of 'laypeople' it is possible to make further divisions into various social categories such as gender, age, or social

---

[4]   Bartlett, *Why Can the Dead Do Such Great Things?*, pp. 103–12.

status. Some individuals, naturally, fall into multiple categories and it must be recognised that there is a fluidity with any such categorising.

Balance of the Sexes

An initial question to ask of the miracle accounts is how balanced the representation of male and female cure-seekers is within the records, and what this might indicate of cult practices and preferences. While each of the hagiographic works considered here was an individual production, and they were created by different hagiographers and produced across the twelfth century, there are certain patterns within the gender balance that appear dominant throughout. Most notably, female cure-seekers seldom outnumber men, even when only taking lay cure-seekers into account.

For the most part, the seven *miracula* represent anything from an even distribution between the two genders to twice as many laymen as laywomen. The only *miracula* to buck this trend is *M. Æbbe* in which there are markedly more female cure-seekers recorded. Further analysis of *M. Æbbe* also reveals a number of younger cure-seekers, either children or youths, thus further decreasing the percentage of adult men recorded as having sought Æbbe's aid. It might be questioned whether the unusual patterns found within *M. Æbbe* are reflective of the unusual nature of the cult centre, and the supposedly misogynist attitude of St Cuthbert at motherhouse Durham Cathedral Priory. Could it be that Æbbe saw a greater number of female cure-seekers owing to Cuthbert's refusal to allow women admittance to the greater part of Durham Cathedral? This might have persuaded some, such as a paralysed woman from Aycliffe, to venture to Æbbe's oratory rather than Cuthbert's tomb.[5] However, she is not the only cure-seeker who travelled from the Durham area; Æbbe also cured a man from Durham of his swollen stomach.[6] *M. Æbbe* makes no explicit mention of Durham directing female cure-seekers to Berwickshire. That said, it is possible that the hagiographer wished to emphasise the cure of women at Coldingham in relation to the restrictions in place at Durham Cathedral.[7] Whether this was done with a sense of competitiveness or reflects a shared ideal between motherhouse and daughter-house is open to debate, but relations between the two institutions were not always convivial.[8]

[5]   *M. Æbbe* IV.38, ed. Bartlett, pp. 64–5. Also see below, p. 181.
[6]   Ibid., IV.30, pp. 58–9.
[7]   For further discussion see Salter, 'Beyond the *Miracula*'.
[8]   Powell, 'Pilgrimage, Performance and Miracle Cures', pp. 83–4.

Table 3.1. Social divisions within the seven *miracula*

	M. Swithuni	*M. Dunstani*	*L. Eliensis*	*M. Moduenne*	*M. Willelmi*	*M. Æbbe*	*M. Jacobi*	**Total**
Lay/Religious								
Lay person	49	17	20	13	77	42	20	238
Religious (male)	1	4	6	0	6	0	4	21
Male/Female (laity only)								
Male	34	8	12	9	40	18	10	131
Female	15	9	8	4	37	24	10	107
Adult/Child								
Adult	40	16	19	11	52	22	17	177
Child or Youth	10	5	7	2	31	20	7	82
Adult/Child (male/female)								
Adult (male)	26	10	14	7	26	8	11	102
Adult (female)	14	6	5	4	26	14	6	75
Child (male)	9	2	4	2	20	10	3	50
Child (female)	1	3	3	0	11	10	4	32
Social status								
Religious (male)	1	4	6	0	6	0	4	21
Noble (male)	6	1	2	0	4	0	4	17
Noble (female)	3	0	2	0	4	3	3	15
Poor (male)	7	0	0	2	5	1	0	15
Poor (female)	5	4	1	1	5	1	0	17
Employment specified (male)	2	1	0	3	10	3	2	21
Employment specified (female)	0	0	2	0	0	0	0	2
Status unclear (male)	19	6	10	4	21	14	4	78
Status unclear (female)	7	5	3	3	28	20	7	73

Discussion of the health complaints brought by both men and women, and the comparisons between the two, received consideration in the previous chapter.[9] This earlier discussion highlighted that eye afflictions were recorded for female cure-seekers more frequently than for their male counterparts. Comparatively, forms of paralysis and illness were recorded in greater numbers among male cure-seekers. For the latter afflictions male cure-seekers account for just over two-thirds of the recorded cases. Male cure-seekers were also recorded with a greater range of health complaints. Parturient concerns, understandably, were the sole category in which only women featured. Were men and boys more prone to illness, or to paralysis, and were women more prone to blindness? Heavier and more demanding manual labour could have caused, or exacerbated, muscular or osteological complaints. Likewise, domestic environments, with open fires and low levels of light, could have impacted on quality of vision. Importantly, loss of sight and paralysis could also be secondary effects of malnutrition, underlying illnesses, or old age and therefore could have impacted on the health of both men and women. Pregnancy can also result in secondary health concerns for women. In *M. Æbbe* an unnamed new mother made the journey to Æbbe's oratory to petition the saintly abbess for a cure for her infant son's paralysis and the blindness in one of her eyes. It is explicitly recorded that 'uehemens angustia partus' ('the fierce anguish of labour') was responsible for her lost sight.[10] Visual disturbances continue to be a recognised symptom of preeclampsia, even if complete blindness is now rare.[11] Of course, it cannot be known whether preeclampsia was the reason for the woman's partial blindness in *M. Æbbe*, but it is important to recognise that the connection was made between her loss of sight and her parturient state.

Many cure-seekers, including the woman above, were recorded in miracle accounts with few personal identifiers. The twelfth-century hagiographies for established cults, such as those of Æthelthryth and Swithun, included less personal information, such as names or social status. Sigal suggested that details including social class for the 'classes populaires' ('popular classes') were rare in hagiography, as hagiographers were more attentive in recording identities for religious men and the aristocracy.[12] Whether such details were not specified by the cure-seeker (or at least not recorded by the shrine-keeper) at the initial reporting of the cure must also be considered. Alternatively, this might have been a purposeful choice on the part of individual hagiographers, not due to any lack of interest but to ensure that focus remained on the miraculous

---

9   See above, pp. 69–72.

10 *M. Æbbe* IV.29, ed. Bartlett, pp. 58–9.

11 C. P. Moseman and S. Shelton, 'Permanent Blindness as a Complication of Pregnancy Induced Hypertension', *Obstetrics and Gynecology* 100 (2002), 943–5.

12 Sigal, *L'Homme et le miracle*, p. 231.

cure and the power of God. The anonymity of cure-seekers might have also enhanced the 'everyman' sense of universal appeal that the cult centres wished to champion. It is also possible that this was very much a personal preference for the hagiographers. For new cults there are higher percentages of named cure-seekers, as can be seen in *M. Willelmi* and *M. Jacobi*. The inclusion of such details indicates that the hagiographers in these instances saw it as important to identify the recipients of the saints' aid; presumably as this added weight to the claims of the efficacy of the saint in question. *M. Willelmi* is notable in this respect, as there were monks within the Norwich community who were initially dubious of William's sanctity.[13] Thomas of Monmouth clearly felt the need to include as much detail as possible, from personal characteristics to previous attempts to find cure via other medical avenues, in order to emphasise the boy-martyr's saintliness.

Rich and Poor

Miracles prove particularly fascinating when they allow a glimpse into issues such as social standing or provide personal details such as the cure-seeker's name or their occupation. References to affluent or impoverished cure-seekers are uncommon within these accounts. Nevertheless, comparing the two, where they do appear, and the types of affliction recorded in relation to these cure-seekers, has the potential to reveal the differences and similarities of health concerns affecting those at either end of the financial, and social, spectrum (Table 3.2).

Table 3.2. Comparative afflictions of higher- and lower-status cure-seekers*

	Higher-status	Lower-status
Blindness and other eye afflictions	3	10
Bodily paralysis (partial or full paralysis, 'humps', curvature of the spine or knees, etc.)	5	8
Complaints relating to bodily pain (internal organs or limbs, or both, but with no reference to sickness or paralysis)	1	0
Difficult labour	1	0
Ear and speech impediments (deafness and muteness)	0	1
'Illness' (unspecific but including sickness, fever, etc.)	13	2

[13]   Thomas of Monmouth, *M. Willelmi* II.1, II.9–12, ed. Jessop and James, pp. 57–62, 89–96.

	Higher-status	Lower-status
Injuries (accidents, incidents, animal bites/stings/ attacks or other unfortunate events resulting in bodily damage)	1	1
'Leprosy'	0	1
Mental health complaints (madness, possession, epilepsy, etc.)	2	2
Muteness and other speech impediments	2	0
Tumours, swellings and growths (including 'cancer', 'gout', dropsy)	1	0
Unexplained weakness/feebleness (no obvious reference to illness or paralysis)	1	0
Total	30	25

* This table includes all mentions of such members of the laity, including children and youths whose social status, or that of their parents, was recorded. Higher-status cure-seekers include those clearly recorded as nobles, knights, statesmen, or recorded as wealthy. Lower-status individuals include those who are explicitly described as being poor or impoverished.

Immediately obvious when considering this matter are the differences in the numbers of those cured of eye afflictions or illness; the former being more prevalent among the accounts of poorer cure-seekers, the latter being more frequently recorded in relation to those of more privileged positions. These two afflictions aside, there is little to differentiate the complaints brought by the nobility and the poor to the seven cults in question. Finucane's analysis suggested that there were differences in the ailments upper- and lower-class cure-seekers were shown to have brought to the shrines, meaning that the analysis of these seven *miracula* is noteworthy for indicating that our saints were not seen to have specialised in either one particular cure or in curing one class of cure-seeker.[14] Nevertheless, social status must have impacted upon day-to-day circumstances that could have resulted in certain individuals being more prone to certain complaints. Paralysis, more dominant among the poor, could be indicative (like eye afflictions) of a poor diet. Tony Waldron's analysis of the skeletal evidence of diet and nutrition has revealed the impact both insufficient (and excessive) diets had on the body, with a deficient diet having an especially damaging effect.[15] In a similar vein, for those who relied

---

[14] Finucane, *Miracles and Pilgrims*, pp. 143–5.
[15] T. Waldron, 'Nutrition and the Skeleton', in *Food in Medieval England: Diet and Nutrition*, ed. C. M. Woolgar, D. Serjeantson and T. Waldron, Medieval History and Archaeology (Oxford, 2006), pp. 254–66 (258–63).

on physical labour rather than those of more affluent means, it might be questioned whether paralysis was cause for greater concern considering the physiological stresses of manual labour.[16] Regarding high-status cure-seekers it is also worth considering Finucane's argument here that upper-class pilgrims found admitting physical impairment shameful, although the presence of even a few cases within the *miracula* counteracts this somewhat.[17] The miracles are not devoid of accounts of noble persons who are severely impaired.[18]

While physical impairment might be affected by societal circumstances, the high proportion of wealthy cure-seekers healed of illness is curious and raises the question of whether those of higher status suffered from these complaints more frequently. This seems unlikely. More likely was that the nobility had greater liberty to search for a remedy for such a complaint. The peasantry, even when not tied to the land, were more limited in their freedom and finances to travel, and to procure medical assistance. Conversely, one extremely wealthy man from London first travelled to St Augustine's, Canterbury, where he found remedy for one of his gout-swollen feet, before Swithun cured the other foot.[19] *M. Swithuni*'s hagiographer noted that the man 'inuectus equo' ('was carried by horse') to Canterbury, a luxury many cure-seekers would have been unable to afford.[20] Of course, the search for miraculous healing was not a leisure activity, but this account does highlight that some would have greater flexibility, in their time and finances, to search for their desired cure.

Among the accounts of wealthier cure-seekers, the miracles regularly record that various avenues of healthcare were attempted before turning to the saints. Leofmær, a knight from Barningham, had been unwell for fifteen days with an incapacitating illness that physicians could not cure.[21] Leofmær followed the advice of Æthelthryth – relayed to him by a woman from Barningham – that he should make a candle with a wick that had been passed around the bed he was lying on. The wick had not quite circled the bed when he began to recover. Once recovered, Leofmær ensured that the candle was made. He then travelled to Ely and placed it at Æthelthryth's altar, dedicating himself to the saintly abbess.

---

[16] Metzler, *Disability in Medieval Europe*, p. 161.

[17] Finucane, *Miracles and Pilgrims*, pp. 149–50.

[18] For example, *L. Eliensis* III.36, ed. Blake, pp. 274–6, trans. Fairweather, pp. 332–5.

[19] *M. Swithuni* 13, ed. Lapidge, pp. 658–9.

[20] Ibid. It should be noted that Lapidge uses 'horseback' rather than 'horse' here, but I have chosen the more literal translation in this instance.

[21] *L. Eliensis* III.36, ed. Blake, pp. 274–6, trans. Fairweather, pp. 332–5.

That a well-established saint's cult at a cathedral priory, such as Æthel-thryth's at Ely, was attractive to a range of cure-seekers, including potential patrons like Leofmær, is perhaps not surprising. New foundations also gar-nered popular support from a range of lay devotees. Yarrow has shown that William of Norwich had a number of higher-status supporters, including 'domina' ('Lady') Mabel de Bec.[22] The presence of the nobility within *M. Jacobi* might similarly be anticipated owing to Reading being a royal foundation with continued royal interest throughout the twelfth century.[23] *M. Jacobi*, like the other *miracula*, does include a range of cure-seekers, as Ward and Yarrow have also noted.[24] Yet, it is striking that the hagiographer was attentive in recording personal details for the six higher-status cure-seekers recorded: two knights, Robert of Stanford and Ralph Guibin; Mauger Malcuvenant, the sheriff of Surrey; and three noblewomen, Goda (wife of a Herefordshire knight), Ysem-bela (wife of Sewel, Lord of Curridge), and Aquilina (daughter of Reginald de Courtenay and wife of Gilbert Basset).[25] Reference is also made in passing to the viewing of James's reliquary by the earl of Gloucester, his wife, and 'pluribusque non mediocris proceribus potentie' ('several great and powerful lords').[26] Ward's comment that all levels of society were represented within *M. Jacobi* notwithstanding, the absence of explicit references to poverty within the accounts is striking.

The absence of any direct mention of poverty, though, does not mean that the poor were not present, rather that closer reading of the accounts is required to find anecdotal evidence of their interaction with St James and his cult centre. When another Ysembela – this one being the paralysed daughter of a fisherman called John who was thrown out by her stepmother – returned home unsuccessfully from Canterbury (unwilling to follow James's advice to visit Reading), she turned to her 'amita' ('[paternal] aunt').[27] On hearing Ysem-bela's story, the woman told her niece, 'Nummum quem solum habeo accipe et ex eo cum Rading ueneris candela tibi eme' ('Take the only coin I have and

[22] Thomas of Monmouth, *M. Willelmi* III.11, ed. Jessop and James, pp. 135–6; Yarrow, *Saints and Their Communities*, p. 161. Also see below, p. 187.

[23] Yarrow, *Saints and Their Communities*, p. 201.

[24] Ward, *Miracles and the Medieval Mind*, p. 116; Yarrow, *Saints and Their Communi-ties*, p. 198. Also see K. Leyser, 'Frederick Barbarossa, Henry II and the Hand of St James', *English Historical Review* 90 (1975), 481–506 (498–9).

[25] *M. Jacobi*, fol. 171va–b, 172rb, 174va–b, 175ra; Kemp, 'The Hand of St James' I, VII, XVII, XXI, XXIV, XXIVa, 6–7, 8–9, 13, 16–17.

[26] *M. Jacobi*, fol. 173ra; Kemp, 'The Hand of St James' XI, 10–11.

[27] *M. Jacobi*, fol. 174va; Kemp, 'The Hand of St James' XX, 15.

when you get to Reading buy yourself a candle with it').[28] The donation of this only coin subtly implies that Ysembela and her aunt were both lacking in funds. Judging by the description given in the account of her relationship with her stepmother, Ysembela was unlikely to find any assistance there, and John, her father, is conspicuously absent from the account. Whether he would have seen Ysembela as a burden, like her stepmother did, cannot be known but the picture painted is one of a family with little financial means. Perhaps it is in this light that the stepmother's attitude might be understood. Impoverished parents were certainly at a disadvantage when it came to supporting their impaired children, but the miracle accounts highlight that attempts were still made by the majority to secure their offspring's good health.[29]

Ysembela's plight and lack of familial support stand out due to her being a 'puella' ('girl').[30] However, adult poor and impaired cure-seekers could also be seen as a burden on the community. M. Swithuni records, with some sympathy, the predicament of three blind 'muliercule' ('little women') from the Isle of Wight who lived in 'miserande paupertatis' ('miserable poverty').[31] The three, unnamed, women heard about the miracles of Swithun and their neighbours agreed to help transport them across the Solent. On reaching the mainland, however, the women were abandoned without a guide and without enough money to purchase even one meal. As fortune would have it, they met a deaf cure-seeker who was also on his way to Winchester, and he took on the role of guiding them. On their arrival at Swithun's tomb, all four petitioned the saint and the women received their sight and the man his hearing; the latter's cure being referred to as payment for the charitable services undertaken.[32]

As Metzler has argued, caution must be used in emphasising impairments as an inconvenience, for any level of society. In her analysis of a broad range of miracles, Metzler discovered that it was 'comparatively rare' to find evidence of impairment being a burden, at least from the perspective of others.[33] Similarly rare within the miracles were reports of mockery by the able-bodied.[34] The accounts from M. Swithuni and M. Jacobi reflect this, in that they show sympathy for the three blind women and Ysembela, and they celebrate the

[28] Ibid.
[29] Finucane, The Rescue of the Innocents, p. 57.
[30] M. Jacobi, fol. 174rb; Kemp, 'The Hand of St James' XX, 14.
[31] M. Swithuni 6, ed. Lapidge, pp. 652–3.
[32] Ibid., pp. 654–5.
[33] Metzler, Disability in Medieval Europe, pp. 163, 165.
[34] Ibid.

considerate acts of the deaf man and Ysembela's aunt in progressing the cure-seekers' journey, thus emphasising the virtue and importance of charity.[35] What then do the miracle accounts reveal about cure-seekers from each end of the social spectrum? First and foremost, their presence within the hagiographies is symbolic of the saints' wide-ranging appeal in much the same way as the variety of cures was, as discussed in the previous chapter. These local saints were not specialists and had the potential to aid any deserving devotee regardless of their social standing or complaint. Secondly, while there were some differences in the complaints recorded as having been brought to the saints depending on social standing, these were not as varied as might have been expected. Where those of lower social standing were more dominant it is likely that lifestyle and occupational hazards had a part to play. Analysing these accounts also emphasises the fact that few cure-seekers were overtly referred to in terms of social status, thus suggesting some level of middle ground that was not seen to be noteworthy, in contrast to extreme wealth or poverty. The hagiographers' input in the *miracula* here is worth considering; *M. Jacobi*, as noted, paid greater attention to the personal details for wealthier cure-seekers who, in turn, might have become benefactors to the royal abbey.

Names and Occupations

Each of the seven case studies includes at least one named cure-seeker, and at least one reference to a cure-seeker's occupation. Although these details are not directly connected to the healthcare aspect of the cure-seeking process, this information offers further insight into the individuals whose experiences of holy healing survive within these sources and can therefore assist in building a broader picture of the cure-seekers.

Considering the named individuals recorded within these miracles, of whom there are ninety-six, reveals a broad range of forenames and the occasional use of a surname or moniker in order to further identify the individual.[36] Reviewing the hagiographies in chronological order of their production also illustrates the introduction of Norman and continental forenames and, in turn, a decline in the number of Old English names. Of course, it must be remembered that the hagiographies for established cults contained accounts that occurred before the Conquest. However, such names also lingered into the twelfth century: *M. Willelmi* records cure-seekers such as Blythburgh, who became swollen after being bitten by a viper, alongside Robert, son of William

---

[35] *M. Swithuni* 6, ed. Lapidge, pp. 652–5; *M. Jacobi*, fols. 174rb–174va; Kemp, 'The Hand of St James' XX, 14–16.

[36] Appendix 1, pp. 215–16.

de Crachesford, who was 'cerebri turbati laborantem insanis' ('troubled with the insanity of a disturbed mind').[37]

As noted, *M. Willelmi* and *M. Jacobi* appear to have been particularly interested in recording these more personal aspects. Such a practice could be indicative of a growing interest in documenting specific details during the latter half of the century, or evidential of the fact that both were new cults attempting to establish themselves. Both suggestions have merit, but the fact that *M. Æbbe*, produced at around the same time as *M. Jacobi*, does not follow the same patten, highlights that this cannot be taken as a general trend. Hagiographical preferences cannot be discounted in the decision to include or exclude this more detailed information. As stated, there were various reasons why a hagiographer may or may not have included certain personal details.

Analysis of lay occupations proves equally interesting owing to the diversity among the employments recorded.[38] Occupations are also potentially informative with regard to a cure-seeker's affliction. *M. Moduenne* records two individuals who were involved in the rebuilding of the church roof at Burton Abbey. Both men, a carpenter and a workman, were saved from serious injury, if not death, when they fell from the scaffolding while working on the roof beams: a reminder of the dangers involved in the building of these great church structures.[39]

The miracles also include cure-seekers working in domestic service. A range of terminology is used to describe those in service: 'seruiens' ('servant'); 'domesticorum' ('domestic servant'); 'ministrare solebat' ('used to serve'); 'servulam' ('young, female servant'); and 'famulam' ('female servant').[40] In addition to those working in more domestic environments, Gilbert, the hound-keeper of a northern nobleman, and Reimbert, seneschal to the abbot of Battle Abbey, can also be considered as working in this 'service industry'.[41] A number of administrators, in the form of clerks, are also referred to. Some of these clerks are recorded as having been employed by specific individuals, including the

---

[37] Thomas of Monmouth, *M. Willelmi* VI.15, VII.3, ed. Jessop and James, pp. 251–3, 265.

[38] Appendix 2, p. 217.

[39] Geoffrey of Burton, *M. Moduenne* 50, ed. Bartlett, pp. 210–13.

[40] *M. Swithuni* 51, 54, ed. Lapidge, pp. 684–5, 688–91; Eadmer of Canterbury, *M. Dunstani* 25, ed. Turner and Muir, pp. 204–5; *L. Eliensis* I.48, III.31, ed. Blake, pp. 59–60, 265, trans. Fairweather, pp. 79–80, 319. Regarding 'domesticorum', Lapidge translates this as 'domestic servant' rather than the more literal (but less eloquent) '[servant] of domestics'; I have kept the same wording as Lapidge here.

[41] *M. Jacobi*, fols. 173vb–174ra; Kemp, '*The Hand of St James*' XVIII, 13–14; Thomas of Monmouth, *M. Willelmi* VII.1, ed. Jessop and James, pp. 263–4.

unnamed clerk of the sacrist of Canterbury Cathedral, who fell ill while the sacrist was conducting family business in Norfolk, and was healed by William (as was the sacrist's palfrey).[42] More unusual are the mentions of a musician and a needle-seller in *M. Æbbe*, the latter of whom was also an 'adolescens' ('adolescent').[43]

The fact that mentions of lay employment occur in all seven hagiographies permits a better understanding of those who sought the saints' aid. Many of the jobs mentioned, when not domestic, relate to industries and services that would be associated with urban environments, the four references to Norwich's 'money men' being one example of this.[44] Owing to the diverse range of occupations, comparative analysis of these cure-seekers would not indicate any overall trends in work-related complaints. Nevertheless, acknowledging the range of employment recorded within the miracles allows for greater appreciation of the individuals who sought out the saints and their brand of healthcare. Of course, when it comes to employment and vocation, there is one group within the miracle accounts who cannot be ignored: the religious men.

Monks and Clerics

Representing only twenty-one cure-seekers, it might appear that there would be little to say regarding the cure-seeking religious men who sought out saintly healing. However, their minimal presence, and complete absence from *M. Moduenne* and *M. Æbbe*, is intriguing. Even in the minority, or because of this minority, their presence within the hagiographies is revealing of the places and processes of miraculous cure-seeking. Equally revealing is that there is not a single account in which the religious individual was a nun, despite three of the saints being women of the Church.

Within the five *miracula* where monks and clerics were recorded as the recipients of healing miracles, the frequency of their presence varies greatly. In *M. Swithuni* only one of the fifty cure-seekers was a man of the Church. The prior of Abingdon had been blind for fifteen years and had received no help from physicians before being cured through Swithun's intercession.[45] In contrast, Æthelthryth is credited with the healing of six churchmen in *L. Eliensis*, as is William in *M. Willelmi*. Owing to the length of *M. Willelmi*,

---

[42] Thomas of Monmouth, *M. Willelmi* III.29, ed. Jessop and James, pp. 160–1.

[43] *M. Æbbe* IV.6, IV.36, ed. Bartlett, pp. 38–41, 58–9.

[44] Thomas of Monmouth, *M. Willelmi* III.22, IV.3, IV.13, VI.3, ed. Jessop and James, pp. 154–5, 168–9, 182–3, 223. Also see Yarrow, *Saints and Their Communities*, pp. 161–2.

[45] *M. Swithuni* 29, ed. Lapidge, pp. 668–9.

this equates to less than a tenth of all William of Norwich's cure-seekers. In contrast monks and clerics represent almost a quarter of all cure-seekers in *L. Eliensis*. Incidentally, *L. Eliensis* also contains eight religious men who, rather than benefiting from Æthelthryth's care, brought divine punishment upon themselves in retribution for harm inflicted on Ely Cathedral and its community, including its patron saint.[46]

This combination of cure and punishment is paralleled in the recording of the laity who were, likewise, the recipients of both. The similarity between the representation of these religious men and their lay counterparts within the miracles, as further discussed below, raises a question of why monks and clerics should be so infrequently represented within these *miracula*. That the hagiographers wished to promote the saints' connection to, and protection of, the laity could explain why so few monks and clerics feature in these *miracula* collections. But it must be remembered that the texts under consideration here were produced in Latin and thus were not in a format that would have allowed immediate dissemination to the laity. That is not to say that there were not vernacular hagiographies, as Bartlett has discussed, indeed these appear in Irish and Old English at an early date, however these texts were likely for personal use not public promotion.[47] It is also not true that monks or clerics would have been without health complaints, including difficulties such as joint problems that were the result of their onerous daily routines and restricted diets.[48] Clearly, as was also the case with a number of lay cure-seekers, some religious men first investigated other avenues of healing. That monks had better access to healthcare within the monastery is possible, but it is still curious that so few should be recorded within these miracles when the descriptions of those few who *are* included in these accounts reveal that their experiences of ill health and affliction were not dissimilar to those of the laity.

As noted, in many ways the representation of these religious men is little different from accounts of laypeople. Monks and clerics who were miraculously healed – sometimes having sought other medical aid first – similarly placed their trust in the healing powers of the saint, sometimes following a vision, sometimes having come to the site of the tomb or altar. Despite being a man of the Church, Abbot Osbert of Notley Abbey, whom we met in the previous

---

[46] *L. Eliensis* I.49, III.92, III.120, III.121, III.138, ed. Blake, pp. 60–1, 338–41, 369–70, 370–1, 385–7, trans. Fairweather, pp. 80–2, 415–19, 457–8, 458–60, 476–8.

[47] Bartlett, *Why Can the Dead Do Such Great Things?*, pp. 578–86.

[48] Horden, 'Sickness and Healing', p. 414. Also see: R. Gilchrist and B. Sloane, *Requiem: The Medieval Monastic Cemetery in Britain* (London, 2005), pp. 209–13; Patrick, *The 'Obese Medieval Monk'*.

chapter, was not granted any preferential treatment by St James.[49] Owing to
Osbert's 'grauissima occulorum egritudine' ('grievous affliction of the eyes')
he had been unable to rest due to the pain.[50] With medical intervention only
exacerbating the problem, one of his canons advised he make a vow to visit
Reading 'sanctumque Jacobum pereg[ri]nationis sue muneribus ueneraturum'
('and honour St James with the service of his pilgrimage').[51] On making his
vow, Osbert immediately found his discomfort eased and subsequently made
the journey to Reading to fulfil his vow.

The process of cure followed by Osbert mirrors that of many lay cure-seekers. A sick layman was similarly cured on making ready for his visit to
Swithun's shrine.[52] In both cases it was simply the act of preparing to journey
to the saint which was required for the healing to occur, regardless of whether
this action was undertaken by a layman or a monk. Both men are thus given
the cure they desire on the proviso that they will follow through with their
promise to fulfil their vow; and, as cure comes first, the journey can be made by
able-bodied individuals who, presumably, were able to complete the journey in
less time than it would have taken had they still suffered from their afflictions.
On arrival, thanks were given to the saint and to God, thus fulfilling the vows
previously made.

If a vow were not kept, and no journey made, the saints could show their
displeasure. A young man suffered from a second broken arm after he failed
to fulfil his promise of visiting Reading after James cured his first injury.[53]
This contract-like vow worked as a basic principle across the board, and was
a practice open to all, religious or lay. Indeed, this was a route of cure-seeking
open to all, which emphasises the perceived universality of the saints and their
brand of therapy. Saints could help cure anyone and anyone could undertake
the process of cure-seeking. This was key in the structure and practice of medieval healing cults.

The range of afflictions shown to be brought to the saints, analysed in the
previous chapter, made it evident that these seven saints were not perceived as
being specialists in the cure of any one ailment. Rather, as this chapter reveals,
they were celebrated for their ability to manifest a broad range of cures to a
broad range of cure-seekers. As with the overall pattern of healing, illnesses

[49] *M. Jacobi*, fol. 174ra–b; Kemp, '*The Hand of St James*' XIX, 14. Also see above,
pp. 74–6.
[50] *M. Jacobi*, fol. 174ra; Kemp, '*The Hand of St James*' XIX, 14.
[51] Ibid.
[52] *M. Swithuni* 8, ed. Lapidge, pp. 654–5.
[53] *M. Jacobi*, fols. 174vb–175ra; Kemp, '*The Hand of St James*' XXII, 16.

and paralysis feature frequently in the cases of religious men, with such a case absent only from *M. Swithuni* (Table 3.3). Oral complaints, predominantly toothache, are also a prominent feature; religious men account for over half of cases recorded within the seven *miracula*. Complaints of this nature, as touched upon in Chapter 2, could be indicative of the better diet afforded to those living within the cloister. Better diet might also explain why there are fewer accounts of eye affliction here than was seen as part of a general trend across the case studies.[54] Although it might be considered that close reading of religious texts would likely have resulted in the deterioration of eyesight over time within monastic environments.

Table 3.3. Afflictions recorded for monks and clerics

	M. Swithuni	*M. Dunstani*	*L. Eliensis*	*M. Willelmi*	*M. Jacobi*	**Total**
Blindness and other eye afflictions	1	0	0	0	1	2
Bodily paralysis (partial or full paralysis, 'humps', curvature of the spine or knees, etc.)	0	1	1	0	1	3
Complaints relating to the mouth (toothache, ulcers, etc.)	0	0	2	1	0	3
'Illness' (unspecific but including sickness, fever, etc.)	0	2	1	2	1	6
'Insomnia'	0	0	0	1	0	1
Lower body complaints (dysentery, piles)	0	0	0	1	0	1
'Mental health' complaints (madness, possession, epilepsy, etc.)	0	1	1	0	0	2
Tumours, swellings and growths (including 'cancer', 'gout', dropsy)	0	0	1	1	1	3

A more unusual inclusion among the miraculous cures of the monks and clerics is the sole case of insomnia recorded across these seven *miracula*. The account, recorded by Thomas of Monmouth, relates to the oldest monk of Norwich Cathedral Priory, another Thomas.[55] As a result of suffering from a long-standing 'imbecillitate' ('weakness'), Thomas had been moved to the

---

[54] For more on monastic diet see B. Harvey, *Living and Dying in England, 1100–1540: The Monastic Experience* (Oxford, 1993), pp. 34–6, 38–41.

[55] Thomas of Monmouth, *M. Willelmi* III.10, ed. Jessop and James, pp. 134–5.

priory's infirmary where, for three days, he had been unable to sleep.[56] This had caused him great distress. Thomas of Monmouth notes that the elder Thomas felt particularly distressed at night as he was 'nec ad modicum oculi eius ualebat quiescere' ('unable to rest his eyes even for a moment').[57] Being so affected by his insomnia, Thomas prayed to William of Norwich for the recovery of his lost sleep, his insomnia not his long-term weakness being his main concern. On finishing his prayers, Thomas fell silent and fell asleep. On waking, refreshed, Thomas called out and gave thanks to God and to William. No mention is made, either by Thomas in his prayers, or in describing his recovery, of his long-term infirmity, a complaint which likely related to his old age. It was the lack of sleep that caused him concern and emotional, if not physical, discomfort. This unusual finding within the *miracula* highlights the close-knit nature of the cloistered community. Despite the rarity of such reports within the miracles, troubled sleep surely would not have been unusual within monastic communities. In Thomas's case, it is possible that this was exacerbated by his long-term weakness, which resulted in a great deal of bedrest and allowed for little activity. Particularly interesting within this account is the recognition that physical complaints could result in emotional distress. It was the latter that acted as the catalyst for Thomas's prayers, and the cure was deemed successful when he awoke feeling revived.[58]

The issue of age will be returned to later in this chapter, but it is worth considering how the level of familiarity within a monastic community might reflect the more interpersonal nature of these accounts of miraculous cure-seeking recorded within the hagiographies. Records such as that of Thomas and Abbot Osbert suggest an intimacy between hagiographer and cure-seeker that allowed for a greater level of personal detail to be provided. These accounts also indicate that religious men had access to other forms of healthcare, be that the long-term care of the infirmary for Thomas, or the use of ointments in the case of Osbert. Both also indicate the greater availability of a variety of healthcare practices to monastic communities, some of which were undoubtedly less accessible to certain members of the lay community either due to a lack of similar infrastructure or a lack of financial means.

Access to healthcare within monasteries might be another explanation for why so few religious men are recorded within the hagiographies. This access to medical care, not to mention access to respite and a better diet, might have staved off some of the afflictions that were more prevalent outside the cloister.

[56] Ibid., p. 135.
[57] Ibid.
[58] Ibid.

Moreover, monks, at least by the twelfth century, were less likely to be involved in rigorous manual labour that could put stress upon the body or pose a risk of accidents. Also worth acknowledging is that, even within monastic communities, not all stories of miraculous cure were likely to be recorded in *miracula* and some reports might have been kept alive via word of mouth, just as an oral culture for relating tales of the miraculous must have existed beyond the monastery. The limited presence of religious men within the *miracula* therefore, is not necessarily indicative of a lack of connection between religious men and saints or a lack of reliance on the saints in times of need. Archbishop Lanfranc himself benefited from Dunstan's intercession when he was severely ill.[59] Rather, this is a more complex issue and the understandings and experiences of healthcare in the cloister constitute a topic worthy of much greater research on its own merits. After all, as highlighted by Kerr, it was not as if members of religious communities were immune to ill health.[60] Indeed, the rigours of the monastic routine, and the need to wake for the night offices, meant a number of monks suffered from insomnia, just as the elder Thomas of Norwich had.[61]

A further point worth considering, and to be returned to below, is that the monks within these miracle stories came from both the cult-centre community and other institutions. This offers a tantalising glimpse into the intricate, and important, networks that existed between religious communities. However, this raises an important question: what about nuns? It would not be expected for nuns to appear in great numbers, but it might be assumed that the miracles would include some reference to them. Yet they are significant in their absence.

Religious Women

Nuns, in accordance with restrictions, led a more secluded life and thus venturing out from the cloister was an unlikely practice.[62] Yet, absence from the cloister in order to seek the aid of a saint would surely not be seen as deviant. After all such restrictions did not prevent some nuns from leaving their confines for less spiritually-rewarding activities, and evidently this theoretically strict enclosure was not always the reality.[63] Lack of evidence within the hagiographies, however, leaves the issue open to question. Have nuns been

---

[59]   Eadmer of Canterbury, *M. Dunstani* 21, ed. Turner and Muir, pp. 192–5.
[60]   Kerr, *Life in the Medieval Cloister*, p. 97.
[61]   Kerr, 'Health and Safety', 6.
[62]   Kerr, *Life in the Medieval Cloister*, p. 69.
[63]   Ibid., pp. 69, 135–6; M. Goodrich, *Worcester Nunneries: The Nuns of the Medieval Diocese* (Chichester, 2008), pp. 43, 51, 59.

purposefully excluded by hagiographers, or did nuns not seek the aid of the saints? Both seem unlikely and there is evidence that female monastics did find cure via saints, but within the walls of their convents, and that other forms of healing were also available to them. The hagiography *Liber S. Gilberti*, relating to the founder of the Gilbertine Order, supports this in recording an incident involving a nun from Chicksand Priory.[64] Mabel Stotfold tripped on entering the nunnery's kitchen and dislocated her foot.[65] The nuns could not remove her shoe due to the swelling and had to cut it from her foot. Various remedies were then tried, including 'tam trahendo, tum inplastra ponendo' ('putting [Mabel's] foot in both traction and in plaster'), but this only increased her suffering.[66]

Mabel's cure came over a year later. Having lost hope of any cure, one doctor stated that the only option was to amputate her foot which 'nigrum esse ad similitudinem ueli sui' ('was as black as her veil').[67] Mabel requested that a candle be made to her measurements that was to be used for St Gilbert. Along with the candle, Mabel was taken to the church, and a liturgical towel, used by Gilbert at his death, was placed on her foot and she stayed in vigil until the day of Gilbert's feast. While asleep Mabel saw men in albs enter the church and approach the altar, followed by Gilbert, dressed in priestly robes. Gilbert turned and blessed her three times and signalled for her to rise; following the third blessing she woke and stood. On standing, Mabel fell on her face while attempting to reach Gilbert, but this proved her cure was complete. Mabel's recovery was thus secured via saintly means, but within the privacy of Chicksand Priory. Her account was described on oath and with the additional testimony of her prioress, Christina, who had bound the swollen foot with the liturgical cloth and had observed the decreased swelling afterwards.

L. Gilberti includes seven accounts of the miraculous cure of nuns, found in both the formal and informal miracle collections.[68] Nuns, unsurprisingly, were not excluded from holy healing, but importantly they would not have been expected to travel outside their monasteries to secure this assistance. These limitations sit in contrast to the religious men recorded in our *miracula* who, as noted, were not just monks of the cult centre but monks and clerics from external institutions too (Table 3.4). This reinforces that, like rules regarding

---

[64] *The Book of St Gilbert* (hereafter *L. Gilberti*), ed. and trans. R. Foreville and G. Keir, OMT (Oxford, 1987).

[65] *L. Gilberti* Formal Miracle 17, ed. Foreville and Keir, pp. 284–9.

[66] Ibid., pp. 286–7.

[67] Ibid.

[68] Ibid., Formal Miracle 10, 14–17, Informal Miracle 6, 12, ed. Foreville and Keir, pp. 276–7, 280–9, 310–15, 316–17.

enclosure, different expectations towards miraculous cure were conventional for monks and nuns. Analysis highlights that two-thirds of the religious men within these miracle accounts were members of the cult centre. However, the five *miracula* to include religious men also all contained at least one account of an 'external' monk or cleric. In the case of *M. Swithuni* the only account relating to a monk is the account of the prior of Abingdon whose sight was restored by Swithun on visiting the saint's shrine.[69] The representation of monastic mobility and the lack of nuns in these *miracula* is intriguing but, as Bailey noted, clerics were relatively free to travel and, while monks would have been dissuaded from this unless for business, there were acceptable reasons for them to leave their cloisters.[70] Nuns, however, were thought to have been in greater danger (physically and morally) than monks when travelling, and the imposition of stricter restrictions on their travel might aid in explaining their lack of presence within these *miracula*.[71] Importantly, while it is perhaps surprising that there are so few reports of 'in-house' monastic miracle cures, these restrictions also provide a reason why other religious men might appear so seldom within our seven *miracula*.

Table 3.4. Monks and clerics from the cult centre
and those from other institutions

	Monks from the cult centre	Monks and clerics from other institutions
M. Swithuni	0	1
M. Dunstani	3	1
L. Eliensis	5	1
M. Willelmi	4	2
M. Jacobi	2	2
Total	14	7

The presence and representation of monks and clerics, and the lack of nuns, is a topic that deserves further discussion. Suffice to say those religious men who did seek out the aid of Swithun, Dunstan, Æthelthryth, William and James

---

[69]   *M. Swithuni* 29, ed. Lapidge, pp. 668–9.

[70]   A. E. Bailey, 'The Rich and the Poor, the Lesser and the Great', *Cultural and Social History* 11 (2014), 9–29 (17).

[71]   Ibid., 18; Kerr, *Life in the Medieval Cloister*, p. 69; D. Webb, *Pilgrimage in Medieval England* (London, 2000), p. 240; D. Webb, *Medieval European Pilgrimage*, European Culture and Society (Basingstoke, 2002), pp. 90–2.

(and undoubtedly many more whose accounts did not make it into the final *miracula* collections) found their cures in similar ways to their lay counterparts. The afflictions they brought were likewise diverse, with dental complaints being prominent alongside more expected ailments such as paralysis and illness. Moreover, just like the laity, religious men of various ages sought out holy healing, from younger monks such as Æthelweard at Canterbury who was possessed by a demon, to the aforementioned, elderly Thomas at Norwich who was so affected by his lack of sleep.[72] Finding evidence of these more vulnerable cure-seekers, the young and the old, is however not always an easy feat.

Younger and Older Cure-Seekers

Definitions of age must be understood within contemporary social and cultural contexts. Indeed, definitions of ageing even within one period are far from clear-cut, as is evidenced by the varying 'Ages of Man' theories circulating in the high Middle Ages.[73] Nevertheless, it is clear that there was an interest in recognising various stages of life and the hagiographies focused upon here are no exception to this. From the hagiographers' perspectives, including accounts of cure-seekers with a range of ages – in addition to both genders and a broad social range of cure-seekers – further emphasised the universality of the saints' charity and their popular appeal. This also highlights that those who sought saintly intervention through cure-seeking also believed in this universality and did not perceive there to be barriers to miraculous cure based on social or personal circumstances, or age.

A number of medievalists have already highlighted the importance of considering medieval childhood and old age, including Nicholas Orme, Joel Rosenthal, and Shulamith Shahar.[74] The study of premodern childhood, in particular, has progressed since Philip Ariès's well-known, and now widely disputed, argument against the existence of childhood in premodern cultures.[75] Finucane and Lett have considered the accounts of children within posthumous

---

[72] Eadmer of Canterbury, *M. Dunstani* 19, ed. Turner and Muir, pp. 182–9; Thomas of Monmouth, *M. Willelmi* III.10, ed. Jessop and James, pp. 134–5.

[73] For discussion of the 'Ages of Man', see: Burrow, *The Ages of Man*, pp. 5–54; E. Sears, *The Ages of Man: Medieval Interpretations of the Life Cycle* (Princeton, 1986), pp. 16–37. For an archaeological perspective see R. Gilchrist, *Medieval Life: Archaeology and the Life Course* (Woodbridge, 2012), pp. 32–67.

[74] Orme, *Medieval Children*; J. T. Rosenthal, *Old Age in Late Medieval England*, The Middle Ages Series (Philadelphia, 1996); S. Shahar, *Childhood in the Middle Ages* (London, 1990); S. Shahar, *Growing Old in the Middle Ages: 'Winter clothes us in shadow and pain'*, trans. Y. Lota (London, 1997).

[75] P. Ariès, *Centuries of Childhood*, trans. R. Baldick (London, 1996), pp. 31–47.

miracles, with both noting the importance of familial relationships, and Lett also arguing that sons were favoured.[76] Recently issues of premodern childhood health and healthcare have been addressed by Kuuliala, who used canonisation records to investigate children's health in the late medieval period, and Hannah Newton, who produced a thoughtful study of children's health in early modern England.[77] Further discussion of this topic, with consideration of the experiences of younger and older cure-seekers, would undoubtedly be a worthy and extensive study. But what can the miracle reports reveal about the complaints and experiences of those cure-seekers whose 'age identity', at either end of the age spectrum, was made evident by the hagiographers?

Children and Youths

All seven *miracula* contain accounts relating to pre-adult cure-seekers, in total accounting for just over a third of all lay cure-seekers, and thus indicating the recognised importance of these younger individuals among those who sought the saints' aid. The hagiographers were clearly keen to promote saints as carers for the young. It was recognised that children, and childhood, differed from adulthood. Children were seen to be playful, and youths (especially boys) were often seen as reckless. These characteristics were supported by humoral theories on ageing. The Hippocratic *Regimen* and later works, including Bede's *De temporum ratione*, followed a four-stage model that aligned each age with the predominance of one of the humours.[78] Bede noted that children were cheerful and tender-hearted due to the fact blood was most prevalent in childhood; in adolescence this gave way to the predominance of red bile that resulted in youthful leanness, boldness, and irritability.[79]

That there were varying stages of development in pre-adulthood was also reflected in the variety of terminologies which could be used to describe children and youths. This range of expressions is reflected within the miracles with terms such as 'infantulus' ('infant') and 'nuper nato' ('newly born'), highlighting the miraculous cure of the very young, and 'adolescens' ('adolescent') and 'iuuenis' ('youth'), marking out those of a more pubescent or nearly-adult age.[80]

---

[76] Finucane, *The Rescue of the Innocents*, p. 55; Lett, *L'Enfant des miracles*, p. 161.

[77] Kuuliala, *Childhood Disability and Social Integration*; H. Newton, *The Sick Child in Early Modern England, 1580–1720* (Oxford, 2014).

[78] Bede, *De temporum ratione* 35, trans. Wallis, pp. 100–1; Hippocrates, *'Regimen'* I.xxxii–xxxiii, in Hippocrates, Heracleitus, *Nature of Man*, trans. Jones, pp. 224–95, 272–81.

[79] Bede, *De temporum ratione* 35, trans. Wallis, pp. 100–1.

[80] Thomas of Monmouth, *M. Willelmi* III.9, ed. Jessop and James, p. 134; *M. Æbbe* IV.29, ed. Bartlett, pp. 58–9; *M. Swithuni* 11, ed. Lapidge, pp. 656–7; Geoffrey of

For adolescent girls, the language has an additional undertone of marking them out as 'uirgo' ('virgin'), thus indicating their pre-sexual status.[81] This status, Bailey noted, had secular and spiritual connotations, but the key factor was that the term indicated an unmarried girl or woman.[82] Specific ages are only occasionally recorded within the accounts, with hagiographers preferring the use of broader and more fluid language, including 'puer' ('boy') and 'puella' ('girl').[83] A little more vague, but implying parental, and often paternal, dependency are the terms 'filius' ('son') and 'filia' ('daughter').[84] In the majority of such accounts the narrative implication is that the cure-seeker is not yet an adult, although in a minority of cases this line appears more blurred.[85] The presence of this varied language within the hagiographies makes it easier to identify younger, pre-adult cure-seekers and highlights their presence among the individuals cured by miraculous means.

Most of the miracles involving younger cure-seekers reveal that parents were greatly concerned with the health and welfare of their offspring. Seeking cure for a child was an act of parental love not just for the present, but also one of concern for the future. Serious impairments and disfigurements could have a great effect on an individual, making them dependent on family. Friends proved similarly concerned with the well-being of their acquaintances: one 'iuuenis' ('youth'), mute since birth and suffering from a curvature of the shoulders for eleven years, was carried to Dunstan's shrine by friends.[86] Although impairments gained later in life could prove a burden, the lifelong care

---

Burton, *M. Moduenne* 48, ed. Bartlett, pp. 200–5.

[81] Thomas of Monmouth, *M. Willelmi* II.7, ed. Jessop and James, pp. 79–85. For connections between sexual identity and the female body see: H. Leyser, *Medieval Women: A Social History of Women in England, 450–1500* (London, 1996), p. 93; K. M. Phillips, *Medieval Maidens: Young Women and Gender in England, 1270–1540*, Manchester Medieval Studies (Manchester, 2003), pp. 24–30.

[82] A. E. Bailey, 'Wives, Mothers and Widows on Pilgrimage: Categories of "Woman" Recorded at English Healing Shrines in the High Middle Ages', *Journal of Medieval History* 39 (2013), 197–219 (209).

[83] *M. Swithuni* 47, ed. Lapidge, pp. 682–3; *M. Æbbe* IV.13, ed. Bartlett, pp. 52–3. For discussion of the language used in *M. Willelmi* with regard to defining children and youths, see R. J. Salter, 'Minors and the Miraculous: The Cure-Seeking Experiences of Children in Twelfth-Century English Hagiography', in *Kids Those Days: Children in Medieval Culture*, ed. L. Preston-Matto and M. A. Valante (Leiden, 2021), pp. 67–94.

[84] For example: *M. Swithuni* 5, ed. Lapidge, pp. 652–3; *M. Æbbe* IV.17, ed. Bartlett, pp. 52–5.

[85] Salter, 'Minors and the Miraculous', pp. 70–3.

[86] Eadmer of Canterbury, *M. Dunstani* 5, ed. Turner and Muir, pp. 162–5.

required by an individual who suffered since birth must have been a greater responsibility still. Due to the possible impact this could have on the quality of an individual's life, and their independence, it is unsurprising that so many desired a cure or that cases of paralysis and sensory impairments feature so heavily in the accounts of younger cure-seekers: these afflictions account for approximately sixty per cent of the miracles recorded for children and youths.

Sudden illness, however, could prove to be a pressing concern with a greater risk of fatality. It was just as important for a saint to be able to cure these afflictions, especially for the young and vulnerable, such as the infant son of Radulfus:

> infantulus filius Radulfi [...] ad mortem egrotabat et iam hore supreme mors sola supererat. Vnde patri consultum est et matri ut in longum et latum ad mensuram pueri festinantissime candela fieret, factam sancto Willelmo pro filii sospitate uouerent, et procul dubio statim puerum incolumem incolumes reciperent [...] prout dictum est, candela conficitur, et paternis delata manibus ad sepulcrum sancti martiris uotaliter offertur. Regrediens pater filium se reperire gaudet incolumem quem pauloante dimiserat morientem.

> (the infant son of Radulfus [...] was sick unto death and his last hour was at hand. So his father and mother were advised that a candle of the length and breadth of the little boy should be made with the utmost haste, and that when it was made they should offer it to St William for the restoration of their son, and that without doubt they would receive back their son safe and whole [...] straight away the candle was made, and having been brought by the father's hands it was offered as a votive offering at the sepulchre of the holy martyr. The father on his return rejoiced to find his son safe whom a little while before he had given up for dead.)[87]

Illnesses could quickly escalate, and a number of the accounts of sickness, such as that above, emphasise that the sufferer was close to death.[88] Without access to antibiotics or vaccines, and with a remedy needing to be fast-acting, it is no wonder that parents put their faith in the saints, or that *miracula* would wish to champion the successful recovery of ill children. Modern faith in medicine, and medical advice, might thus be seen in a similar light. In both instances medieval and modern parents place their faith in the abilities of 'higher powers', be those powers spiritual or scientific. The saints were figures

---

[87] Thomas of Monmouth, *M. Willelmi* III.9, ed. Jessop and James, p. 134.

[88] Ibid. For another example, see *L. Eliensis* III.42, ed. Blake, pp. 280–1, trans. Fair-weather, pp. 340–2.

in which medieval society had faith and the hagiographies reflect the fact that cults were seen, universally, to be places of healing, be the sufferer lay or religious, rich or poor, old or young, or disabled or sick.

The Elderly

Evidence of elderly cure-seekers is less easily distinguishable within the miracles. In part this might be due to an understanding that bodily health does decline with age. Indeed, in terms of humoral theory, the concept of the ageing body becoming colder and, after a period of moistness, also beginning to dry out, fits well with what might be considered as the visual elements of the ageing process.[89] It could also be questioned whether older individuals would be as willing, or as able, to undertake a cure-seeking journey. If such a journey was made, would older cure-seekers have benefited from that visit if their complaint was caused by ageing? It is also worth asking how older cure-seekers were identified in contrast to other adults, if at all, within the miracle accounts.

Unlike children and youths for whom there was a vast range of terminologies that could be employed, elderly cure-seekers are linguistically less discernible within miracle accounts. There are only seven cases in which older, lay, cure-seekers can be identified, fewer surely than the number who did try to secure saintly assistance. Interestingly, six of these more senior laypeople were women.[90] Only one report, found in *M. Moduenne*, refers to an older male cure-seeker: an unnamed pensioner of a local nobleman named William.[91] That ageing men did not seek out the saints' intercessory aid as frequently appears unlikely, and it must be considered that terminology and social identity came into play here. As with younger female cure-seekers, defined through their sexual immaturity and virginal status, older women were identified, societally and linguistically, in relation to their experience and maturity.[92] A noblewoman whose sight was restored by Swithun is referred to as 'matrona' ('matron'), a term that carries with it a sense of status that implies a level of seniority.[93] *M. Dunstani*, likewise, refers to a matron from London who had

[89] Bede, *De temporum ratione* 35, trans. Wallis, pp. 100–1.
[90] *M. Swithuni* 9, 42, ed. Lapidge, pp. 654–5, 676–9; Eadmer of Canterbury, *M. Dunstani* 7, 26, ed. Turner and Muir, pp. 164–7, 204–7; Thomas of Monmouth, *M. Willelmi* IV.11, V.23, ed. Jessop and James, pp. 181–2, 217–18.
[91] Geoffrey of Burton, *M. Moduenne* 45, ed. Bartlett, pp. 184–7.
[92] Leyser, *Medieval Women*, p. 93.
[93] *M. Swithuni* 9, ed. Lapidge, pp. 654–5.

suffered with a serious illness.[94] Eadmer of Canterbury also emphasised the advanced age of a blind woman, identifying her as 'anus quaedam' ('a certain old woman') who sought her cure 'in senectute' ('in [her] advanced age').[95]

The most intriguing and insightful of the accounts to record the experiences of elderly cure-seekers, though, is that of Alditha in her second appearance within *M. Willelmi*.[96] In her previous cure-seeking, Alditha, the wife of Toke the chandler, was cured from a long-standing illness.[97] In her second appearance, Alditha is referred to as the 'olim uxor' ('former wife') of Toke, and her affliction, that of the loss of her hearing, appears connected to her advancing age:

fidei ductu ad memoratum sancti martiris sepulcrum uenit, ac surdiciei sue remedium petiit. Ex multo etenim tempore obsurduerant aures adeoque inualuerat incommodum, ut nisi tuum illius auribus os applicares ab ipsa nequaquam audiri posses. Unde et in publicam prodire uerebatur, et non nisi domesticorum utebatur alloquiis. Timebat enim ualde ne surdiciei sue ibprobrium aliene quandoque noticie prodiret in risum

([Alditha] came, led by faith, to the tomb of the holy martyr, and implored relief from her deafness; for during a long time her ears had been growing deaf, to such an extent that you could only make yourself heard by putting your lips close to her ear. She was consequently afraid to go out, and only talked to her own family, fearing lest the reproach of her deafness should be detected by others, and bring derision upon her.)[98]

Alditha's sense of embarrassment and fear that she would be mocked for her inability are evident and led her to become isolated from her community. It is hard not to feel for Alditha in her suffering due to her mortification at her increasing deafness, and because of what must have been a progressively lonely existence. Her consequent emotional response was surely not unique. Other individuals must have similarly found themselves increasingly cut off from their communities because of their impairments. Community support might also prove difficult to secure, as the three blind women from the Isle of Wight found when they were abandoned on their way to Swithun's shrine at Winchester.[99]

[94] Eadmer of Canterbury, *M. Dunstani* 26, ed. Turner and Muir, pp. 204–7.
[95] Ibid., 7, pp. 164–5.
[96] Thomas of Monmouth, *M. Willelmi* V.23, ed. Jessop and James, pp. 217–18.
[97] Ibid., III.14, p. 147.
[98] Ibid., V.23, p. 218.
[99] *M. Swithuni* 6, ed. Lapidge, pp. 654–5.

Like Alditha, all but one of these older women suffered with ill health or a sensory impairment, such as loss of sight or hearing. That ageing individuals were at risk of such complaints as illnesses or deteriorating vision or hearing is to be expected, but that they still sought remedies for these complaints is noteworthy. The one account not to fall into these categories is a unique account within these seven *miracula* as it refers not to an issue of personal health, but to a wolf attack in which the elderly woman was saved by Swithun from serious bodily harm or worse.[100] Due to her advanced age, the woman was unable to fend off the wolves and, reportedly, was dragged out of her house by the pack. Evidence for wolves in high medieval England is not easy to find, however there is proof for their continued albeit decreasing presence in the late eleventh and twelfth centuries; their extinction in England was almost certain by the fifteenth century, as Aleksander Pluskowski has discussed.[101]

Attacks by animals are rare within the *miracula*, nevertheless their inclusion is a reminder that not all injuries or afflictions were caused by underlying health concerns or accidents. The implication in the account of the wolf attack in *M. Swithuni* is that due to her sex, advanced age, and the nature of the aggressors, this was an individual, seemingly living alone, who was unable to defend herself. This highlights an underlying vulnerability among elderly individuals especially those without familial or communal networks of support. This sense of vulnerability can also be observed in the accounts of younger cure-seekers; again these were individuals who (ideally) had familial support. Young individuals were also at risk from accidents or animal attacks, as Finucane and Orme have both discussed.[102] Considering the recognised vulnerabilities of society's oldest and youngest, it is not surprising that the miracle accounts would champion their presence among the cure-seekers who sought holy healing. Nor should it be a surprise that individuals of all ages would seek out saintly assistance to rectify their health complaints.

*   *   *

This chapter had a simple starting point: to establish who the individuals recorded within the case-study *miracula* were. Understanding the people

---

[100] Ibid., 42, pp. 676–9.

[101] A. Pluskowski, 'The Wolf', in *Extinctions and Invasions: A Social History of British Fauna*, ed. T. O'Connor and N. Sykes (Oxford, 2010), pp. 68–74. Also see A. Pluskowski, *Wolves and the Wilderness in the Middle Ages* (Woodbridge, 2006), pp. 18–39.

[102] Finucane, *The Rescue of the Innocents*, pp. 101–49; Orme, *Medieval Children*, pp. 98–100.

represented in these accounts of posthumous miracles is vital in order to consider not just the range of afflictions believed to have been cured through the saints' merits, but also the processes and experiences of miraculous cure-seeking. Of course, establishing who our cure-seekers were requires accepting the nature of the *miracula* as edited collections that were produced to advertise, celebrate and promote the cults and the merits of the saints.

The process of analysing the miracles follows the methodology set out by previous scholars in this field, namely Finucane and Sigal.[103] With the focus here being on a select group of case studies it is possible to consider wider trends and to pick up on, and follow, the stories of certain individual cure-seekers. In terms of the trends that the miracles present it is impossible to overlook the high proportion of lay individuals recorded and that, generally, it was male cure-seekers who were in the majority. The cure-seeking of younger individuals was also well recorded within the hagiographies, accounting for just over a third of all healed cure-seekers within the seven works.

The level of detail provided within these sources for the cure-seekers, as noted, does vary. Some hagiographers, such as Thomas of Monmouth, were keen to include as many personal details as possible, including names, and even occupation. Why some miracle accounts included more or less personal detail will always be open for debate as the reasons could stem from various causes, such as the length of time the cult had been established or the stylistic preferences of individual hagiographers. Where these details are included, though, it is possible to build a broader picture of the cure-seeker and their background. One group of individuals who stand out among the cure-seekers, and for whom it is possible to consider the strains of their daily life and the toll this took on their health, are the religious men. Despite featuring to a lesser extent than their lay counterparts, the inclusion of monks and clerics in the majority of these *miracula* highlights that they had recourse to the saints' brand of healing. Further investigation into religious interaction with the saints' cults also revealed that, while not present within the seven *miracula*, nuns were not averse to seeking divine assistance for corporeal complaints. However, due to stricter rules regarding their enclosure, religious women were unlikely to undertake cure-seeking that would take them outside their monastic community, as *L. Gilberti* revealed. In contrast, the men identified were not always monks of the associated monastery, and the 'other' religious men were both monastic and secular ecclesiastics, thus suggesting that monks were permitted greater freedoms in visiting other institutions. Further research into religious

---

[103] See above, pp. 14–15.

communities and their experiences of healthcare and, especially, holy healing would evidently prove a valuable addition to the study of medieval medicine.

This chapter has emphasised the crucial role of the laity within the cults of the saints. Lay support, or the lack thereof, could make or break a cult. While it is evident that a number of individuals first sought medical assistance from more earthly practitioners, many of the cure-seekers recorded in these accounts would have had limited access to, or resources for, sustained medical treatment. Indeed, even monks like Abbot Osbert found that this could be a costly affair and that there was every chance that prescriptions would be ineffective or even exacerbate symptoms.[104] Of course, miracle stories naturally emphasise the effectiveness of the divine, as accessed through the saints. This was, after all, a form of healing that stood above temporal efforts and could supply remedies for seemingly incurable complaints. The wide range of cure-seekers recorded within the *miracula*, therefore, is evidence of sufferers having exhausted their other options and of individuals being willing to trust in a higher power of healing. Age, social status, and sex all emerge as significant, although subtle, factors within these collections of healing miracles. However, external factors must have also influenced decisions to seek out miraculous healing and it must be asked what distances cure-seekers were willing to and likely to cover in the process of securing the saints' aid.

---

[104] See above, pp. 74–6.

4

From Near and Far: The Geography of the Cults and the Distance Travelled

In taking the next step on the journey to the shrine, and following the previous chapter's establishment of who our cure-seekers were, this chapter addresses the geography of the cults. Considering the distance travelled by cure-seekers, as represented in the miracles, through statistical and literary analysis, provides better insight into the geographical scope of the cults. While local supporters were the primary demographic of cure-seekers, well-established and popular cults had the potential to attract widespread attention. As a result, it might be expected that hagiographies, in their promotion of their saint, would emphasise reports where journeys of longer length were made. An interesting issue therefore arises with regard to the representation of travel and geographic locale.

The geographical reach of the cults of saints has been a feature of studies produced since Finucane's *Miracles and Pilgrims*. The importance of the reach of saints, for Finucane, was that it provided insight into the spread of the cult. Although his analysis revealed that cults found greater support in the local vicinity, Finucane noted that within the closing accounts in many *miracula* there were higher numbers of pilgrims from further afield, and concluded that this showed both the developing scope of the cult and also a dying down of interest in the cult's immediate vicinity.[1] That a hagiographer might wish to promote the increasing influence of their saint's cult is understandable, although whether this should mean that interest closer to home was declining is worth querying. Just because there was an increase in accounts relating to those who were at a greater distance from the cult does not mean that there was a decrease in local devotion. Ward's *Miracles and the Medieval Mind* and, more recently, Yarrow's *Saints and Their Communities* have also seen the merits of considering the importance of geographic scope in understanding the shape of the cult. Both, like Finucane, recognised the value of the cults to their immediate area. For Ward, the shift in the saint's patronage, from protector to

---

[1] Finucane, *Miracles and Pilgrims*, pp. 161–2, 171.

healer, in the high Middle Ages reflected the changing relationship between the saints and their local communities.[2] Yarrow too considered this element of care in highlighting that William's cult might have acted as an extension of the bishop of Norwich's own pastoral care.[3] Correspondingly, Emily M. Rose noted that Thomas of Monmouth emphasised local lay support for William's cult as monastic endorsement alone would not have been enough.[4] Support from both the local laity and the monastic community was required. In the studies of Finucane, Ward and Yarrow, discussion was kept broadly to pilgrims and devotees as a general group, even if miracle accounts were a key source of analysis. The present analysis differs, focusing specifically on those who received miraculous cure and their distance from the site of their healing. The chapter that follows will then take up the journey to the shrines themselves to consider the experience and practicalities of travel.

Analysing Geographic Range

Calculating Distance

When Finucane undertook his study of the distances between the shrines and 'origin-site[s]', the distance between the two was measured 'as the crow flies', in a straight line from initial location to the site of the cult centre.[5] However, such measurements do not account for topography. It is extremely rare that travel is ever undertaken in a perfect straight line unless on an old Roman road. Further and fuller discussion of the practicalities of travel follow in the next chapter, but in calculating the distances it is important to consider that it is rare for a route to be so direct. In analysing the distance between the origin-site and the cult centre, and as many English roads today follow older routes, calculations here have been made by mapping recommended walking routes.[6] These measurements provide a guide to the likely distances that would have been covered. However, these calculations are made with the caveat that tracing the exact journeys undertaken is not possible as such details are absent within the miracle accounts. For example, when travelling to a shrine a pilgrim might have diverged from their route for sustenance or shelter, taken a wrong

---

[2]   Ward, *Miracles and the Medieval Mind*, p. 67.

[3]   Yarrow, *Saints and Their Communities*, p. 154.

[4]   E. M. Rose, *The Murder of William of Norwich: The Origins of the Blood Libel in Medieval Europe* (Oxford, 2015), p. 120.

[5]   Finucane, *Miracles and Pilgrims*, p. 161.

[6]   This was achieved by using Google Maps, <https://www.google.co.uk/maps/> [accessed 15 July 2020].

turning, or found their route diverted for reasons beyond their control. What is presented here, therefore, is a considered estimate based upon the available information provided by the hagiographers.

Within this overarching caveat four further points are worth noting. First, that it is rare for accounts of international cure-seekers to provide more information than their country of origin. The exception to this within our case studies is *M. Æbbe* for which all but one of the Scottish cure-seekers are provided with specific origin-sites. With Coldingham situated in the Scottish Borders, this level of insight is perhaps unsurprising, but for most international, continental, cure-seeking pilgrims it must be accepted that calculating specific distances is not possible.

The second point to consider is the role of secondary locations. Æbbe's cult, as noted, involved two locations that were roughly two miles apart: the oratory at Kirk Hill, and the church of Coldingham Priory. As the final chapter reveals, the majority of *M. Æbbe*'s cure-seekers found their cure at the oratory and then returned to the priory. From the perspective of calculating travel, the short distance between the two locations does not adversely affect the analysis, but it is a point worth acknowledging. More notable are instances in which an entirely separate shrine location, at another institution, is referred to. *M. Swithuni* records four healing miracles that occurred at Swithun's statue in Sherborne Abbey's church.[7] *M. Dunstani* includes one reference to a cure credited to a chasuble belonging to Dunstan held by Westminster Abbey.[8] *M. Jacobi* refers to miracles at a cross erected in Bucklebury (twelve miles west of Reading).[9] Sherborne and Westminster evidently had connections to Swithun and Dunstan, and must be treated as locations in themselves. The Bucklebury Cross, likewise, was established in St James's honour following a mass held by Abbot Roger of Reading which resulted in the communal cure of a plague outbreak.[10] The wooden cross, along with Swithun's statue and Dunstan's chasuble, thus acted like a secondary relic at a secondary cult centre.[11] In these six accounts, distance has been measured from the origin-site to this secondary location.

The third point to acknowledge is that, in the majority of instances, the cure-seekers made their journey to the cult centre prior to their cure, but others made the journey post-cure in order to honour the saints and complete their

---

[7]   *M. Swithuni* 44–6, 53, ed. Lapidge, pp. 680–3, 686–9.

[8]   Eadmer of Canterbury, *M. Dunstani* 26, ed. Turner and Muir, pp. 204–7.

[9]   *M. Jacobi*, fol. 173va; Kemp, '*The Hand of St James*' XVI, 12–13.

[10]   *M. Jacobi*, fols. 173rb–173va; Kemp, '*The Hand of St James*' XIV, 11–12.

[11]   *M. Jacobi*, fol. 173va; Kemp, '*The Hand of St James*' XV, 12.

cure-seeking process. Both are considered here, as both made the journey; so too are those for whom there is no evidence of a journey to the shrine being made. The latter were likely to have travelled to the shrines after their cure to fulfil a vow even if this was not recorded in the miracle: after all, their miraculous cure had been reported to the cult centre. In comparison to Finucane's *Miracles and Pilgrims*, which looked outward from the shrine, the focus here is reversed and more practically minded and looks towards the shrine: how far from the saints' cults did these cure-seekers reside? Localised interest, as previous scholarship has shown, is predominant, but what of those who came from further afield, what types of distances did they cover, and do all seven *miracula* reveal similar patterns in this respect? It must be remembered that most cure-seekers were impaired in some manner and it must be questioned as to whether this also impacted on their choice of saintly physician.

The final point that requires consideration is the way that miracles record distances for English cure-seekers. Thomas of Monmouth was very meticulous in recording origin-sites, but other hagiographers provide less definitive descriptions for the distance traversed. In *M. Jacobi*, hound-keeper Gilbert was noted as being from 'aquilonalibus Anglie' ('northern England').[12] Two women in *M. Swithuni* were reported as being from 'occidentali regione' ('the west region') of England.[13] One woman in *M. Moduenne* was recorded as having come from 'longinquo' ('far away').[14] Accounts such as these, along with those that provide no mention of origin-site, have been categorised here as 'distance unknown'.

But what about those with slightly more detail? Where a specific county was recorded, but not a specific origin-site, a midpoint within the county is used to measure the distance covered. This provides the fairest estimate of the distance. Where places are named but not easily identifiable, care has been taken. A woman from Collingbourne was cured by St James of a long-standing complaint, but it is unclear whether she came from the village of Collingbourne Ducis or Collingbourne Kingston.[15] That the two Collingbournes are less than two miles from each other means that the distance between them and Reading is similar, at roughly thirty-seven miles for each.

Other place names are more ambiguous owing to the commonness of the name. A mute adolescent, with his parents, made a journey to Ely from

[12] *M. Jacobi*, fol. 173vb; Kemp, 'The Hand of St James' XVIII, 13.
[13] *M. Swithuni* 22, ed. Lapidge, pp. 664–5.
[14] Geoffrey of Burton, *M. Moduenne* 50, ed. Bartlett, pp. 212–13.
[15] *M. Jacobi*, fol. 173ra; Kemp, 'The Hand of St James' XI, 10–11.

Bradeford.[16] Bradeford is likely now known as Bradford – coming etymologically from 'broad ford' – and there are now nine locations in England of this name, spelled this way in medieval records.[17] With such a commonplace name it is not possible to say which was meant. In Blake's edition of *L. Eliensis*, the suggestion is even made that 'Bradeford' might be Bradford Farm, Stuntney, a location less than two miles from Ely.[18] Considering the localised nature of these seven cults, which this chapter reveals, it seems likely that the account refers to this latter location. Nevertheless, as there is no additional information to identify this Bradeford, it is not possible to provide a measurement for this account.

Local and Mid-Distance Travel

Where distances can be calculated, the greatest concentration of cure-seekers was within the immediate vicinity of the cult centre (Table 4.1). Origin-sites within a twenty-mile radius of the cult centres represent just under two-fifths of the cure-seekers recorded within these accounts. A local man was made mad while attending funeral games in Winchester, causing him to blaspheme and be tormented for the next three days.[19] Lambert, a *homunculus* (man of restricted stature), and a servant of Lanfranc, was cured of his decreasing eyesight by Dunstan.[20] A parishioner from Ely was punctured in the ribs by a wooden stake after falling into a hedge and, after a year of increasing poor health (and with no resolution from physicians), he was cured by Æthelthryth.[21] A woman who had been blind for seven years 'de uicino uenit' ('came from the neighbourhood') to Æbbe's oratory where she was cured after the abbess appeared to her and touched her on the forehead and eyes.[22] In *c.* 1155, a woman from Earley made the journey of three miles to Reading Abbey after she became 'morbo tumescan[s] ydropico' ('swollen with the disease of dropsy') and was cured in the abbey church's presbytery.[23]

---

[16]   *L. Eliensis* I.45, ed. Blake, p. 58, trans. Fairweather, p. 79.

[17]   *The Cambridge Dictionary of English Place-Names: Based on the Collections of the English Place-Name Society*, ed. V. Watts (Cambridge, 2004), p. 77.

[18]   *L. Eliensis* I.45, ed. Blake, p. 58 n. 3; P. H. Reaney, *The Place-Names of Cambridgeshire and the Isle of Ely*, English Place-Name Society 19 (Cambridge, 1943), p. 221. There are no other Bradfords close to Ely, but they can be found in Devon, Dorset, Lancashire, Northumberland, Somerset, Wiltshire and Yorkshire (West Riding).

[19]   *M. Swithuni* 41, ed. Lapidge, pp. 676–7.

[20]   Eadmer of Canterbury, *M. Dunstani* 25, ed. Turner and Muir, pp. 204–5.

[21]   *L. Eliensis* III.58, ed. Blake, p. 305, trans. Fairweather, p. 373. Also see above, p. 27.

[22]   *M. Æbbe* IV.28, ed. Bartlett, pp. 58–9.

[23]   *M. Jacobi*, fol. 171vb; Kemp, 'The Hand of St James' II, 7.

Table 4.1. Distances from origin-sites to the cult centres of the cure-seekers

	M. Swithuni	M. Dunstani	L. Eliensis	M. Moduenne	M. Willelmi	M. Æbbe	M. Jacobi	**Total**
English cure-seekers								
Local								
5 miles or under	5	6	9	7	33	8	6	74
6–20 miles	4	4	3	1	14	0	2	28
Mid-distance								
21–50 miles	8	0	1	0	23	1	7	40
Long distance								
51–100 miles	4	0	3	0	2	1	3	13
101 miles or over	2	0	1	0	4	4	3	14
Foreign cure-seekers								
Mid-distance								
Scotland	0	0	0	0	0	5	0	5
Long distance								
France	2	0	0	1	0	0	0	3
Germany	0	1	0	0	0	0	0	1
Normandy	1	0	0	0	0	0	0	1
Scotland	0	0	0	0	0	3	0	3
Wales	0	0	0	0	0	1	0	1
Distance unknown	24	10	9	4	7	19	3	76

As distance between origin-site and the cult centre increases, there is a decline in the number of cure-seekers recorded. Nevertheless, despite lower numbers, individuals at a mid-distance from the saints' shrines do feature in the majority of the miracle stories and are especially notable in William's hagiography. *M. Willelmi* is, in fact, a fascinating case study; Thomas of Monmouth was diligent in the recording of origin-sites for many of the accounts compiled in William's *miracula* with forty-three different place names provided.[24] The

---

[24] Appendix 3, pp. 219–21.

majority of these named origin-sites are within mid-distance, or a fifty-mile radius, of Norwich. Six accounts record identifiable locations further afield, with three places being named but ambiguous. Importantly, most cure-seekers who lived within five miles of Norwich Cathedral came from the city itself, with three other origin-sites named within *M. Willelmi* (each referred to once). Among these residents was the son of Gurwan, a Norwich tanner, who was cured after a message was relayed from St William via a woman from London.[25] The woman, roughly 110 miles away in the capital, received three visions before coming to Norwich to pass her message on to Gurwan. In reporting the miracle, *M. Willelmi* records that she knew nothing of Norwich prior to this and presumably this also meant she knew little of William either. This would explain why three visions were needed before she was willing to act, especially considering that relaying this message entailed travelling some distance. Regardless of the peculiar manner in which this message was delivered to Gurwan, this account highlights how awareness of the boy-martyr was relatively localised, at least in the early days of his cult.

Those external to Norwich, as Yarrow observed, predominantly came from a cluster of villages that surrounded the city.[26] *M. Willelmi*'s patterns, while amplified in the meticulous recording of place names, reflect trends seen in all seven sources. A similar clustering occurs in *M. Swithuni* with six cure-seekers coming from the Isle of Wight, only one of whom made the journey to Winchester following their cure.[27] The Isle of Wight was under English jurisdiction, and not a great distance from Winchester. The difference here, compared to the clusters of cure-seekers near Norwich, was the necessity for islanders to cross open water, putting the Isle of Wight cure-seekers into a unique category of mid-distance travellers.

That saints should prove to have had such a localised cure-seeking focus is in keeping with the saints' identities as patrons and protectors, and even friends, to their communities, both monastic and lay.[28] This was not unique to English cults, and can be seen in contemporary pilgrimage practices in, for example, southern Italy as well.[29] In addition to individual locals finding their cure, the miracles also record occasions when the saints protected and cured their communities from dangers faced by the community as a whole.

---

[25] Thomas of Monmouth, *M. Willelmi* IV.2, ed. Jessop and James, pp. 167–8.

[26] Yarrow, *Saints and Their Communities*, pp. 152, 168.

[27] *M. Swithuni* 6, 36, 54, 55, ed. Lapidge, pp. 652–5, 672–5, 688–95.

[28] Bartlett, *Why Can the Dead Do Such Great Things?*, pp. 221–2.

[29] P. Oldfield, *Sanctity and Pilgrimage in Southern Italy, 1000–1200* (Cambridge, 2014), pp. 226, 239–40.

Abbot Roger's aforementioned mass (and use of the water of St James) at Bucklebury is a good example of this.[30] Additionally, when a plague struck Reading resulting in the death of members of the lay community and thirteen of the abbey's brethren, the monks processed James's hand around the town.[31] During the procession, *M. Jacobi* records, 'in plateis autem ponebantur infirmi in domorum autem limitibus emortui' ('the sick were laid out in the streets, the dead being kept indoors') in order that they might see, and be cured by, the reliquary during the procession.[32]

It was within the local area that one was likely to find the greatest awareness of the saint and of the miracles it was reported that the saint had performed. The further away from the cult centre, the less frequent the chance of a cure-seeker. However, among the case studies, only *M. Dunstani* and *M. Moduenne* are without English cure-seekers whose origin-site was over twenty-one miles from the cult centre. The remaining *miracula* all included individuals from further afield. News would spread quickly through the community, especially in urban locations. Such reports would permeate outward from the shrine through families and neighbours, and pilgrims and other travellers who might have witnessed the miraculous cure, seen evidence of the saint's power at the shrine (for example, abandoned crutches hanging on the walls), or heard tell of it.[33]

That pilgrims, including cure-seekers, heard oral testimony of saintly merits and facilitated their transmission is evidenced in Eadmer of Canterbury's *Miracula S. Oswaldi*.[34] Written shortly after *M. Dunstani*, and at the request of Worcester Priory, this is a short collection of accounts that complements Eadmer's *vita* of Oswald. Oswald interceded on behalf of a penitent 'Saxiconis' ('Saxon'), freeing and healing him from the iron bonds that had damaged his skin.[35] Following the miracle, Eadmer notes that the man returned to his own lands 'praedicaturus suis et aliis quam misericordi oculo Deus illum respexerit' ('intending to preach to his own people and others, telling with what merciful gaze God had looked upon him').[36] As evidence of the penitent fulfilling his preaching promise, the following account records that a second penitent

---

[30] *M. Jacobi*, fols. 173rb–173va; Kemp, 'The Hand of St James' XIV, 11–12.

[31] *M. Jacobi*, fol. 172ra; Kemp, 'The Hand of St James' IV, 7–8.

[32] Ibid.

[33] Finucane, *Miracles and Pilgrims*, p. 156.

[34] Eadmer of Canterbury, *Miracula S. Oswaldi*, in Eadmer of Canterbury, *Lives and Miracles of Saints Oda, Dunstan and Oswald*, ed. and trans. A. Turner and B. Muir, OMT (Oxford, 2006), pp. 290–323.

[35] Ibid., 2, pp. 294–5.

[36] Ibid., 2, pp. 296–7.

arrived in Worcester within a few days. His decision to seek out Oswald's aid, Eadmer tells us, was due to the 'diuulgata fama' ('dissemination of the news') of the previous miracle which had come to his notice.[37] On securing his release from his own iron bonds, this second man left Worcester and, presumably, took the story of his miraculous liberation (and that of the Saxon) with him.

In addition to the dissemination of miracle reports by those who had experienced, or witnessed, these occurrences at the shrine it is worth considering the discussion provided by Finucane regarding the establishment of Thomas Cantilupe's cult and the dissemination of his miracles at the close of the thirteenth century.[38] Nearby Herefordshire villages, Finucane highlighted, were drawn into a local 'pilgrimage network'.[39] In addition to the oral testimony of those who were cured, weekly markets brought villagers into Hereford making them potential messengers of local news.[40] Many nearby villages would have also been predisposed towards their local cult centre (and thus cult), owing to episcopal, abbatial or monastic manor ownership, and the duties of the almoner in the outlying communities.[41] Potential cure-seekers might be further persuaded of the merits of a local saint by family, friends and neighbours who encouraged visiting or praying to the saint. Such encouragements are also recorded in our seven *miracula*. A paralysed youth living on the estate of the sheriff of Hampshire was advised by friends to seek Swithun's aid; and Adam, son of John, the bishop's chamberlain, was inspired by his friends to seek William's assistance with his long-standing fever.[42] Importantly, in the case of Hereford, Finucane noted that on the occurrence of a miracle the cathedral bells would be rung, the miracle announced in the nave and the *Te Deum* sung by the clergy and assembled laity.[43] The ringing of church bells is particularly noteworthy for being an indicator of the miraculous that would have immediately drawn attention from those outside the cult centre, and might even be

---

[37] Ibid., 2, pp. 298–9.

[38] R. C. Finucane, 'Pilgrimage in Daily Life: Aspects of Medieval Communication Reflected in the Newly-Established Cult of Thomas de Cantilupe (d. 1282), Its Dissemination and Effects upon Outlying Herefordshire Villagers', in *Walfahrt und Alltag in Mittelalter und früher Neuzeit. Internationales Round-Table-Gespräch, Krems an der Donau, 8. Oktober 1990*, ed. G. Jaritz and B. Schuh (Vienna, 1992), pp. 165–218.

[39] Finucane, 'Pilgrimage in Daily Life', p. 170.

[40] Ibid., p. 176.

[41] Ibid., pp. 171–6.

[42] *M. Swithuni* 56, ed. Lapidge, pp. 694–7; *M. Willelmi* V.4, ed. Jessop and James, p. 191.

[43] Finucane, 'Pilgrimage in Daily Life', pp. 168–70.

heard by those in surrounding areas. Such methods of dissemination would have spread outwards from the cult centre, through local communities and, in the case of the Saxon man at Worcester, beyond that too.

The spread of miracle stories would have been important in terms of attracting cure-seekers who might otherwise be persuaded to visit competitors. East Anglia provides a key example of the level of regional competition between shrines. Ely, despite being an established centre with a well-renowned saint in Æthelthryth, has a scarcity of mid-distance travellers. This could reflect the competition from neighbouring saints, Edmund at Bury to the south-east, and Ivo at Ramsey twenty miles to the west, who would have been potential contenders for cure-seekers' attention.[44] From the mid-twelfth century the rapid development of William's cult at Norwich would have introduced another potential local rival. Ramsey Abbey, importantly, was situated between Ely and Ermine Street (also known as the Great North Road). This ancient road, to be discussed in the following chapter, was still used by those travelling between London and northern England.[45] Such a route might well have been used by one blind woman who travelled from London to Coldingham.[46] Despite this close competition, which might have impacted on mid-distance pilgrims, Ely did attract cure-seekers from outside East Anglia, with *L. Eliensis* recording a handful of longer-distance cure-seekers.

In the later twelfth century there was one national competitor against whom all cult centres had to contend: Thomas Becket. This sense of competition did not escape the hagiographies, although references are often subtle, focusing on the success of the title saint rather than the failure of Becket (or other holy figures). Indeed, sometimes the saints guided cure-seekers to their colleagues. Gaufrid of Canterbury first sought Becket's aid for his toothache only for St Thomas to tell him to go to William's shrine, which he did after his cure.[47] No doubt was cast over Becket's abilities, rather it was the martyred archbishop himself who directed Gaufrid to Norwich. In a strange development, Gaufrid was then joined for part of his 138-mile journey by both Becket and St Edmund, reaching Norwich the day after he set off.[48] The implication here is that the competition between the saints was merely friendly rivalry. Conversely, St James appeared to one cure-seeker, Ysembela, at Canterbury

44 Webb, *Pilgrimage in Medieval England*, pp. 25, 42.
45 See below, pp. 148–9.
46 *M. Æbbe* IV.2, ed. Bartlett, pp. 32–5.
47 Thomas of Monmouth, *M. Willelmi* VII.19, ed. Jessop and James, pp. 289–94. Also see above, pp. 72–3.
48 Ibid., VII.19, pp. 292–3.

instructing her to come to his shrine at Reading, arguing that she would find no cure for her paralysis from Becket at Christ Church.[49] As a side note, it is worth highlighting that despite their abbey being a royal foundation, Reading's monks had a complex relationship with Becket (who had dedicated the abbey church in 1167) and they came to own a number of his relics.[50]

Crossing the Country and Beyond

While local support was an important feature among cult devotees, the miracles often highlight that their saints also appealed to cure-seeking pilgrims from further afield. Here those who travelled unknown distances must also be brought into the discussion. Only *M. Swithuni* and *M. Æbbe* record less than a fifth of their cure-seeking pilgrims as local. However, both contain high numbers of individuals for whom no distance can be calculated, and it is likely that many of these cure-seekers travelled less than twenty miles. That so many accounts do not refer to the origin-site of the cure-seeker is striking and could be the result of two possible explanations. First, that cult centres were less concerned with recording information regarding journeys than might be expected. The miracle was of the greatest importance. Alternatively, it could be suggested that many of those for whom no journey is mentioned were unlikely to have travelled far. It would surely be important, to both the cure-seeker and the recorder of a miracle, to provide details of longer and more challenging journeys, as this would illustrate the influence of the saint. When no details were recorded, could it be that the journeys were not considered noteworthy? There is merit in this second suggestion, and if this is accepted then what emerges is that most cure-seekers made journeys to shrines within no more than a few days' travel of their homes.

While a decrease in the number of cure-seekers as distance from the shrine increased is not unexpected, only *M. Dunstani* and *M. Moduenne* contain no definitive references to longer-distance English cure-seekers. Yet, Dunstan does cure a German pilgrim, Clement, of the wounds caused by his penitential irons, and Modwenna does the same for a French penitent.[51] Even if fewer in number, the posthumous hagiographies do include cure-seekers who lived more than twenty miles from the shrine (including fourteen who originated

[49] *M. Jacobi*, fol. 174rb–174va; Kemp, 'The Hand of St James' XX, 14–16.
[50] For further discussion see: R. Koopmans, 'Thomas Becket and the Royal Abbey of Reading', *English Historical Review* 131 (2016), 1–30; R. Baxter, *The Royal Abbey of Reading*, Boydell Studies in Medieval Art and Architecture (Woodbridge, 2016), pp. 61–2.
[51] Eadmer of Canterbury, *M. Dunstani* 8, ed. Turner and Muir, pp. 166–7; Geoffrey of Burton, *M. Moduenne* 51, ed. Bartlett, pp. 216–19.

from over 100 miles away in these case studies), and this is significant. That cure-seekers might undertake longer journeys highlights the importance of other travel and cure-seeking factors in the choice of saint. Following instructions or advice (divine or temporal) to seek out a specific saint or 'calling in' to a shrine while travelling through the area, are both features found in accounts of these longer journeys. In both instances, although for differing reasons, the distance of the shrine from home becomes a less significant factor in the cure-seekers' decision to find a cure.

In one noteworthy account, a cleric 'debilem corpore et multimoda infirmitate oppressum' ('infirm in the body and worn down by many sorts of illness') was recorded as having first visited Bury before securing Modwenna's assistance at Burton following a vision in which he was advised to do so.[52] The distance between the two sites is 122 miles, but *M. Moduenne* does not specify whether Bury was not also the cleric's origin-site. This would fit the patterns for cure-seeking practices – that the first choice of saint was most likely local – but it is possible that a lengthy journey had already been undertaken by the cleric in order to reach Bury. However, *M. Moduenne* was focused on Modwenna's ability to cure what Edmund would not. This is another indication of inter-cult rivalry but it also suggests that some cure-seekers were willing to undertake long-distance journeys to find a cure.

Two further noteworthy longer-distance cure-seekers are recorded within *M. Jacobi* and involve named girls from Sussex and Essex who appear to have both travelled to Reading alone.[53] Alice the daughter of a clerk from Essex, and Ysembela the daughter of John the fisherman from 'Estonie' near 'Seford', were both affected by paralysis following time spent out of doors.[54] Alice was attacked by a demonic figure on returning from the sheepfold; this resulted in a short-term madness and the fusion of her left arm to her chest.[55] Ysembela became paralysed down the left side of her body after sleeping outside in the summer.[56] In both cases the girls looked for remedy elsewhere before being directed to Reading following visions of St James. Alice's account provides

[52] Geoffrey of Burton, *M. Moduenne* 50, ed. Bartlett, pp. 212–15.

[53] *M. Jacobi*, fols. 172rb–172vb, 174rb–174va; Kemp, 'The Hand of St James' VIII, XX, 9–10, 14–16.

[54] 'Seford' is possibly Seaford, East Sussex. 'Estonie' might be Easton, however there is no evidence of an Easton in Sussex today. There are Eastons in Dorset, Hampshire, Huntingdonshire, Lincolnshire, Norfolk, Northamptonshire, Somerset, Suffolk, Wiltshire and Yorkshire (East Riding), but none of these would seem likely locations as Ysembela's 'Estonie'.

[55] *M. Jacobi*, fol. 172rb–172vb; Kemp, 'The Hand of St James' VIII, 9.

[56] *M. Jacobi*, fol. 174rb; Kemp, 'The Hand of St James' XX, 14.

no details of the places she first visited, merely that she 'a finibus suis egressa circuiuit terram et perambulauit eam per sanctorum loca querens remedium et salutis solatium' ('left home and went round the land seeking from the shrines of saints a cure and aid to health').[57] Having been unsuccessful, Alice 'pertesa miserie et plena amaritudine repatriauit et in acta desperauit' ('returned home worn out with grief and full of bitterness and gave up in despair').[58] Once home, a certain woman, to whom James had appeared with a message for Alice, informed the girl that she should travel to Reading.[59] Alice then journeyed to Reading Abbey where she found her cure.

St James, however, had to appear multiple times directly to Ysembela instructing her to go to Reading. Ysembela was reluctant to make the journey, preferring instead to remain at Becket's tomb, despite the apostle's warning that she would find no cure there.[60] Importantly, and unusually for miracle stories, Ysembela's reasons for staying in Canterbury were recorded within *M. Jacobi*, allowing for valuable insight into the concerns that might govern the cults and cult centres chosen by cure-seekers:

Vidit itaque Sanctum Iacobum in uisu ad se uenientem [. . .] Qui dixit ei quid his moraris quid hic queries. Cui illa Salutem meam quero et Sanctum Thomam expecto. Apostolus respondit. Nequaquam hic salute accipies sed uade Rading ad monasterium meum et ibi conualesces. At illa Rading non uidi et monasterium tuum nescio. Et quomodo possum illuc ire cum sim debilitate et infirma uie nescia et egeria. Certe non ibo nec me ineassum ultra fatigabo. Iterum et iterum institit apostolus admonando ut Rading ire profecto asserens quod ibi et non alibi conualesceret. At illa admonenti contraria promitterra incredula uisa sibi cum apostolo litigare et sese Rading non ituram affirmare.

(And in a dream she saw coming towards her St James [. . .] He said to her, 'What are you waiting here for? What do you seek?' 'I am in search of a cure', she replied, 'and I am waiting for St Thomas.' The apostle answered, 'You will certainly not receive a cure here, but go to Reading, to my monastery, and there you will be healed.' 'But' she said, 'I have not seen Reading, nor do I know your monastery. And how can I go there when I am crippled and weak, ignorant of the way and penniless? No, I shall not go nor will I tire myself out any more to no purpose.' The apostle insisted again and again,

---

[57]   *M. Jacobi*, fol. 172va; Kemp, '*The Hand of St James*' VIII, 9.
[58]   Ibid.
[59]   Ibid.
[60]   *M. Jacobi*, fol. 174rb; Kemp, '*The Hand of St James*' XX, 15.

urging her to go to Reading and declaring that she would be healed there and nowhere else. But she rejected his advice and refused to believe his promises, seeing fit to argue with the apostle and to maintain that she would not go to Reading.)[61]

Ysembela appeared not to have recognised St James or trusted the advice given. Furthermore, she had concerns over the fact that Reading was unknown to her, meaning that not only did she not know the way, but that she had not heard of the monastery or of James's miracle working at Reading. Ysembela was also reluctant to travel due to her paralysis and lack of money when she was unconvinced of the benefits of this undertaking. Caution over the unknown destination was a key factor in Ysembela's unwillingness, but importantly, so was her wariness over the journey itself. Her paralysis would mean any journey would take some time to complete and her lack of funds placed her in a vulnerable position. Moreover, it must be remembered that Ysembela, like Alice, was recorded as having been a child, and age may also have been a factor in this. An adult might be more willing to make such a journey, but Ysembela was young, naive about locations further away and, understandably, more concerned with her welfare than with respecting the apostle.

Ysembela's account provides a rare glimpse into concerns that could have affected travel. Nowhere else in these seven *miracula* was this sentiment disclosed, yet these trepidations surely played upon the minds of many if not all cure-seekers, no matter which saint they sought or how long they spent on this undertaking. Such apprehensions are worth bearing in mind when considering the journeys undertaken by cure-seekers and pilgrims as they reveal important, practical, reasons why localised journeys were favoured.

Concern over travelling while impaired might also explain why some cure-seekers undertook the process of making a vow and only completed their promise to visit the shrine after receiving their requested remedy. Such was the case for Robert de Alta-Ripa, a knight from Arundel.[62] Robert made the journey to Ely, covering 125 miles, after being cured of a serious illness. This illness 'in fastidium et contemptum verteretur' ('turned [him] into an object of disgust and contempt') and left him looking like a corpse.[63] In a vision Æthelthryth told him to mend his ways and come to Ely with a candle. He was then to continue to Santiago de Compostela. On Æthelthryth's departure he found himself cured and made his way to Ely where, *L. Eliensis* notes,

[61] Ibid.
[62] *L. Eliensis* III.42, ed. Blake, pp. 280–1, trans. Fairweather, pp. 340–2.
[63] *L. Eliensis* III.42, ed. Blake, p. 280, trans. Fairweather, p. 341.

'fraternitatem accepit' ('[he] received the brotherhood'); no further mention was made of travel to Spain.[64]

As noted in Ysembela's account, some cure-seekers had no knowledge of saints and shrines in other regions of the country. It was only through James's continued insistence that Ysembela eventually made the journey which led to her cure. Conversely, others who traversed great distances had been wandering from shrine to shrine for some time, or found themselves in the region for other purposes, such as a needle-seller in *M. Æbbe* who came from Barry, Angus.[65] The statistics reveal that there was a general trend of cure-seeker numbers declining as distance increased. These general trends ring true for all seven hagiographies with the notable exception of *M. Æbbe*. Long-distance travel, meanwhile, was represented by fourteen per cent of the accounts. *M. Æbbe* also offers the only examples of travel from elsewhere in the British Isles, with eight Scottish cure-seekers, and one Welsh. Further discussion of the Scottish cure-seekers, below, sheds invaluable light on the borderland nature of Æbbe's cult and explains why foreign cure-seekers are so notable in this hagiography. Every other foreign cure-seeker recorded in these *miracula* came from continental Europe. These continental travellers predominantly came from Normandy and France, the exception being Clement in *M. Dunstani*.[66] Not every *miracula* recorded foreign visitors, and no clear pattern emerges from the statistics for this group. For example, Canterbury and Winchester were both southern cult centres near major ports but *M. Dunstani* only records one foreign visitor and makes, surprisingly, no mention of Norman or French cure-seekers.

M. Moduenne, despite its compact size, includes one account of a French penitent pilgrim; this is the final miracle in the hagiography and was added to Geoffrey's collection by Prior Jordan shortly after the abbot's passing.[67] The Frenchman arrived late one night having been wandering from place to place. He had been bound with irons and the one which remained had cut off the blood flow to his arm and had worn through his skin. Jordan recorded: 'Ego [...] ad eiusdem monasterii ualuas ueniens, inueni quendam pre foribus excubantem habitu peregrinum et pauperem, loquela et cultu alienigenam' ('I [...] came to the gates of the monastery and found a man lying on the ground outside. He was dressed like a poor pilgrim and his speech and appearance

[64] Ibid.
[65] *M. Æbbe* IV.36, ed. Bartlett, pp. 62–5.
[66] Eadmer of Canterbury, *M. Dunstani* 8, ed. Turner and Muir, pp. 166–7.
[67] Geoffrey of Burton, *M. Moduenne* 51, ed. Bartlett, pp. 216–19.

showed him to be a foreigner').[68] What specifically about his appearance showed him to be an 'alienigenam' was not documented, yet his clothing might have included those items already associated with pilgrimage: the scrip, staff and sclavein. The detailed description of this man's appearance is reflective of its being Jordan's first-hand testimony. This also suggests that such an arrival was an unusual occurrence for Burton, meaning that these details stood out to Jordan. The lengthy account of the miracle appears to confirm that Modwenna's cult was rarely frequented by those from further afield, either within England or from elsewhere in Europe.

While unsurprising that Modwenna's cult appealed primarily to a regional audience it is surprising that, despite the international status of James, *M. Jacobi* makes no reference to any cure-seekers from overseas. However, it must be remembered that despite James's apostolic identity, his cult at Reading never took off, although James's scallop shells became a frequent symbol for the abbey from the thirteenth century onwards.[69] The only accounts to refer to France are the fatal punishment of Matthew of Boulogne, and the passing mention of Henry II crossing the Channel in an account involving the healing of a canon from Merton Priory.[70] The canon, Roger Hosatus, was cured when two of the Reading monks visited Merton whilst returning the hand to Reading. Two further accounts refer to overseas journeys: Prince John's trip to Ireland (when a member of the prince's retinue broke his arm); and Peter de Leuns's previous, and unrelated, pilgrimage to Santiago de Compostela with his father.[71]

The most important feature of Roger Hosatus's cure was that James's hand was in transit. Reading's main relic, unlike those of the other case-study saints, was a small, entirely transportable, object. Of course, even when monastic institutions housed the tomb of the saint it did not mean that they were without smaller reliquaries. At Worcester a portable shrine for Oswald was carried around the city in times of communal crises.[72] As mentioned, James's reliquary was carried through Reading during a severe plague, with Abbot Roger also taking the reliquary to Bucklebury for the same purpose.[73] It was due to this portability that Reading was concerned over the hand's safety and kept

---

[68] Ibid.

[69] Koopmans, 'Thomas Becket and the Royal Abbey of Reading', 26–7.

[70] *M. Jacobi*, fol. 175ra–b; Kemp, '*The Hand of St James*' XXV–XXVI, 17–18.

[71] *M. Jacobi*, fols. 174vb–175ra, 175ra–175vb; Kemp, '*The Hand of St James*' XXII, XX-VII, 16, 18–19.

[72] Eadmer of Canterbury, *Miracula S. Oswaldi* 8–10, ed. Turner and Muir, pp. 314–21.

[73] *M. Jacobi*, fols. 172ra, 173rb–173va; Kemp, '*The Hand of St James*' IV, XIV, 7–8, 11–12.

it out of reach of the public visiting the shrine. Evidence of this can be noted in both a reference to devotional focus being on the painted image of James at the altar, and in the cure of the woman from Collingbourne who was permitted to view the reliquary because she arrived concurrently with William, the second earl of Gloucester (cousin to Henry II), who had permission to see the relic.[74] That the relic appears to have been difficult to access, and often on loan to the king, highlights the important perceived connection between the saint and their cult centre. Indeed, Frederick Barbarossa's request to Henry II for the relic to be returned could imply that the hand was still seen to be the king's possession, which could explain the limited access given at Reading and its occasional departure.[75] It was enough for cure-seekers to know that the hand was in the guardianship of the abbey. Those who visited were still connecting with the saint, even if the object was not visible. While no continental cure-seekers visited Reading, there were a range of cure-seeking pilgrims who came from the local area and further afield within England.

The representation of local cure-seekers within miracle accounts assists in presenting the saints, first and foremost, as being concerned with the welfare of their own people; this aided in rooting the saints, via their relics and shrines, to their cult centres and local communities. The hagiographers, seemingly, did not seek to present the cults as national, or international. What was of greater importance was to highlight the power of the saints *in situ*; through the miracles bestowed upon those who came to their shrines and through their care more broadly of those under their protection.

The pattern of cure-seeking was that often sufferers would first seek the assistance of their local saint; only if no cure was forthcoming might cure-seekers have ventured further afield. There was a level of interdependence between cult and local community and, while the few cure-seekers from some distance might aid in spreading the word of the saint's abilities, on a daily basis focus was on the saint's 'own' people. If a cure could be found in a nearby location, what reason would there be for any sufferer to seek a remedy further away? Only direct intervention through visions or counsel, or presence in a locality for other purposes, would appear to override this.

Æbbe's Scottish Cure-Seekers

Considering 'localness' in relation to the northernmost of our seven cult centres is particularly revealing. Coldingham's location in the Scottish Borders provides one notable difference from the other cults as foreign cure-seekers

---

[74] *M. Jacobi*, fol. 173ra; Kemp, '*The Hand of St James*' XI, 10–11.
[75] Leyser, 'Frederick Barbarossa, Henry II and the Hand of St James', 25–6.

are a more notable presence here owing to there being several Scottish cure-seekers recorded in *M. Æbbe*. Their presence in the miracles requires further exploration, however, as some of these Scots might have been considered as relatively local cure-seekers.

M. Æbbe's hagiographer was an English monk from Durham Cathedral Priory who was based at the dependent daughter-house. *M. Æbbe* was keen to promote the 'Englishness' of the saint and in so doing play down any Scottish claims to her cult and her identity.[76] The result of this, interestingly, is that among the eight cure-seekers from Scotland only one was referred to purely as 'Scoticus nacione' ('Scottish by nation'), a term that, as Bartlett highlighted, was used in reference to Gaelic-speaking individuals from north of the Forth.[77] *M. Æbbe* provides details of the origin-sites for the remaining seven, including the one other officially named as being a cure-seeker 'de Scocia' ('from Scotland'), a youth from Barry, Angus.[78] Of the remaining six, five lived within fifty miles of the priory, with origin-sites named as: the Edinburgh area; the province of East Lothian; Newbattle, Midlothian; Seton, East Lothian; and Mersington in Berwickshire.[79] The remaining cure-seeker travelled from Lanark, a distance of 100 miles from Coldingham (Table 4.2).[80]

Table 4.2. Distances from origin-site to the cult centre of Æbbe's Scottish cure-seekers

	M. Æbbe
Scottish cure-seekers	
Mid-distance	
21–50 miles	5
Long distance	
51–100 miles	1
101 miles or over	1
Distance unknown	1

[76] C. Whitehead, 'A Scottish or English Saint? The Shifting Sanctity of St Aebbe of Coldingham', in *New Medieval Literatures 19*, ed. P. Knox et al. (Cambridge, 2019), pp. 1–42 (5).

[77] *M. Æbbe* IV.39, ed. Bartlett, pp. 64–5.

[78] Ibid., IV.36, pp. 62–3.

[79] Ibid., IV.5, IV.6, IV.12, IV.34, IV.35, pp. 36–41, 50–1, 60–3.

[80] Ibid., IV.26, pp. 58–9.

That the majority of *M. Æbbe*'s Scottish cure-seekers came from south of the Forth, and indeed were closer to Coldingham than motherhouse Durham Cathedral Priory (eighty-eight miles south), alters how the cult is perceived. Within the wider Scottish Borders area Æbbe held appeal and was able to attract a number of cure-seekers, either through her own merits or through providing a suitable stopping place for those travelling further; the latter being the case for a paralysed man from 'Edenburgensium finibus' ('the Edinburgh area') who was returning from an unsuccessful pilgrimage to Canterbury.[81] Having stopped in Berwick, and having been advised to seek out Æbbe's shrine at Kirk Hill, he spent fifteen days in Coldingham before undertaking the journey to the oratory itself. The distance between Coldingham and Kirk Hill is two miles, but this journey, owing to his paralysis, took him the majority of the day, and resulted in the hagiographer commenting that he moved 'testudinis emulans tarditatem' ('like a slow tortoise').[82] As presented in *M. Æbbe*, Æbbe's cult therefore appears to have been relatively localised in nature, much like our other six cults. This also suggests that the Anglo-Scottish frontier (which fluctuated throughout the Middle Ages) meant less to those living in the Borders than might be expected of the more politically minded.

Who Travelled When?

Before or After

There were two typical processes for cure-seekers to follow in their search for miraculous healing. The first was to make the journey to the shrine ahead of their cure. The second was to complete the cure-seeking process by journeying to the shrine after the cure had been acquired through the making of a vow. The importance of these two processes, and particularly travel prior to the cure, was reflected within the miracle reports (Table 4.3). Almost three-quarters of the cure-seekers in the case-study hagiographies visited the saints' cult centres prior to their cure. This shows there was emphasis placed on the shrine as a space of divine intercession and highlights that this was the preferred process for cure-seeking pilgrimages. Those individuals who made the journey only after their cure include a number who were bedridden and were physically incapable of making the journey ahead of time. A man cured by Swithun had previously been paralysed and unable to leave his bed for many years.[83] Leofmær, a knight from Barningham, had been bedridden with an illness that

---

[81]   Ibid., IV.5, pp. 36–7. Also see above, pp. 84–5.
[82]   Ibid., pp. 38–9.
[83]   *M. Swithuni* 8, ed. Lapidge, pp. 654–5.

resulted in the loss of his sight, speech and hearing for fifteen days.[84] Edward Haver and his daughter were both cured of fever at home through the water of St James, and then made a journey of thanks to the abbey.[85]

Table 4.3. Point at which travel was undertaken by the cure-seeker or another on their behalf

	M. Swithuni	*M. Dunstani*	*L. Eliensis*	*M. Moduenne*	*M. Willelmi*	*M. Æbbe*	*M. Jacobi*	**Total**
Journey by the cure-seeker								
Journey made prior to cure	41	15	20	13	63	42	14	208
Journey made to fulfil a vow after the cure	5	1	5	0	9	0	7	27
No journey by cure-seeker								
On behalf of the cure-seeker before cure	0	0	0	0	5	0	1	6
On behalf of the cure-seeker after cure	0	0	0	0	2	0	0	2
No travel, or no evidence of travel	4	5	1	0	5	0	2	17

Two others notable for having travelled to the shrine after a resolution to their health concerns are the parturient women. Both Bothilda and Aquilina found their relief through thaumaturgic waters imbued with the saints' powers and, owing to the nature of their health concerns, had to delay their thanksgiving visit to the shrines.[86] Bothilda, wife of Girard (the monk's cook), had been in labour for fifteen days and found no medicines were able to comfort her or induce the baby.[87] Her remedy came when she took the fern leaf she had collected from William's tomb in the monk's cemetery and mixed this with holy water. Before drinking, she called out to William and, having drank her concoction, she immediately gave birth to a boy. Thomas of Monmouth notes

---

[84] *L. Eliensis* III.36, ed. Blake, pp. 274–6, trans. Fairweather, pp. 332–5. Also see above, p. 98.
[85] *M. Jacobi*, fol. 172ra–b; Kemp, '*The Hand of St James*' V–VI, 8. Also see below, p. 186.
[86] See above, pp. 68–9.
[87] Thomas of Monmouth, *M. Willelmi* II.6, ed. Jessop and James, pp. 78–9.

that, after some time, Bothilda gave thanks to God and William for her safe delivery. Presumably, this pause between the birth and her arrival at the shrine was owing to the period of purification required of all women post-labour (this was recognised as lasting for approximately a month).[88] Aquilina, the wife of Gilbert Basset, similarly undertook a delayed journey to the shrine after a four-day labour and an eventual stillbirth.[89] Various attempts had been made to alleviate Aquilina's suffering but neither the doctors and midwives, nor the precious stones sent by Henry II, were of any use. *M. Jacobi* notes that this was because the foetus had not moved into the correct position and 'ex transuerso uentris uersatus matris aluum sibi hereditauerat ibi sepulcrum' ('had turned across [Aquilina's] belly and made the mother's womb its own tomb').[90] On drinking the water of St James, sleep came over Aquilina and she gave birth with no pain. On waking, she had a tall candle made and sent to Reading Abbey. After the 'dies purificationis sue' ('days of her purification'), Aquilina travelled to the shrine herself.[91]

Delay in making a post-healing visit was less acceptable for others. Indeed, the saints keenly reminded those who hesitated in making good their vows either by appearing to them to hurry their journey or, more punitively, through returning the affliction until the vow was completed and the visit made. Several cure-seekers fell foul of the saints in this manner including a woman struck with a second illness by Swithun, and the youth who suffered a second broken arm when he failed to journey to James's shrine.[92] In both instances, the return of the affliction acted as the reminder needed, and on making the promised journey the saints relieved the recurrent complaint.

The process of making a vow and recovering prior to the journey to the saint's shrine, while less frequently recorded, was clearly a recognised and accepted cure-seeking process. Such a process could be just as effective. One other account in the miracles that falls within this category requires some thought. Twelve-year-old John, a monk at Ely, suffered from a bad ulcer that had caused 'per cuncta membra illius pruriginem scaturire faceret, officium ipsis auferret et motum' ('itching to spread generally though all his limbs and deprived him of the use of them and their movement').[93] He was so affected

[88] Leyser, *Medieval Women*, p. 130.

[89] *M. Jacobi*, fol. 174va; Kemp, '*The Hand of St James*' XXI, 16.

[90] Ibid.

[91] Ibid.

[92] *M. Swithuni* 10, ed. Lapidge, pp. 656–7; *M. Jacobi*, fols. 174vb–175ra; Kemp, '*The Hand of St James*' XXII, 16. Also see above, p. 105.

[93] *L. Eliensis* III.130, ed. Blake, p. 379, trans. Fairweather, p. 469.

that he could neither eat or drink by himself nor make the sign of the cross, and his fellow monks had given up hope in his recovery. While sleeping in the infirmary, John was visited by Æthelthryth who promised that he would recover, but not at Ely. Rather John was to go to Bury St Edmunds. Intrigued, the young monk followed Æthelthryth out of the infirmary and to her shrine where he began to keep vigil. When he bowed his head in prayer, 'omne virus, quo interius torquebatur, evomuit et, postea evigilans, sanus effectus' ('he vomited up all the poison by which he was being inwardly tormented and, after sleeping, found himself to be well again').[94] After being cured through Æthelthryth's intercession at Ely, he made his way to St Edmund's shrine in order to complete the process and secure his new-found good health. *L. Eliensis* makes it clear that it was Æthelthryth's intercession that resulted in John's cure, so why this process necessitated a journey to Bury and the shrine of St Edmund, some twenty-five miles away, is unclear. Nevertheless, John clearly recognised the importance of following the advice of Ely's saintly patron and fulfilled his vow to visit Bury.

Remote Cure-Seeking

It was rare that cure-seekers would not make the journey to the shrine themselves, whether that was before or after their cure. Nevertheless, the miracle accounts do include nine instances in which the journey was made on behalf of the cure-seeker. These journeys might have been seen as having a certain similarity to proxy pilgrimages, where the individual arranged for another to undertake the physical journey on their behalf. Such proxy pilgrimages were often made in wills, and involved international journeys to locations like Rome or Jerusalem, but cure-seeking pilgrimages remained closer to home and were more likely to be undertaken before the cure.[95] Often, as with cure-seekers who came to the shrine after their cure, these individuals were bedbound and could not have made the journey themselves. Among *M. Willelmi's* accounts of this nature are four cases in which the afflicted individual was a child. In these instances, it was the parents who undertook visiting the shrine on behalf of their unwell offspring. Radulfus's infant son was sick and close to death before his father offered a votive at the shrine.[96] Gurwan the tanner had already lost five sons before his sixth was cured of an eighteen-week illness after a candle

---

[94] Ibid.

[95] Finucane, *Miracles and Pilgrims*, p. 46.

[96] Thomas of Monmouth, *M. Willelmi* III.9, ed. Jessop and James, p. 134. Also see above, p. 114.

was presented at William's shrine on the boy's behalf.[97] William also received a candle from William Polcehart and his wife when doctors were unable to cure their son's illness, and at the moment of the candle's donation the boy recovered.[98] The daughter of Bartholomew de Creak was suffering from a burning fever when her mother made a candle 'propriis fieri manibus' ('with her own hands').[99] As soon as the candle was made, the girl's fever abated and the candle was then offered at William's tomb. All four children were severely ill and it is little wonder that they were unable to travel to the shrine themselves, or that their parents showed such concern over their health.

While some cure-seekers had the journey to the shrine undertaken on their behalf, the miracles also include a small number of cases that make no reference to any journey having been made to the cult centre at all. Considering the saints were not above backtracking on the provided cure when vows were not fulfilled, it must be asked why this small but notable group of individuals appear to have remained remote cure-seekers, and how the reports of their miraculous cure came to be known by the hagiographers. In some accounts, such as that of Ralph Gibuin, a knight cured by St James of a severe fever, the hagiographer frustratingly offers no details of how, or where, the cure came about.[100]

Other accounts reveal that news of holy healing reached the cult centres via post-cure testimony. Pilgrims might bring with them news of multiple miraculous cures. Following the cure of Walter, a priest at Tivetshall, and his family from a grave illness, Thomas of Monmouth was informed by Walter of their cure (although *M. Willelmi* provides no further details of the other family members).[101] In other instances news travelled through the network of monastic houses. Following Dunstan's orders, an infirm woman from London was cured at home after the monks of Westminster Abbey sent her Dunstan's chasuble, which was in their possession.[102] No mention was made of the woman then travelling to either Westminster or Christ Church following her recovery. Nevertheless, it must be assumed that the Westminster community were informed of the miracle on the return of the chasuble. As the woman did not then report this herself by coming to Canterbury, it is likely that the Westminster community relayed the news of this miracle to the Canterbury

---

[97] Ibid., IV.2, p. 167. Also see below, p. 198.

[98] Ibid., V.18, pp. 209–10.

[99] Ibid., III.25, p. 157.

[100] *M. Jacobi*, fol. 175ra; Kemp, 'The Hand of St James' XXIVa, 17.

[101] Thomas of Monmouth, *M. Willelmi* IV.12, ed. Jessop and James, p. 182.

[102] Eadmer of Canterbury, *M. Dunstani* 26, ed. Turner and Muir, pp. 204–7.

Cathedral monks. Similarly, a monk named Byrhtmaer took a portable relic of Æthelthryth's tunicle to the house of William of Flanders when his young son was sick and close to death.[103] The boy recovered after Byrhtmaer ordered that he be wrapped in the tunicle. Most telling is *M. Swithuni*'s report of the cure of a French noblewoman. The woman had been struck by a sudden illness which caused her pain and resulted in a loss of speech (she also reportedly did not drink anything for twenty days).[104] An English priest who happened to be in the area told the woman's husband of Swithun's miracles and urged the husband to keep vigil with a lit candle for his wife, praying to Swithun. This, the priest said, could be achieved in 'ecclesia aliqua' ('any church'), and once this had been undertaken the man returned home to find his wife's health restored.[105] Again, there was no mention that either husband or wife came to Winchester, and it must be understood that this miracle was either reported by the priest or reported through other means to the Winchester monks.

Such accounts highlight one of the most pungent arguments made by Finucane: that there were many cure-seekers who believed themselves to have been the recipients of miraculous healing beyond those recorded in the miracles.[106] Among these unrecorded cure-seekers were likely a number who were cured away from the shrine, including those cured at home. Cult centres and the saints' shrines were undoubtedly perceived to be centres of saintly intercessory abilities, as will be further discussed in Chapter 6. Nevertheless, and while local support was key, the influence of some saints did spread further than might at first be thought. Swithun, of course, had a well-established cult and one that was located at a centre within reasonable distance of an important port, and such factors must have undoubtedly benefited any knowledge of him on the Continent. Nevertheless, for most cure-seeking pilgrims, making a journey to the shrine – either to request aid or to make good on a promised vow – was evidently an important part of the process and experience of securing holy healing.

*   *   *

This chapter analysed the distances travelled to the shrines as part of the cure-seeking process. It was expected that there would be greater numbers of local cure-seekers, and this generally proved to be correct. While such a

---

[103] *L. Eliensis* III.59, ed. Blake, p. 306, trans. Fairweather, p. 375.

[104] *M. Swithuni* 33, ed. Lapidge, pp. 670–1.

[105] Ibid.

[106] Finucane, *Miracles and Pilgrims*, p. 13.

result was anticipated, in-depth consideration established just how central the relationship was between saints and their communities. That saints should appeal to their nearby communities was the result of multiple factors. It was logical that a sufferer wishing to find holy healing would first exhaust all the local options before seeking the aid of saints further afield. This choice was respectful to the resident patron saint, but it was also practical. Able-bodied cure-seekers would have found journeys of great lengths to be both time consuming and challenging, and this problem would have increased if the sufferer were impaired or in ill health. Equally, spurning a local saint who protected the sufferer's community would be improper unless other factors intervened.

Further study of travel and travel experiences follows in the next chapter. However, it is important to recall the concerns voiced by Ysembela to St James. Both her faith and the disabling nature of her affliction gave her reason to remain at Canterbury, but she was also unaware of James's cult and Reading Abbey. Ysembela did not know how to get there and was anxious about undertaking the journey while in poor health and without having the finances to do so. Navigation and geographical knowledge must also have played a vital role in the travel choices made by cure-seeking pilgrims. While some roads and trackways did cut across the country, life for the majority was lived at a local level. Familiarity with long-distance routes was unlikely unless such knowledge was an occupational requirement.

Some of those who sought cure further afield appear to have done so on the advice of family and friends, or even the saints. Indeed, it was due to the advice of friends that a blind woman travelled from London to St Abb's Head with her young daughter as a guide. Others who covered longer distances travelled to multiple shrines prior to securing saintly intercession, and this resulted in extensive time on the road. This is particularly evident in accounts involving penitents suffering from wounds caused by iron bonds. Both Clement in *M. Dunstani* and the French pilgrim in *M. Moduenne* were exiles and had been to numerous shrines before finding relief.

This chapter exposes a surprisingly high percentage of accounts that do not name the cure-seeker's origin-site. While it can be reasonably assumed that many of these cure-seekers were locals, it was important that they remained listed as travelling 'unknown' distances in order to highlight the paucity of details provided within the miracle stories in these instances. It is striking that there appears to have been so little interest in recording these details, particularly at established cult centres. What remains unknown is when this information was discarded. Was it in the initial record or in the hagiographer's editing? That the recording of the miracle itself was the most important feature is hardly surprising, but certain hagiographers, notably Thomas of Monmouth, put greater stock in including additional details.

Yet, written records of miraculous cure at the shrine were only one means by which news of holy healing was noted and circulated. For many, word of mouth would have been important in advertising the powers of a saint; and dissemination of previous miraculous successes clearly drew in other hopeful cure-seekers. News would have spread more quickly through the local area, and into the surrounding villages, through the actions of cure-seekers and witnesses, but also potentially by monks and clerics and by the laity who were active in the area. Dissemination of the reports of miracles is thus inextricably connected to the geographic scope of the cult and provides one explanation for the local nature of our seven cults.

If an individual did undertake a longer journey to seek the aid of a specific saint, what was their motivation? Can it be assumed that the journey was undertaken only because the individual had heard of the saint's abilities, or were other factors involved? A journey might be made after the failure of another saint or because the individual had other reasons to be in that area. While the distances can be measured, motivations only become apparent through textual analysis, thus highlighting the importance of utilising this multi-methodological analysis.

By considering the distances covered by cure-seekers, this chapter has revealed the importance of a saint's local appeal and the necessity of some form of travel to the shrine – predominantly before healing – for the majority of cure-seekers. The need to travel might appear an obvious one, but it does not often appear in discussions of the processes and experiences of cure-seeking pilgrimage. As such, it is important that further attention is given to this topic. The choice of saint was not made solely out of a sense of spirituality but also with practical reasons in mind and Ysembela's concerns are particularly noteworthy for their valuable insight. What then might a cure-seeker have expected in setting out for the shrines, and did Ysembela's concerns match the realities of travelling on England's roads?

5

The Road to Recovery:
The Experience of Seeking Cure

That a visit to a saint's shrine required travel is an evident but often over-looked part of these cure-seeking pilgrimages. Yet, this is an important part of the cure-seeking process. For some, the journey to the shrine would have been relatively straightforward. For others, these journeys might require travelling beyond the familiar or spending prolonged periods of time on the road. Ysembela's comments to St James, mentioned in the previous chapter, reveal the trepidations some had before undertaking longer-distance jour-neys.[1] Even those travelling relatively short distances might have had anxieties over the journey, especially if their affliction had a detrimental effect on their mobility. Paralysis and blindness, notably, would have been limiting even over a short distance; while those who were described as sick were often said to be unable to leave their beds prior to their miraculous cure, suggesting that cov-ering even a short distance would be near impossible, except with considerable help. Nevertheless, pilgrimages were made, and these journeys contributed to the overall cure-seeking experience.

As the miracle accounts focus on the result – the successful cure – addi-tional contemporary evidence must be consulted to establish what travel in twelfth-century England was like. To understand the road network, and travel on this network more broadly, consideration of the legal concerns and regu-lations, and the accounts of contemporary travellers, is essential. Taking these sources into account, alongside the miracles, allows for a greater contextual understanding of a very necessary part of the cure-seeking process.

Travel has been an understudied area of the pilgrimage experience, at least for English pilgrimage. Recently though there has been growing interest in considering pilgrims within the pilgrimage landscape. Of note is Martin Locker's study of four English pilgrimage routes that may have been traversed by a hypothetical pilgrim.[2] Locker's research was chronologically broad, with a

---

[1] *M. Jacobi*, fols. 174rb–174va; Kemp, '*The Hand of St James*' XX, 15. Also see above, pp. 132–3.

[2] M. Locker, *Landscapes of Pilgrimage in Medieval Britain* (Oxford, 2015), pp. 21, 29.

greater emphasis on the later medieval centuries. His field work, and attention to the sensory experiences of the journeys, provides a fascinating angle from which to consider pilgrimage. Noteworthy are Locker's studies of the pilgrimage from Ely and to Winchester, which offer a thoughtful consideration of the local landscapes and of the, often ancient, road networks which ran through these regions.[3]

England's Road Network

In an article on England's medieval roads, Frank Stenton noted that much of the infrastructure consisted of prehistoric tracks and the remains of Romano-British roads.[4] Stenton and, later, Brian Hindle both argued that there was little evidence to suggest any deliberate road building during the medieval period.[5] Travellers going by road in the twelfth century, therefore, primarily relied on the surviving routes that had served the country for many centuries, be these well-used local tracks or the great road networks that crossed the country. Reliance on a pre-existing road system is understandable, given the costs in labour and land associated with creating new roads. There was also, however, growing demand for roads, a system integral to the country's economy, meaning that this lack of investment is peculiar.[6]

High-medieval traffic consisted of drovers and merchants, various officials (ecclesiastical and secular), the king and his court, and pilgrims. Indeed, pilgrims would have been a substantial presence on England's roads, especially at certain times of the year and on certain routes to major shrines.[7] With such requirements for travel it is unsurprising that there was considerable use of pre-existing Roman roads, some of which remained paved.[8] Roads also developed from often-used tracks, as long-term common usage led to them

---

[3]   Ibid., pp. 27–61, 62–97.
[4]   F. Stenton, 'The Road System of Medieval England', *The Economic History Review* 7 (1936), 1–21 (6).
[5]   Ibid., 6; B. P. Hindle, 'The Road Network of Medieval England and Wales', *Journal of Historical Geography* 2 (1976), 207–21 (208). For a detailed discussion of bridges and their development in the Middle Ages, see D. F. Harrison, *The Bridges of Medieval England: Transport and Society, 400–1800*, Oxford Historical Monographs (Oxford, 2004).
[6]   Stenton, 'The Road System', 4; Hindle, 'The Road Network', 208; B. P. Hindle, *Roads, Tracks and Their Interpretation*, Know the Landscape (London, 1993), p. 52.
[7]   Hindle, 'The Road Network', 208.
[8]   For more on the construction of Roman roads see H. E. H. Davies, 'Designing Roman Roads', *Britannia* 29 (1998), 1–16.

becoming recognised as rights of way.[9] Unlike the surviving Roman roads, these roads were not marked by paving or even boundary markers. Instead they were often no more than compacted mud-tracks, much like the footpaths that still cover the countryside today. These routes, Hindle summarises, came to have a status through their customary and regular usage as rights of way rather than through any physical markers or boundaries.[10] This lack of physical definition meant that multiple routes often ran side-by-side, with new paths forged when tracks became obstructed or impassable.[11] That ease and practicality influenced the development of routes is further evidenced by the Anglo-Saxon practice of establishing tracks that ran along the course of a valley basin, rather than on the higher ridgeways.[12]

In contrast to these more fluid tracks, the Roman roads stood as relatively unchangeable structures, and might have proved a more welcome option to all travellers, including cure-seekers. As former Roman settlements, several English towns and cities are located on this ancient road system, thus making the routes to these locations easier to map. Winchester was accessible via multiple roads including one that ran from Silchester, which itself was positioned on the road from London to Cirencester.[13] Roads from the ports of Dover, Lympe, Richborough and Reculver all led to Canterbury and then on to London. From Cambridge a road led into the Fens close to Ely, while Caistor St Edmund (situated close to the later city of Norwich) was the termination point for the road leading north from Colchester. Reading, Burton and Coldingham were non-existent as settlements during this earlier period, but they lay close to, or on, Roman roads. Burton-on-Trent is situated approximately midway between Wall and Little Chester, and Reading lies just ten miles north of Silchester. The Roman road from Learchild terminates at Berwick-upon-Tweed and could have been used by those travelling to Coldingham (a mere eleven miles further north); similarly, Ermine Street passes through Newstead *en route* to Edinburgh.

Of the many ancient roads used in medieval England, though, four stand out. These roads – Ermine Street (or the Great North Road), Watling Street, the Icknield Way, and the Fosse Way – have come to be known as the 'Four

[9]   Hindle, 'The Road Network', 208.
[10] B. P. Hindle, *Medieval Roads*, Shire Archaeology 26 (Princes Risborough, 1982), p. 6.
[11] Ibid.
[12] Locker, *Landscapes of Pilgrimage*, p. 70.
[13] *Ordnance Survey Historical Map: Roman Britain*, 6th edn (Southampton, 2010).

Highways', or the 'King's Highways'.[14] These had been major roads in the infrastructure of Roman, and even pre-Roman, Britain and remain prominent features of the landscape today. Their importance was due to their positioning and the level of royal protection granted to those who travelled on them.

The Four Highways

Henry of Huntingdon was the first to express the notion of the 'Four Highways' in his *Historia Anglorum*.[15] Henry named and provided the terminus points for each of the four roads, concluding that these four roads were the 'principales calles Anglie' ('principal highways of England').[16] He praised them for being 'multum quidem speciose, sed nec minus speciose, sanciti edictis regum scriptisque uerendis legum' ('very broad as well as splendid, [and] protected by the edicts of kings and by venerable law codes').[17] Conversely, the contemporary *Leges Henrici Primi* did not regard royal protection as having been exclusive to these four roads.[18] *L. Henrici* was not an official legal document. However, it is a record of laws, many of which pre-dated Henry I's reign, that were still relevant in twelfth-century England.[19] *L. Henrici* contains laws that concerned the safeguarding of the 'via regia' (royal roads) and 'herestrete' (highways or army roads) and implies that all highways were under royal jurisdiction.[20] *L. Henrici* therefore indicates that, at least theoretically, there was a level of protection granted to travellers on all highways, while also recording that the *viae regiae* were to be kept at a suitable width, indicating that these were by no means inconsequential roads.[21]

Despite *L. Henrici*'s implication that all highways were under royal jurisdiction there is no clear specification of *which* roads were considered highways. Evidently not every road could claim this status. Henry of Huntingdon

---

[14] For a map see A. Cooper, 'The King's Four Highways: Legal Fiction Meets Fictional Law', *Journal of Medieval History* 27 (2000), 351–70 (353).

[15] Henry of Huntingdon, *Historia Anglorum: The History of the English People* I.7, ed. and trans. D. Greenway, OMT (Oxford, 1996), pp. 22–5. Also see Cooper, 'The King's Four Highways', 355–7.

[16] Henry of Huntingdon, *Historia Anglorum* I.7, ed. Greenway, pp. 22–5.

[17] Ibid.

[18] *Leges Henrici Primi* (hereafter *L. Henrici*), ed. and trans. L. Downer (Oxford, 1972); A. Cooper, 'The Rise and Fall of the Anglo-Saxon Law of the Highway', *The Haskins Society Journal: Studies in Medieval History* 12 (2002), 46–9.

[19] *L. Henrici*, ed. Downer, pp. 5–7.

[20] Ibid., 80.3a, pp. 248–9. '*Herestrete*' can also refer to 'army roads', see: Cooper, 'The Rise and Fall', 59; Stenton, 'The Road System', 2–3.

[21] *L. Henrici* 80.3, ed. Downer, pp. 248–9.

suggests that it was only the Four Highways which were protected, while *L. Henrici* suggests that any road which could be deemed to be a 'highway' might be covered by these laws. And what about those roads not covered? The *Leges Edwardi Confessoris*, actually compiled *c.* 1136, and never intended for official use, contains references to royal roads similar to *L. Henrici*.[22] Particularly important is that this law code acknowledged that not all roads were equal and, like *Historia Anglorum*, the king's peace only covered the Four Highways. Other roads were the responsibility of the county, and fines were to be paid locally.[23] These county roads were undoubtedly well-known and well-used by local travellers, and would lead onto the main streets within the towns, while also acting as extensions to the national road network.

Little is known of the local roads and byways used during this period. As their use was a day-to-day necessity rather than a legal or fiscal matter, evidence of these paths was never accurately recorded. *Mappae Mundi* had been produced since the seventh century, but these were hardly designed for practical navigation.[24] It was not until the mid-fourteenth century that the first 'roadmap' of Britain was produced. The Gough Map (named after antiquarian Richard Gough) shows a slightly misshapen Britain populated with little towns that are labelled and connected by rivers and fine red lines, seemingly depicting roads.[25] While produced in the later Middle Ages it is possible to identify our seven cult centres on the map, suggesting they were still worthy of note. The old cathedral cities of Canterbury, Ely and Winchester are predictably prominent, as are Norwich and Reading. On a smaller scale are Coldingham and Burton-on-Trent. The latter is identified only by a small structure resembling a house, although a church depicted nearby might represent Burton Abbey. Unlike Burton-on-Trent, the other six locations, including the priory at Coldingham, are all clearly identified as places with religious houses, and are depicted with spired churches.

Questions have been raised about the nature of the red lines of the Gough Map and whether these do indicate roads. It is difficult to imagine what else the markings represent, but certain major routes, including London to Dover,

---

[22]   Cooper, 'The King's Four Highways', 357.

[23]   *Leges Edwardi Confessori* XII.9–10, in B. O'Brien, *God's Peace and King's Peace: The Laws of Edward the Confessor*, The Middle Ages Series (Philadelphia, 1999), pp. 158–203 (170–3); Cooper, 'The King's Four Highways', 358.

[24]   J. Williams, *Mappa Mundi and the Chained Library: Treasures of Hereford Cathedral*, 2nd edn (Norwich, 2005), p. 2.

[25]   N. Millea, *The Gough Map: The Earliest Road Map of Great Britain?*, Treasures from the Bodleian Library (Oxford, 2008); *Linguistic Geographies: The Gough Map of Great Britain*, <http://www.goughmap.org/> [accessed 24 June 2020].

were not illustrated. Indeed, few of the Roman roads are depicted.[26] Whether or not the Gough Map's network of roads is taken at face-value, it is clear that, as Stenton stated, little had been done to progress the overall road infrastructure.[27] This, together with the absence of maps and widely-recognised pilgrim routes, would mean that inexperienced travellers could face major difficulties with navigation, especially if they ventured beyond their local area.

Known Routes and New Paths

Known routes were surely helpful if the destination lay on, or close to, such a road. But it is important to remember Ysembela's concerns in *M. Jacobi*. Despite Reading being situated close to the Roman road from London to Cirencester (which ran through Silchester ten miles to the south), Ysembela's preference – having not heard of Reading and being unsure of the way – was to remain at Canterbury.[28] The prominence of local cure-seekers within the hagiographies, particularly evident in *M. Moduenne*, suggests that even cult centres located on ancient roads would not necessarily attract a high number of long-distance pilgrims and travellers if the location were more remote. This highlights an easily overlooked point: not only was a road required but so was knowledge of the road, which in turn would depend upon the numbers of people who had reason to use it.

Pilgrimage centres which had centuries of history to fall back upon were at an advantage. Canterbury, in particular, with its many roads leading to Kentish seaports and up to London, was well placed. Additionally, routes which were in more frequent use, especially those which were used by royal messengers or merchants and traders, would also act as a magnet for various hospitality trades. In other instances, journeys might be diverted from a direct path to pass a monastic *hospitium* that would allow the traveller a place to recuperate. This hospitality, however, was not limitless, and monastic customaries and statutes expressed practical limits on the time guests might stay. At Abingdon Abbey guests were permitted two nights' accommodation, but smaller houses with fewer resources might limit stays to a single night.[29] Such institutions were likely to be located in or close to towns or along major roads, and even parish churches would offer some respite for a weary pilgrim.[30] Less-frequented

[26] Millea, *The Gough Map*, p. 14.
[27] Stenton, 'The Road System', 6.
[28] *M. Jacobi*, fols. 174rb–174va; Kemp, 'The Hand of St James' XX, 15.
[29] Kerr, *Monastic Hospitality*, pp. 184–5.
[30] Locker, *Landscapes of Pilgrimage*, p. 50.

routes were unlikely to offer the same degree of hospitality. This in turn could discourage their use by long-distance travellers.

Yet, it should be recognised that pilgrims, particularly those seeking miraculous cure, travelled for distinctive reasons and might seek out less-frequented destinations. Here the evidence of the fifth book of the *Codex Calixtinus*, better known as *Iter pro peregrinis ad Compostellam* (*The Pilgrim's Guide to Santiago de Compostela*), is useful.[31] Believed to be the work of Aimery Picaud, a monk of Parthenay-le-Vieux, Poitou, and dated to the early twelfth century, the *Compostella* is thought to be the first purpose-made 'tourist guide'. It directed pilgrims from France through the mountainous regions of northern Spain to Galicia in the west.[32] For obvious reasons, the *Compostella* is not evidence of the experiences of English pilgrims. Nevertheless, the description of this well-known, well-used, way suggests there would be no trouble finding lodgings on routes that were frequently used, although Picaud is far from complimentary about the hospitality a pilgrim could find in certain regions of northern Spain.[33] By the later Middle Ages, larger ecclesiastical institutions in England were running inns for travellers, highlighting how demand for accommodation had grown.[34] Accommodation also offered pilgrims the chance to meet, and possibly pass on the news of their own journeys and the shrines they had visited, or planned to visit.

Hospitals, discussed in Chapter 1 with regard to healthcare and welfare, are worth returning to here for their importance to travellers, and particularly pilgrims.[35] While monastic institutions played a crucial role in establishing their own facilities for guests, *hospitia* would also be found along, or close to, roads.[36] Indeed, the majority of medieval hospitals in Kent were founded along the aforementioned Watling Street, a point that indicates the high usage of this ancient road and also the understood requirement for such establishments for travellers.[37] Watson has suggested that by *c.* 1200 most people in England would have been as familiar with these institutions as with monasteries.[38] Because these *hospitia* offered shelter, travellers might well have planned their journeys, or limited

---

[31]   Aimery Picaud, *The Pilgrim's Guide to Santiago de Compostela* (hereafter *Compostella*), ed. and trans. W. Melczer (New York, 1993).

[32]   Ibid., pp. 32, 134 n. 3, 140 n. 31.

[33]   Ibid., pp. 87, 140 n. 29.

[34]   Webb, *Pilgrimage in Medieval England*, p. 225.

[35]   See above, pp. 56–9.

[36]   Sweetinburgh, *The Role of the Hospital*, p. 242.

[37]   Webb, *Pilgrimage in Medieval England*, p. 224.

[38]   S. Watson, 'The Origins of the English Hospital', *Transactions of the Royal Historical Society* 16 (2006), 75–94 (76).

the distance covered in one day, in order to make use of their hospitality.[39] Such shelter must have been particularly appreciated when travelling in poor weather as this would have provided a dry place to spend the night.

Landscape and Weather

Whan that Averylle with his shoures soote
The droughte of March hath perced to the roote [. . .]
So prikryh hem nature in his corages –
Thanne longen folk goon on pilgrymages[40]

Thus begins Geoffrey Chaucer's prologue to *The Canterbury Tales*, highlighting the expectation that pilgrimages were likely to commence with the first signs of spring. The warmer weather of spring and summer would improve road conditions, and the days grew longer. The timing also suited the pattern of the agricultural year, with April and, later, July proving timely months for travel: the former coming before farm labour began in earnest and the latter being before the harvest.[41] Such practical benefits and considerations for travel would have been apparent to the cure-seeking pilgrims just as they would have been to other travellers. That is not to say that cure-seekers and other pilgrims did not journey at all during the winter months, but they would likely find their journeys hampered to a greater extent by inclement weather and limited hours of daylight.[42] The marshy Fens around Ely would become less passable, while rivers could become swollen and flooded in the colder and wetter months. Seasonal weather conditions, such as fog, could present additional complications.[43] As hagiographies rarely refer to the details of travel or weather conditions, the testimony of a well-known twelfth-century traveller becomes relevant.

[39] This point has also been made by Wendy Childs, see W. R. Childs, 'Moving Around', in *A Social History of England, 1200–1500*, ed. R. Horrox and W. M. Ormrod (Cambridge, 2006), pp. 260–75 (262).

[40] Geoffrey Chaucer, *A Variorum Edition of the Works of Geoffrey Chaucer, 2. The Canterbury Tales: The General Prologue*, ll.1–12, ed. M. Andrew et al., 1 vol. in 2 parts (Norman, OK, 1993), Part 1, 125–210.

[41] Locker, *Landscapes of Pilgrimage*, pp. 163–4.

[42] Webb, *Pilgrimage in Medieval England*, p. 222. Regarding royal travel, which does appear to have continued in the winter months, see B. P. Hindle, 'Seasonal Variations in Travel in Medieval England', *The Journal of Transport History* 4 (1978), 170–8 (177).

[43] Locker, *Landscapes of Pilgrimage*, pp. 55, 163. It was not until the seventeenth century that the Fens began to be drained, see H. C. Darby, *The Draining of the Fens*, 2nd edn, Cambridge Studies in Economic History (Cambridge, 1956).

Gerald of Wales recounts, in *Itinerarium Kambriae*, that winter was a time for strong winds, and at the aptly named Newgale Sands, in 1171–72, strong winds blew 'praeter solitum pro callae vehementia sabulosis australis Kambriae litoribus solo tenus sabulo nudatis' ('with such unprecedented violence that the shores of South Wales were completely denuded of sand').[44] Gerald's recollections of his own travels through Wales in 1188, as part of Archbishop Baldwin's crusade-preaching posse, make it clear that the travelling party were challenged by the topography of the Welsh landscape. At the River Neath near Margam the tidal sands acted like quicksand and Gerald almost lost his only pack-horse.[45] After this the companions crossed the Neath by boat as the fords were treacherous due to monthly shifts in tidal patterns, and heavy rain, affecting where the fordable passages were to be found.[46] Gerald later reveals the difficulties of traversing the mountainous landscape of the Caernarfon valley: the steep incline required the horses to be dismounted and for the journey to proceed on foot.[47]

Gerald's experience of travel in Wales might not be typical of journeys taken across the British Isles – the specific topographical features of differing landscapes must be kept in mind – yet his experience of the weather and varying landscapes is enlightening. The risks of quicksand are reflected in the Bayeux Tapestry's depiction of William's campaign against Conan of Brittany.[48] The infamous account of King John's lost treasure in the Wash highlights how treacherous tidal changes could be.[49] Traversing steep terrain was also a challenge faced by those seeking Æbbe's assistance at her oratory at Kirk Hill.[50]

Ely was a similarly challenging location to reach due to the need to cross the Fens. The marshes provided many locals with a livelihood but were also

---

[44]   Gerald of Wales, *Itinerarium Kambriae* (hereafter *Itinerarium*) I.13, in Gerald of Wales, *Itinerarium Kambriae et Descriptio Kambriae*, ed. J. F. Dimock, RS 6 (London, 1868), p. 100; Gerald of Wales, *Itinerarium Kambriae* (*Itinerarium*) I.13, in Gerald of Wales, *The Journey through Wales and The Description of Wales*, trans. L. Thorpe (London, 1978), p. 157. It should be noted that Dimock's edition provides the Latin text for *Itinerarium*, and Thorpe provides a modern translation.

[45]   Gerald of Wales, *Itinerarum* I.8, ed. Dimock, pp. 72–3, trans. Thorpe, pp. 130–1.

[46]   Ibid.

[47]   Gerald of Wales, *Itinerarum* II.6, ed. Dimock, p. 125, trans. Thorpe, p. 184.

[48]   D. M. Wilson, *The Bayeux Tapestry: The Complete Tapestry in Colour: With Introduction, Description and Commentary* (London, 1985), plates 19–20.

[49]   P. Webster, *King John and Religion*, Studies in the History of Medieval Religion 43 (Woodbridge, 2015), p. 173.

[50]   *M. Æbbe* II, ed. Bartlett, pp. 8–9.

prone to flooding and could prove hazardous to those inexperienced with the local terrain. Despite this, *L. Eliensis*'s accounts of healing miracles make no mention of how cure-seekers found their way to Ely. Nevertheless, *L. Eliensis*'s chronicle-like second book demonstrates that crossing the Fens was not without challenge. Particularly noteworthy is the recording of William I's conflict with Hereward 'the Wake', in 1070–71.[51] While *L. Eliensis*'s author was acquainted with his marshy surroundings, William and his men, armed and mounted on horses, were not. In recording their struggles with the marshes *L. Eliensis* highlights the hazardous and changeable nature of the land that surrounds Ely and its cathedral.[52]

Despite the unstable and potentially treacherous Fens, *L. Eliensis* proves that cure-seekers did manage to reach Æthelthryth's tomb. A major reason for this success was the causeways built to and from Ely. One causeway of note is that which ran between Ely and Soham, just less than six miles away.[53] The causeway was created after St Edmund appeared to a farmer from Exning, twelve miles south of Ely. The saintly king stated that he wanted a causeway: 'qua dominam mean beatissimam Æðeldreðam adire queam' ('by which I may go and visit my lady, the most blessed Æthelthryth').[54] On the orders of Bishop Hervey, John, one of Ely's monks, took up the challenge of constructing the causeway.[55] This occurred under Hervey, appointed to the episcopate by Henry I, and was thus a twelfth-century initiative. Causeways through the Fens would certainly aid travellers who wished to visit Ely. No shrine could succeed without a trustworthy, identifiable road or track. The advice of locals, as Wendy Childs noted, must have also been beneficial for those who did not live within the immediate area, as too would way-markers that could aid in signposting routes.[56]

That poor weather could prevent, or slow, travel has been discussed by Paul Brand in his study of late medieval excuses for not travelling to court; flooding (barring or destroying the road to court) is often found among the excuses.[57] Such reasons for not travelling can also be found in *miracula*. The son and

[51] D. Roffe, 'Hereward (*fl.* 1070–1071)', in *ODNB*, <https://doi.org/10.1093/ref:odnb/13074> [accessed 18 July 2020].
[52] *L. Eliensis* II.109, ed. Blake, pp. 190–1, trans. Fairweather, p. 225.
[53] *L. Eliensis* III.32, ed. Blake, p. 266, trans. Fairweather, p. 320.
[54] Ibid.
[55] Ibid.
[56] Childs, 'Moving Around', pp. 264–5.
[57] P. Brand, 'The Travails of Travel: The Difficulties of Getting to Court in Later Medieval England', in *Freedom of Movement in the Middle Ages: Proceedings of the 2003 Harlaxton Symposium*, ed. P. Horden (Donington, 2007), pp. 215–28.

daughter of one local cure-seeker, the paralysed Margery de Honimer, put off the journey to Thomas Cantilupe's shrine for two months – despite living less than five miles from Hereford – due to concerns over the health of their mother, requiring time to raise money, and the necessity of waiting for the most suitable time to go.[58] Whether the latter related to waiting for better weather or for a time when it was acceptable to leave the seasonal cycle of rural labour is unclear, but evidently there was a need to plan the journey around personal circumstances.[59] Similar necessities might well have stalled, or even prevented, the journeys of other cure-seekers as well.

This local knowledge was vital since unpaved roads and tracks were at risk of deterioration and damage during poor weather. Those who could wait for the better weather of the warmer seasons therefore were likely to do so. The lack of attention to these factors within the miracle stories is not because such factors were negligible, but because the focus is upon the miracles themselves. Equally absent from our seven *miracula*, although an issue that must have been of concern to those on England's roads at this time, were any mentions of those threats that did not improve with the arrival of the drier months.

A More Human Threat

On some journeys it was not the weather or the terrain, but a more human threat that presented itself. Apprehensions regarding thieves and assailants are evident in *L. Henrici*.[60] There were also concerns raised over the risk to the morality of those who might be corrupted during their time away from their parish. Women were seen to be particularly at risk. Such apprehensions could have put off some cure-seekers and pilgrims from making journeys, especially into areas of the country with which they were less familiar.

The seven hagiographies make no mention of their cure-seekers having had any such trouble on their journeys. After all, unless the saint had miraculously assisted in protecting a cure-seeker there would be no need to record such a detail. Other sources, again, must be considered to understand these potential threats better. *L. Henrici*'s laws regarding the protection of travellers on the *via regia* show a concern to prevent and punish acts of 'forestel' (an assault by an offender on the road, or who lay in wait along the road).[61] An extreme example of this form of assault can be found in *Itinerarium*. On the road from Carmarthen to the Cistercian abbey of Whitland a messenger came

---

[58]   Finucane, 'Pilgrimage in Daily Life', p. 174.
[59]   Ibid.
[60]   *L. Henrici* 80.2–80.5a, ed. Downer, pp. 248–51.
[61]   Ibid., 80.2, 80.4, 80.4a, pp. 248–51.

to Archbishop Baldwin to report that a young Welshman had been murdered whilst travelling to meet the preaching party.[62] In response, Baldwin had the corpse wrapped in his cloak and 'jugulate juvenis animam pia supplicatione commendavit' ('with pious supplication commended the soul of the murdered youth to heaven').[63] *Itinerarium* implies that this was an unprovoked attack on an innocent messenger. No information about the assailants is provided beyond the fact that twelve archers from the nearby castle at St Clears were punished for the young man's death the following day.[64]

The threat of such a physical assault was clearly cause for concern and many instances of *forestel* were likely the result of attempted roadside theft. This threat of violence is one crucial reason why *L. Henrici* contains clear specifications that highways should be wide enough for two carts to pass.[65] Wider roads allowed for greater visibility so that a traveller could be attentive to potential assailants. Visibility became more challenging when these routes took travellers through woodland where there were ample opportunities for ambush. Attempts to limit woodland assaults were recorded in the *Gesta Abbatum Monasterii Sancti Albani*.[66] One passage refers to Abbot Leofstan's (d. 1064) excessive project for 'vias tutiores' ('safer roads'), through the 'opaca nemora' ('dark woods') on the east edge of the Chilterns between London and St Albans, 'praecipue strata regia, quae "Watlyngestrata" dicitur' ('especially where the royal street, which is called 'Watlyngestrata' [Watling Street], is').[67] Leofstan also had bridges constructed and steep roads levelled out.[68] The chronicle explains the need for this project, as:

> eo tempore per totam Ciltriam nemora spatiosa, dense, et copiosa, in quibus habitabant diversae bestiae, lupi, apri, tauri sylvestres, et cervi, abundanter; necnon, et qui plus nocuerunt, praedones, latrones, vispiliones, exules, et fugitivi

[62] Gerald of Wales, *Itinerarium* I.10, ed. Dimmock, pp. 80–3, trans. Thorpe, pp. 138–41.

[63] Gerald of Wales, *Itinerarium* I.10, ed. Dimmock, p. 82, trans. Thorpe, p. 140.

[64] Ibid.

[65] *L. Henrici* 80.3, ed. Downer, pp. 248–9.

[66] Thomas Walsingham, *Chronica Monasterii S. Albani: Gesta Abbatum Monasterii Sancti Albani* (hereafter *C. Albani*), ed. H. Riley, 3 vols, RS 28 (London, 1867), I, 39–40. Also see Cooper, 'The Rise and Fall', 65–6.

[67] Thomas Walsingham, *C. Albani*, ed. Riley, I, 39–40.

[68] Ibid.

(at the same time through all the Chilterns' spacious, dense and copious forests dwelled in abundance diverse beasts, wolves, boars, wild oxen, and deer; in addition, and more harmful, robbers, bandits, thieves, exiles and fugitives)[69]

Strikingly, the threat posed by the criminals was seen to be the greater danger. Despite Leofstan's attempts, the threat remained for those travelling through this wooded section of Watling Street.[70] Woodland elsewhere also held potential dangers. Blean Forest, between London and Canterbury, became known as a haunt for robbers who preyed upon those travelling to and from Becket's tomb; and Shooter's Hill near London was known for its dangers into the seventeenth century.[71] But were pilgrims a target for thieves? Pilgrims predominantly travelled alone or in small groups, without defences, and made for easy victims, especially if travelling by foot. Laws would have been difficult to enforce in practice, hence the continuous concern over the safety of travelling through wooded areas during this period.[72]

Yet, there was no guarantee an assailant would make a fortune from robbing pilgrims. After all, the pilgrimage ideal was to travel as humbly as possible, relying on the kindness of strangers. Although perhaps not going as far in dispossession of wealth as some in the Church would like, the majority of pilgrims conceded to making their journey in relative poverty.[73] Gerald of Wales stated that any home was open to a weary traveller who sought a bed for the night or merely required refreshment.[74] These ideals, however, did not necessarily fit the realities of twelfth-century travel, as the *Compostella* demonstrates.[75] Various costs would be encountered whilst journeying to a cult centre, from paying for lodgings and refreshments, to giving charitable donations at other churches, or paying for passage across a river. There is evidence for the latter of these within both the *Compostella* and later medieval Plea Rolls. The *Compostella* criticises

---

[69] Ibid.

[70] Ibid., I, 43.

[71] Webb, *Pilgrimage in Medieval England*, pp. 223–4. Blean lies just north of Canterbury, whilst Shooter's Hill is south of the Thames in what is now the Royal Borough of Greenwich.

[72] For additional discussion of this, see: Webb, *Pilgrimage in Medieval England*, p. 223; A. McCall, *The Medieval Underworld* (New York, 1979), pp. 34–5.

[73] J. Sumption, *Pilgrimage* (London, 2002), pp. 168–71.

[74] Gerald of Wales, *Descriptio Kambriae* I.10, in Gerald of Wales, *Itinerarium Kambriae et Descriptio Kambriae*, ed. J. F. Dimock, RS 6 (London, 1868), pp. 182–4; Gerald of Wales, *Descriptio Kambriae* I.10, in Gerald of Wales, *The Journey through Wales and The Description of Wales*, trans. L. Thorpe (London, 1978), pp. 236–7.

[75] Aimery Picaud, *Compostella*, ed. Melczer, pp. 90–6.

the fees charged by ferrymen in northern Spain, arguing that they should only charge those pilgrims who were wealthier and stop demanding payment from every pilgrim to Compostela.[76] Likewise, the Worcester Plea Rolls refer to toll collection in the village of Wychbald.[77] Hugh the toll-gatherer, along with other men from the village, was accused of charging pilgrims for passage through the village. A cart with pilgrims from Gloucestershire was required to pay half a penny, while carts from other counties paid a penny; and one female pilgrim was charged two shillings.[78] The Rolls firmly record that no toll was to be taken from any future pilgrim carts.

Pilgrims, including cure-seekers, would also often purchase candles at the cult centre as a gift to the saint. Ysembela's aunt, who encouraged the journey to Reading, gave her niece her only coin so that Ysembela might purchase the required candle on arrival.[79] This implies that her aunt had previous experience of shrines and shrine practices, and that Ysembela made her journey with very little financial support. Yet, it is hard to believe that Ysembela, a young girl travelling alone, would not have been at risk from thieves, or worse, during her journey.

It should not be presumed that villages or towns were any safer for strangers either. Urban settings presented opportunities for thieves as well as travellers, including pilgrims and cure-seekers, who may have been tempted to engage in immoral behaviour. Stopping for respite might bring the traveller into contact with gambling, drinking and prostitution. Such experiences must have been expected and perhaps even enjoyed by some travellers, including those on pilgrimage. But more vulnerable travellers might also find themselves at risk of exploitation. Concern from the Church over female pilgrims falling into prostitution had been stressed as early as the eighth century by St Boniface to Archbishop Cuthbert of Canterbury.[80] These concerns, as urban centres developed through the Middle Ages, would not have disappeared and neither would the potential for pilgrims to be diverted from their cause. *M. Jacobi* reflects this when recording the miraculous cure of Alice, from Essex, whose

[76] Ibid., pp. 92–3.
[77] 'The Pleas of the Crown at Worcester, 1221', in *Rolls of the Justices in Eyre being the Rolls of Pleas and Assizes for Lincolnshire 1218–19 and Worcestershire 1221*, ed. and trans. D. Stenton, Seldon Society 53 (London, 1934), pp. 441–655 (573–5).
[78] 702 Ibid.
[79] *M. Jacobi*, fols. 174rb–174va; Kemp, '*The Hand of St James*' XX, 15. Also see above, pp. 99–100.
[80] Boniface, *The Letters of St Boniface: Translated with an Introduction* 62, trans. E. Emerton, Records of Civilisation Sources and Studies 31 (New York, 1940), p. 180.

arm had become stuck to her chest.[81] Having been cured at Reading, Alice remained as a laundress at the monastery until 'a quodam fabro seducta et abducta sese meius coniugium resolueret' ('she was seduced and abducted by a certain smith and became his wife').[82] *M. Jacobi's* author clearly sees this as a distraction from the pious occupation of tending to the monks' laundry. Many of those who had made a pilgrimage, especially if the journey were long, would have been in need of finances, either to support their return journey or their living costs in the location they had come to. It is likely that this was the reason behind Alice's initial decision to stay at Reading and work as the abbey's laundress.

The miracles, however, do not present female cure-seekers as being a cause for concern. When analysing hagiographic accounts of female pilgrims, Bailey concluded that far from being discouraging, hagiographers appear to have accepted the idea of female travel even if they did not promote it.[83] Bailey highlights that while most women covered shorter distances than men, many made their journeys with greater levels of disability, thus balancing the pious struggles endured by both sexes.[84] It is not at all surprising, therefore, to find that few women made journeys of considerable distance. Those who did, such as a woman who travelled from near London to Coldingham, with her young daughter as a guide, stand out for this very reason.[85] If women did only travel shorter distances, does this imply that there were indeed apprehensions about female travellers? The very fact that, whilst women are present within the hagiographies, they relied more on their local saints for cure, is suggestive of this. It should also be remembered that none of the accounts focused upon here made any mention of nuns as travellers. The positive approach of the miracle accounts appears to have been in tension with concerns over women travelling, these tensions becoming increasingly apparent in the later Middle Ages.[86]

---

[81] See above, pp. 131–2.

[82] *M. Jacobi*, fol. 172vb; Kemp, '*The Hand of St James*' VIII, 9–10.

[83] Bailey, 'Flights of Distance', 302.

[84] Ibid., 301. Also see Bailey, 'Women Pilgrims and Their Travelling Companions', 115–34.

[85] *M. Æbbe* IV.2, ed. Bartlett, pp. 32–5.

[86] For further discussion of female pilgrims see: S. S. Morrison, *Women Pilgrims in Late Medieval England: Private Piety and Public Performance*, Routledge Research in Medieval Studies 3 (London, 2000), pp. 108–14, 119–22; L.-A. Craig, *Wandering Women and Holy Matrons: Women as Pilgrims in the Later Middle Ages*, Studies in Medieval and Reformation Studies 138 (Leiden, 2009), pp. 21–4, 28–9, 78; D. Webb, 'Women Pilgrims of the Middle Ages', *History Today* 48 (1998), 20–6.

Amongst the morally dubious aspects of travel, the excitements offered by towns ranked highly. A large urban centre, especially for those coming from a rural locale, might well offer the chance for new experiences which, Jonathan Sumption notes, could be enjoyed away from the judgement of neighbours.[87] These moral dangers were also harder for external forces, such as the Church, to defend against. Despite this, hagiographies are, unsurprisingly, far from discouraging of travel. The omission of the possible dangers of the road allows miracle reports to focus on the positive nature of the result – the success-ful cure. Yet, this reluctance to depict the rigours of the journey means that we must look both at the cure-seekers' experiences and beyond the miracle accounts to fully understand how journeys to the shrines were made.

Tracing Travel

We often take for granted that cure-seekers would have used the country's road network to make their journeys. This underlying assumption that travel was undertaken on the roads rather than on the waterways of England could be due to modern preferences, but there is a risk in assuming that travel in the past followed the same pattern. Being aware of possible variations in travel, such as using the waterways, is therefore important.

The Language of Travel

The terminology used in miracles to record journeys to the shrines must be considered to understand how these journeys were completed. The language used in the hagiographies is often relatively ambiguous and, as such, highlights why tracing travel is challenging. Verbs such as *venio* (to come) do not reveal the method of travel. The same can be said for many of the terms deployed in the accounts of cure-seekers, as analysis of *M. Swithuni, M. Dunstani* and *M. Jacobi* demonstrates (Table 5.1). This linguistic ambiguity highlights that it cannot be assumed that journeys to the shrines were made on foot. Only in accounts where a mode of transport is specifically indicated – such as walking, riding, travelling in a cart or barrow, or sailing – can the method of travel be guaranteed. It must also be accepted that certain journeys necessarily required crossing water, as was the case for those travelling to Winchester from the Isle of Wight. In addition to the mode of transport, or lack thereof, this linguis-tic analysis reveals that a number of these terms denote assistance in getting to the shrines. One boy, 'quinquennem etate' ('five years of age'), was simply recorded as having been 'allatum fuisse Wintonie' ('brought to Winchester') by

---

[87] Sumption, *Pilgrimage*, p. 11.

his parents in the hope of finding a remedy for his blindness.[88] Most of these 'guiding' and 'aiding' verbs related to cases of blindness or paralysis, although accounts that involved mad cure-seekers also included such terms. Eadmer of Canterbury used the term 'pertractus' ('drawn to') in recording the miraculous cure of Clement, from Germany.[89] Clement was 'demens actione' ('mad in his behaviour'), and 'petractus' implies that he was forcibly brought to the shrine against his will.[90] What is less clear in Clement's case is whether Clement was drawn, or even dragged, to the shrine by other people or by divine force.

Table 5.1. Terminology used for travel within
M. Swithuni, M. Dunstani, and *M. Jacobi*

Latin verb	English translation	Present in M. Swithuni	Present in M. Dunstani	Present in M. Jacobi
accurro, -ere	to hasten to	✓		
adduco, -ere	to bring to	✓	✓	
adeo, -ire	to go to	✓		
adveho, -ere	to carry	✓		
advenio, -ire	to come		✓	
affero, affere	to bring to	✓		
arrepo, -ere	to creep	✓		
deambulo, -are	to walk	✓		
deduco, -ere	to bring	✓		
defero, -erre	to bring	✓	✓	✓
deporto, -are	to carry	✓		
duco, -ere	to lead	✓		
egredior, egredi	to go from			✓
eo, ire	to go	✓		✓
expono, -ere	to set out	✓		
festino, -are	to hurry	✓		✓
fugio, -ere	to flee	✓		

---

[88] *M. Swithuni* 47, ed. Lapidge, pp. 682–3.
[89] Eadmer of Canterbury, *M. Dunstani* 8, ed. Turner and Muir, pp. 166–7. Also see above, p. 130.
[90] Ibid.

Latin verb	English translation	Present in *M. Swithuni*	Present in *M. Dunstani*	Present in *M. Jacobi*
invenio, -ire	to come upon	✓		
itinero, -are	to travel	✓		
navigo, -are	to sail	✓		
perduco, -ere	to bring		✓	
pergo, -ere	to proceed	✓		
pertraho, -ere	to bring (forcibly)		✓	
pervenio, -ire	to come to		✓	
procedo, -ere	to progress		✓	
propero, -are	to hurry			✓
refero, -erre	to return		✓	
requiro, -ere	to search for	✓		
subsequor, subsequi	to follow			✓
tendo, -ere	to press on			✓
vado, -ere	to go	✓		
venio, -ire	to come	✓	✓	✓

Travel by Water

Did pilgrims take advantage of England's waterways? The existence of natural waterways was often the reason why a settlement was established, and these waterways were of great importance to their local lay and monastic communities. Many goods were carried on the country's waterways as this was more economical.[91] Reading Abbey's wharf, adjacent to the town's wharf, was vital to the monastery and allowed goods to be transported directly into the monastic precinct.[92]

All seven case-study cult centres were located near important bodies of water, and locations such as Ely clearly brought pilgrims into contact with the challenges of traversing watery landscapes. Yet, the only accounts to specifically refer to crossing water were those in which the journey could not be

[91]   Childs, 'Moving Around', p. 265.
[92]   J. W. Hawkes and P. J. Fasham, *Excavations on Reading Waterfront Sites, 1979–1988*, Wessex Archaeology Report 5 (Salisbury, 1997), pp. 11–35, 177–9.

completed without doing so. Within our seven *miracula*, three accounts refer to journeys from the Isle of Wight, and four record journeys from the Continent to England.[93] Two accounts imply no journey was made by those from overseas.[94] A further two accounts refer to travels made in the other direction (neither of which resulted in a cure abroad).[95] Was travel by water simply taken for granted, or were cure-seekers inclined to follow the roadways? Practicalities of cost and access might come into play here, as might the desire to partake in the physical effort of making the pilgrimage by foot.

In considering pilgrims who did navigate waterways it is worth questioning the nature of the boats used. Would boats have been especially hired for the purpose, or would passage be sought on a boat already embarking on that journey? Unlike the well-documented pilgrimages made to Jerusalem from the Italian seaports, it is probable that pilgrimage to these English shrines was less frequent and thus unlikely that there was enough demand for a full-time business of ferrying pilgrims across the Channel or Solent.[96] Conversely, trade between England and the European mainland would have allowed some to find passage across the sea on merchant ships. Landing at Dover, for example, a pilgrim could then progress via Watling Street to London and beyond.

The cure-seekers who travelled from the Isle of Wight to Swithun's shrine are worth consideration here as sea transport was crucial to their journeys and to the island.[97] With no known Roman or Saxon roads, settlements thrived by the waterside at Brading, Yarmouth and Newport, and there must also have been a constant back-and-forth of boats across the Solent for trade and supplies.[98] However, these short journeys were not without the risk of

[93] *M. Swithuni* 6, 35, 36, 48, 55, ed. Lapidge, pp. 652–5, 672–5, 682–3, 690–5; Eadmer of Canterbury, *M. Dunstani* 8, ed. Turner and Muir, pp. 166–7; Geoffrey of Burton, *M. Moduenne* 51, ed. Bartlett, pp. 216–19.

[94] *M. Swithuni* 33, 36, ed. Lapidge, pp. 670–1, 672–5.

[95] Ibid., 16, pp. 658–61; *M. Jacobi*, fols. 175rb–175va; Kemp, 'The Hand of St James' XXVII, 18–19.

[96] J. Sumption, *The Age of Pilgrimage: The Medieval Journey to God* (Mahwah, NJ, 2003), pp. 260–71; Sumption, *Pilgrimage*, pp. 185, 189; N. Ohler, *The Medieval Traveller*, trans. C. Hillier (Woodbridge, 2010), pp. 40–1.

[97] V. Basford, 'Medieval Resource Assessment for the Isle of Wight', Oxford Archaeology (2006), 1–23 (18), <https://oxfordarchaeology.com/images/pdfs/Solent_Thames/County_resource_assessments/Late_Medieval_IOW.pdf > [accessed 18 July 2020].

[98] R. Waller, 'Archaeological Resource Assessment of the Isle of Wight: Early Medieval Period', Oxford Archaeology (2006), 1–8 (7), <https://oxfordarchaeology.com/images/pdfs/Solent_Thames/County_resource_assessments/Early_Medieval_IOW.

shipwreck.[99] As testimony to the dangers of the sea, the Isle of Wight lays claim to the only surviving medieval lighthouse in England. Located next to St Catherine's oratory overlooking Chale Bay, the lighthouse (known affectionately as the 'Pepperpot') was built in the later Middle Ages in response to shipwrecks in Chale Bay: a reminder that even so close to the mainland there were dangers involved with nautical navigation.[100] In order to limit these risks it would make sense if journeys to Winchester began on the north side of the island, perhaps at Newport, before travelling down the River Medina past Cowes, then across the Solent and up the River Test to Southampton. From Southampton the journey to Winchester could be made across land or, perhaps, via the Rivers Test and Itchen. Yet, the only passing reference to Southampton in *M. Swithuni* appears in the account of a crippled Norman nobleman, cared for by Queen Emma, who set out from Winchester 'uiam que ducit ad mare' ('on the road which leads to the sea').[101] This would have been the Roman road, to the west of the Itchen, that ran from Winchester's South Gate to Southampton.[102] It is also likely that the three blind women, abandoned without a guide, disembarked somewhere along the Test, but far enough away from Winchester to have caused them distress at the idea of finding their way without a sighted guide.[103]

Crossing the sea for those on the Isle of Wight or European mainland was clearly essential, but references to England's inland waterways are notably absent within the hagiographies. It remains unclear whether this omission implies that use of the waterways was so common that it was not seen as worthy of reporting, being mundane through its frequency of use, or whether the use of river travel was not undertaken by cure-seekers. The language used within *M. Swithuni*, *M. Dunstani* and *M. Jacobi* proves that it is not definite that all pilgrims came by road. That said, the miracles do include references to cure-seekers who came on horseback; Thomas of Monmouth even included a miracle concerning the healing of a horse.[104] Would the use of boats and ferries not warrant similar mention? The answer to this would surely be that it would, if not in every instance then at least on occasion.

---

pdf> [accessed 18 July 2020]; Basford, 'Medieval Resource Assessment for the Isle of Wight', 17–18.

[99] Basford, 'Medieval Resource Assessment for the Isle of Wight', 18.

[100] Ibid.; D. Tomalin, 'St Catherine's Oratory', *Archaeological Journal* 163 (2006), 51.

[101] *M. Swithuni* 48, ed. Lapidge, pp. 682–3.

[102] Ibid., p. 683 n. 37.

[103] Ibid., 6, pp. 652–5.

[104] Thomas of Monmouth, *M. Willelmi* III.29, ed. Jessop and James, pp. 160–1.

The evidence of the miracle accounts, therefore, although far from conclusive, is that pilgrims and cure-seekers used water transport only when it was absolutely necessary. This is counterintuitive in a period when goods were frequently transported by water; but roads, while slower and more arduous, did not require specialised forms of transport in the way that water did.[105] Furthermore, travel by foot, whilst slow, was free, and any other form of transportation would have required payment, even if it was just to cross a river via ferry. While it could be argued that an unimpaired pilgrim might prefer to take the more challenging route so as to make a show of piety through the suffering they endured on their journey, surely the wish of the cure-seeker would be to succeed in securing a miraculous remedy as quickly as possible? The time taken to travel to a saint's shrine must have greatly influenced the choices made by a cure-seeker when setting out to obtain a miraculous cure.

Travel Times and Longer-Term Travel

The final element of the cure-seeker's journey that requires attention is the time required, and taken, to journey to the shrine. Calculations for the distances that travellers could cover in one day have been made by Sumption as well as by Norbert Ohler and Diane Webb, but there has been little attention given to those who were less mobile.[106] For impaired travellers journeys would have been understandably slower than those made by the able-bodied. At the most severe end of this scale were the paralysed, and those who had no, or limited, sight. It is not surprising, therefore, that some cure-seekers benefited from assistance, either in the form of crutches and barrows, or guidance from family, friends or hired aid. For the visually impaired, the other senses would have also played a vital role on a day-to-day basis. Raven survived by begging and lived off the charity of his neighbours in Tutbury having lost his sight following an illness.[107] On passing Burton one day, presumably whilst begging, he heard the 'tintinnabulum grossum' ('big bell') of the abbey church.[108] Recognising the sound he requested that his guide lead him to the abbey where, following prayers, he was cured by Modwenna.[109] Raven was guided to the church by

[105] Ohler, *The Medieval Traveller*, p. 34.
[106] Sumption, *The Age of Pilgrimage*, p. 251; Ohler, *The Medieval Traveller*, pp. 97–101; Webb, *Pilgrimage in Medieval England*, p. 222.
[107] Geoffrey of Burton, *M. Moduenne* 45, ed. Bartlett, pp. 186–9. Tutbury is just less than four miles from Burton.
[108] Ibid., pp. 186–7.
[109] Ibid. The Latin terms used here come from verbs: 'tractorem' from *traho, -ere* and *tracto, -are* (to draw or pull), and 'ductor' from *duco, -ere* (to lead). The verb *duco* can

his companion, but it was hearing the bells that first directed his attention to Modwenna, and motivated him to seek her assistance. The sound of church bells, not to mention the sight of a church tower, could act as a geographic marker and draw the attention of passers-by. The importance of sound, as well as sight, was not lost on contemporaries and is reflected in the architecture of churches. The eleventh-century bell tower at Cranwich, Norfolk, was designed with 'sound holes' that amplified the sound of the bell.[110]

Raven's reliance on his hearing and a guide would suggest that his eyesight had greatly deteriorated since becoming ill. His guide was most likely a fellow vagrant or family member as Raven could hardly have afforded hired assistance. Conversely, an elderly blind woman, who was abandoned by her guide on a bridge over the Stour, appears to have had hired help.[111] That her guide willingly abandoned her indicates there was not a strong bond between the two. Whatever their relation, a blind cure-seeker who had a guide was at an advantage over those who travelled unaccompanied. The distress felt by the three blind women from the Isle of Wight who were abandoned on the mainland is worth recalling.[112] A guide could ensure that the sufferer was on the right route and could provide some protection to the cure-seeker. Paralysed pilgrims, similarly, were often aided by family or friends, who carried them or brought them in a litter or barrow.[113] Nevertheless, even with assistance, most cure-seekers, regardless of their affliction, were unlikely to be able to cover as much ground as a regular road-user could in a day.

Webb has argued that, despite the quality of their footwear, the nature of the roads and the nutritional limitations of their diets, medieval travellers were robust and could cover two to three miles per hour on foot (about the same as a modern walker could), while a pilgrim on horseback would cover double this.[114] Sumption goes further, suggesting that a pilgrim on horseback could have travelled up to thirty miles a day.[115] Using Webb's calculations, that implies those on foot could walk approximately fifteen miles per day. Childs provides a similar estimate of fifteen to twenty miles for daily travel.[116] Ohler

---

also be found for describing the way the journey to the cult centre is made.
[110] Locker, *Landscapes of Pilgrimage*, p. 48.
[111] Eadmer of Canterbury, *M. Dunstani* 7, ed. Turner and Muir, pp. 164–7.
[112] *M. Swithuni* 6, ed. Lapidge, pp. 652–5. Also see above, p. 100.
[113] For example: Thomas of Monmouth, *M. Willelmi* VI.12, ed. Jessop and James, pp. 244–6.
[114] Webb, *Pilgrimage in Medieval England*, p. 222.
[115] Sumption, *The Age of Pilgrimage*, p. 251.
[116] Childs, 'Moving Around', 260.

took these calculations further still, including a greater range of travellers and travel options, and with slightly more generous calculations for travel times. A pedestrian, argued Ohler, could cover up to twenty-five miles in a day.[117] Of course, these calculations are only an estimate based on able-bodied travellers. Weather conditions, hours of daylight and landscape, as mentioned, let alone the quality of the mount or ability of the walker, would also have affected the distance that could be travelled. In the generally dry and temperate climate of northern Spain, for instance, Aimery Picaud might have covered a greater distance in a day than Gerald of Wales could have achieved in northern Wales. Furthermore, and practically, a traveller might not choose to travel the daily distance they were capable of if that meant passing a suitable place to stay the night. The necessity of finding such lodgings meant that one cure-seeker *en route* to St Andrews diverted at Coldingham and unexpectedly found the cure to his paralysis through Æbbe's intercession.[118]

The need to balance distance covered with suitable rest stops must have especially affected the traveller's decision if the journey to the destination, or return trip, was likely to take more than a day to complete. Yet, such considerations would only apply if the traveller had at least a rough estimate of how long their journey might take, and what respite options there were. Such planning would have been easier for those travelling shorter distances and who knew the local area.

Awareness of distance and estimated travel time initially appears absent within the miracles, possibly because the length of the journey was often not as important as the eventual arrival at the shrine. The account of Gaufrid of Canterbury in *M. Willelmi* stands out for this very reason.[119] Gaufrid suffered from a severe toothache, and in a vision Becket told him to seek William's aid.[120] Gaufrid did so, setting off from Canterbury to Norwich, a journey of approximately 138 miles. On arrival, he claimed to have succeeded in making the journey in only a day due to being accompanied as far as Bury by Saints Becket and Edmund. On the face of it, there was little knowledge of timing. Covering such a distance would undoubtedly take at least a few days. Thomas of Monmouth, however, was clearly aware of how long this journey should have taken. Rather than accept Gaufrid's assertions as given, he made the journey to Canterbury himself to secure testimonies; these supported Gaufrid's claims of his miraculously speedy journey.

---

[117] Ohler, *The Medieval Traveller*, p. 101.
[118] *M. Æbbe* IV.11, ed. Bartlett, pp. 50–1.
[119] Thomas of Monmouth, *M. Willelmi* VII.19, ed. Jessop and James, pp. 289–94.
[120] See above, pp. 72–3.

Thomas of Monmouth's decision to verify the details of Gaufrid's journey for himself provides a clear indication that at least some of the more learned would have had knowledge of how long a journey was likely to take on the twelfth-century roads of England. Monastic communities, who were in contact with other institutions, were likely to have an awareness of the travel times between monasteries. *M. Willelmi* evidences this in recording that the clerk and palfrey of Canterbury Cathedral Priory's sacrist were both cured by William while the sacrist was in Norwich on family business.[121] *M. Jacobi*, likewise, records Abbot Osbert of Notley's visit to Reading after his miraculous cure, and that Reading monks stopped at Merton Priory on returning from taking St James's hand to Henry II before the king crossed to Normandy.[122] The hospitality of the Merton canons to the Reading monks is also a reminder of the importance of the network of monastic houses across the country and the fact that these houses, and their *hospitia*, would have provided rest stops for travelling monks and pilgrims.

Recognition of the slower speeds at which impaired cure-seekers travelled can also be found within a number of miracle accounts. Thomas of York, who suffered from paralysis and had to use crutches, is said to have been 'gradiendo modicum proficiens, longinque peregrinationis itinere multos consumpsit dies' ('journeying slowly, [and] spent many days over his long pilgrimage') to Norwich.[123] A priest's servant from the Isle of Wight who suffered from paralysis was placed on a boat to the mainland, then progressed to Winchester on foot; *M. Swithuni*'s hagiographer noting that the journey took him a fortnight while an able-bodied walker would have made it in a day.[124] A man from the Edinburgh area, who also suffered from paralysis, and had already been to Canterbury, made his way from Coldingham to Kirk Hill slowly like a tortoise, 'a nona diei hora iter protelans in uesperam' ('from the ninth hour of the day until the evening').[125]

Unlike these three men, many cure-seekers, as shown, lived within twenty miles of the cult centre where they were cured. Practical as well as spiritual reasons for requesting a local saint's assistance first must have been important. It is reasonable to assume that cure-seekers would have heard of their local saint's successes and knew how long it took to reach the shrine. Not only was a

[121] Thomas of Monmouth, *M. Willelmi* III.29, ed. Jessop and James, pp. 160–1.
[122] *M. Jacobi*, fols. 174ra–b, 175rb; Kemp, 'The Miracles of the Hand of St James' XIX, XXVI, 14, 18.
[123] Thomas of Monmouth, *M. Willelmi* VII.11, ed. Jessop and James, p. 271.
[124] *M. Swithuni* 54, ed. Lapidge, pp. 688–91.
[125] *M. Æbbe* IV.5, ed. Bartlett, pp. 38–9. Also see above, pp. 84–5.

local saint the patron and protector of their local community, but a journey to the local shrine would take the least time. This allowed for as little disruption as possible to the day-to-day life of the afflicted and, importantly, any guide or companion who accompanied them. The unnamed daughter of a smith from Postwick undertook the five-mile journey to Norwich alone.[126] The round trip could be made in a day, even though on her outward journey she suffered with a long-lasting and severe illness. The lack of parental accompaniment on this journey does not appear to have been due to a lack of parental concern. *M. Willelmi* records that she presented a candle at William's tomb, implying that her cure-seeking was financially supported by her family even if no one was able to accompany her to the shrine; and it is possible that her father's work as a smith kept him from being able to accompany her on the day. Cure-seeking pilgrimages over shorter distances were thus likely to be favoured for various reasons, both practical and pious. The exceptions to this, however, were occasions when cure-seeking pilgrims were directed to specific shrines, or when it took longer to secure a healing miracle, thus resulting in the cure-seeker spending more time on the road to recovery.

Longer-Term Cure-Seekers

Some cure-seekers were willing to undertake seemingly open-ended travel, or multiple trips, or to spend many days at a shrine, in the hope of obtaining saintly assistance. A pensioner from near Burton, spent four days at Modwenna's tomb before being granted his miraculous cure.[127] A smith from Lanark reportedly made three separate journeys to Æbbe's oratory before his sight was restored, while another blind man came to Coldingham with his wife and spent three days in prayer (as, presumably, did his wife) before he was cured.[128] Other cure-seeking pilgrims visited multiple shrines before finally securing saintly assistance. A French penitent pilgrim, cured of the wounds caused by his iron bonds by Modwenna, had visited numerous relics and shrines.[129] Gilbert the 'bernerius' ('hound-keeper') was taken to various shrines by his wife before St James cured him at Reading.[130] One man, cured

---

[126] Thomas of Monmouth, *M. Willelmi* IV.6, ed. Jessop and James, pp. 170–1.

[127] Geoffrey of Burton, *M. Moduenne* 45, ed. Bartlett, pp. 184–7.

[128] *M. Æbbe* IV.26–7, ed. Bartlett, pp. 58–9.

[129] Geoffrey of Burton, *M. Moduenne* 51, ed. Bartlett, pp. 216–19. Also see above, pp. 134–5.

[130] *M. Jacobi*, fol. 173vb; Kemp, 'The Miracles of the Hand of St James' XVIII, 13.

by Swithun, first travelled to Rome in the hope of securing the aid of the apostles.[131]

Some cure-seekers believed that multiple visits to the same saint were required in order to secure saintly intercession. For others, seeking a cure from the same, seemingly unwilling saint, must have seemed a fool's errand. If a saint were unable to grant a cure, what hope was there that a second or third petition would be any more successful? It was surely time to seek assistance from saints further afield. All seven *miracula* include instances in which a cure-seeker visited other shrines prior to finding their cure. In some instances, the individual was directed to their place of healing by family or friends, or on the recommendation of a saint. Others appear to have sought a cure without a finite destination in mind. The number of these longer-term cure-seekers within the hagiographies is small, but they are important in understanding the full range of cure-seeking experiences.

Quinciana was one such long-term cure-seeker. She had suffered from muteness since the age of seven, when she had become lost and spent three nights sleeping in a hollow tree in the woods.[132] Quinciana had married a wealthy man and had three sons, but following Henry II's invasion of Wales she found herself widowed and childless. At around eighteen, after eleven years of mutism, Quinciana turned her attention to the 'corporis salute' ('health of [her] body').[133] Leaving all possessions behind her, she began her pilgrimage 'tam Galliarum quam Anglorum regionem summa egestate comite' ('around both France and England in the utmost poverty').[134] *M. Æbbe* provides no details of where in France and England Quinciana travelled, or for how long she was on the road before arriving at Æbbe's shrine, but the implication is that pilgrimage had become her primary focus. Possibly pilgrimage allowed her to focus her attention on a spiritual purpose. The fact she gave up personal possessions before setting off indicates her willingness to embrace a life of poverty and pilgrimage. There is no indication within *M. Æbbe* that Quinciana was penitent, rather her desire to resolve her muteness is emphasised. Yet, Quinciana's willingness to embrace poverty also highlights that the spiritual and humble nature of the pilgrimage was important to her.

Further study of these longer-term cure-seekers and pilgrims would undoubtedly be beneficial in understanding why they travelled so far from shrine to shrine, sometimes without an obvious finite destination. Did such

---

[131] *M. Swithuni* 16, ed. Lapidge, pp. 658–61.

[132] *M. Æbbe* IV.7, ed. Bartlett, pp. 40–5.

[133] Ibid., pp. 42–3.

[134] 758 Ibid.

pilgrims, perhaps to a greater extent than local pilgrims and cure-seekers, gain more from the journey itself? From a spiritual perspective, a greater time on the road, with limited means of support, would likely draw greater parallels between the individual and the concept of Christ in the wilderness. The longer, and more challenging the journey, the more the pilgrim was tested. Was there a sense, then, that this made for a worthier subject for divine aid? Longer-term pilgrimage might have meant that cure-seekers, such as Quinciana, did not know where their journeys would eventually take them or how long they might find themselves traversing various roads. It also indicates that time was a less concerning factor for some pilgrims.[135]

Considering Quinciana's long-term travel and her decision to undertake this in poverty, it is worth emphasising the penitential aspect of pilgrimage and the spiritual benefits that might be perceived to be gained from longer or more challenging journeys. The concept of an arduous, long-term, and ascetic penitential pilgrimage developed from the Irish monastic tradition.[136] In this tradition, penitents became exiles from their own community, and were expected to accept the hardships of travel as part of their atonement. The Frenchman cured by Modwenna is an example of such a penitent pilgrim.[137] Bailey has noted that twelfth-century *miracula* supported these penitential ideals.[138] The length of the journey was connected to the concept of redemption, with longer distances seen to be more spiritually rewarding.

Although most evident in the accounts of penitents, the perceived penitential nature of travelling to the shrine might also be read into the accounts of those who undertook longer-term or longer-distance journeys. While the recording of Ysembela's concerns is unusual within the miracles, there are miracle stories that implicitly reflect the reluctance of the cure-seeker in setting out on longer journeys.[139] The woman who travelled from London to Coldingham was visited three times by a woman she did not recognise who instructed her 'admonens eam lectum mutare et ulterius sibi quiescendi locum non habere' ('to exchange her bed and no longer have a place to rest').[140] Having refused to do this, the woman was punished with the loss of her eyesight, resulting in her

---

[135] D. Dyas, *Pilgrimage in Medieval English Literature, 700–1500* (Cambridge, 2001), p. 137.

[136] Webb, *Pilgrimage in Medieval England*, p. 234.

[137] Geoffrey of Burton, *M. Moduenne* 51, ed. Bartlett, pp. 216–19.

[138] Bailey, 'Flights of Distance', 294.

[139] Ibid.

[140] *M. Æbbe* IV.2, ed. Bartlett, pp. 32–3. It should be noted that Bartlett translated *mutare* (*muto, mutare, mutavi, mutatus*) as 'abandon'; here I have chosen 'exchange' as a closer translation of the Latin and to reflect that the vision's message was for

travelling to the Kirk Hill oratory. Conversely, those who showed willingness to undertake the journey might find themselves rewarded with their desired cure before having set off, as one man found who was cured by Swithun as the horses were readied for his journey.[141] Thomas of Monmouth's account of Gaufrid's experience, similarly, has a moralistic undertone in emphasising that an arduous journey might not be as daunting with the saints on your side. This chapter focuses on the practicalities and experiences of the cure-seekers' journeys but it should be recognised that such journeys also had a spiritual aspect, and those who did secure their holy healing after travelling some distance, or having spent some time on the road, must have believed that they had proved their spiritual worth through their hardships.

Despite these potential spiritual gains, many cure-seekers appear to have favoured localised travel, and clearly there were various benefits to this decision. Safe travel, even for able-bodied travellers, could not be guaranteed, nor would it have been possible to definitively calculate how long it would take to arrive at the desired destination (let alone complete the round trip). Of course, some travellers would have been more experienced in travelling further afield, but among our cure-seekers these individuals were likely in the minority. Moreover, even a short journey did not promise the cure-seeker a quick cure and, consequently, some undertook multiple journeys or remained at the shrine for multiple days. Every journey, regardless of distance, would have disrupted the daily routine of the cure-seeker and any supporters who accompanied them. For some, responsibilities at home might prevent travelling further afield. It must be understood that experiences of the journey were influenced by the practicalities of travel and by the time spent on the road. The nature of the affliction would have also brought cure-seekers a range of challenges. Quinciana's mutism must have made communication difficult but would not have impacted her mobility as she travelled through England and France. Conversely, Raven evidently had to rely both on the assistance of others and on his other senses to navigate his local environment around Burton.

*   *   *

The previous chapter confirmed that the majority of cure-seekers found their remedy close to home. This, along with the concerns voiced by Ysembela in

---

this woman to exchange the comfort of her bed for pilgrimage. On this latter point see Bailey, 'Flights of Distance', 294.

[141] *M. Swithuni* 8, ed. Lapidge, pp. 654–5.

M. Jacobi, raised questions about the nature of travel and what might be experienced by cure-seekers on the road to recovery. To answer these queries in this chapter, it was necessary to consult a variety of other sources as the miracles alone cannot provide the full picture. The country's road infrastructure, and travel risks, could have affected the potential traveller's decision to journey beyond their local area. Evidently there were various challenges that faced cure-seekers setting off for England's cult centres.

This chapter's investigation into travel offered fascinating insights into this somewhat overlooked aspect of pilgrimage, and specifically cure-seeking, in high medieval England. Much of the road network pre-dated the period, being primarily constructed from surviving Roman roads and ancient trackways. The Roman routes formed a strong backbone to this network, running between Roman settlements such as Winchester, Cirencester, Dover, and Canterbury. Most important was the position of London, through which three of the Four Highways ran. These were the major routes of the country and were so important that they were seen to have the special protection of the king. Those who threatened travellers and those who failed to maintain the highways were at risk of persecution.

Nevertheless, poor weather and criminal behaviour were major problems. Weather conditions would have made journeys difficult or even impossible. Therefore, pilgrims who could wait were likely to favour the fairer weather of spring and summer and the increase in daylight hours. Yet, travel in the warmer seasons would not have prevented perhaps the greatest threat to the traveller, the threat of assault from thieves and outlaws. The *Gesta Abbatum Monasterii Sancti Albani* was striking in the fear voiced concerning the threat of individuals who preyed on travellers at the east edge of the Chilterns. Despite the best efforts of figures such as Abbot Leofstan and the laws of *L. Henrici* against assault on the highways, such dangers remained.

Considering the issues that threatened travellers on the roads, it might be assumed that using the waterways would have offered an attractive alternative. Yet, only in those hagiographical accounts where crossing water was a necessity did mention of such travel occur. This does not prove that all other travellers came by foot. A study of the travel terminology used within three of the seven *miracula* revealed that the hagiographers primarily used terms relating to 'coming' and 'going'; the terminology also emphasised the importance of companionship and assistance. Evidence of how cure-seekers travelled was rare, although specific mention was made of horses, carts, or crutches in some cases. While some travellers owned horses, and almost all could walk to some extent, usage of boats, despite the benefits of water travel, does not appear to have been widespread.

Previous estimations of the speed of medieval journeys reflect what the average able-bodied traveller could hope to achieve. Cure-seekers were often limited in their mobility, and those who must have struggled most were the paralysed and blind. The use of a guide must have been a great advantage and travelling at length without such assistance would have been very demanding. Even the more mobile would have planned their travel around finding lodgings and might not have covered the maximum amount of ground they possibly could in one day. Cure-seekers and their companions would also have been limited in the amount of time that they could spend away from their duties and responsibilities. Therefore, journeying further than the local cult might not have been an option for some cure-seeking pilgrims. Conversely, a few cure-seekers, such as Quinciana, spent much longer, and travelled much further, on their search for miraculous healing.

This chapter's focus on travel offers a new angle for approaching cure-seekers' experiences of travel. The hagiographies, understandably, tend to focus on the miraculous conclusion of the journey, but travel beyond the local, known, and trusted, area was evidently not to be undertaken lightly. No matter the distance, however, most cure-seekers were united in their intended terminus, that destination being the shrines of the saints.

6

Upon Arrival at the Shrine: Cure-Seekers and the Place of Their Cure

The *Regula S. Benedicti* charged Benedictine monasteries with a duty of care and hospitality and, as the previous chapters have established, most cure-seekers travelled to the place of their healing.[1] However, the *Regula S. Benedicti* also impressed the need for a level of separation and the cloistering of the brothers.[2] These concerns were later re-emphasised in the canons of the First Lateran Council and later medieval visitation records, both stressing the need for monastic seclusion. Nevertheless, cure-seekers deliberately sought out the locations in which the saints (or rather their relics) resided and would have expected a hospitable welcome from their hosts. Being welcoming to, and separated from, the laity, monasteries had to balance two juxtaposing duties to fulfil their spiritual and charitable responsibilities. Yet miracle accounts show little concern over the presence of cure-seekers – instead presenting the shrines as being open to all people and at all times – with limited indication of the supervision of, or the boundaries between, sufferers, saints and the monastic community.

We arrive in this final chapter then, along with the cure-seekers, at the shrines of the saints. Of course, it must be understood that the experiences of the churchmen who were miraculously cured, especially those of the cult-centre community, would have differed from those of the lay cure-seekers. But what would the majority of cure-seekers have expected on arrival at the shrines?[3] To address this, the question of where in the monastery cure-seekers sought their cure must be asked. We must also consider the regulation and reception of lay visitors, and the matter of whether cure-seekers were seen to be 'guests'

---

[1] *Regula S. Benedicti* 53, ed. McCann, pp. 118–21.

[2] Ibid., 66, pp. 152–3.

[3] In addition to the discussion of cure-seekers' experiences of the shrines here, a newly-published article by Bailey promises to be illuminating on this topic: see A. E. Bailey, 'Reconsidering the Medieval Experience at the Shrine in High-Medieval England', *Journal of Medieval History* 47.2 (2021), 203–29.

of the monastery. It must be recognised that Benedictine monasteries like our seven cult centres were, to an extent, independent institutions. Consequently, the ways that monasteries approached the issue of lay presence might well differ. Those that were established, larger and located in urban centres such as Canterbury, Ely and Winchester, which were visited by numerous travellers, would have been more practised in handling lay visitors than smaller, rural monasteries. Conversely, establishments such as Burton, with a principally local focus, could have developed stronger relations with the local laity. Reading had a special duty of hospitality written into its foundation charter, while Norwich permitted lay access to William's tomb in the monks' cemetery and chapter house (prior to the translation to the cathedral itself). Meanwhile, despite Æbbe's cult developing across two physically separated locations, there was connection between the two and interaction at both sites between cure-seekers and Coldingham's monks.

Beyond 'Sacred Space'

When addressing lay presence within the monasteries, it is important to acknowledge the work that has been undertaken in recent decades regarding theories of space and in particular 'sacred space'. Conceptualising and understanding space largely stems from the fundamental work of Marxist philosopher and sociologist Henri Lefebvre.[4] Lefebvre separated space into three categories – physical, social and mental – all of which had clearly recognised characteristics.[5] Lefebvre sought to define and analyse the urbanisation of the European landscape, thus sparking medievalists' interest in this topic as a category of historical analysis.[6] Lefebvre emphasised that considering space in isolation was 'an empty abstraction' and that actual spaces are always multivalent; sacred space is, therefore, not solely abstract and should be understood as inhabiting physical and social spaces as well.[7]

Megan Cassidy-Welch took up this discussion with regard to medieval sacred spaces.[8] Cassidy-Welch perceived that spatial use and practices shape

4   H. Lefebvre, *The Production of Space*, trans. D. Nicholson-Smith (Oxford, 1991). For discussion see M. Cassidy-Welch, 'Space and Place in Medieval Contexts', *Parergon* 27 (2010) 1–12 (1).
5   Lefebvre, *Space*, pp. 11–12.
6   Ibid., p. 269; Cassidy-Welch, 'Space and Place', 1–2.
7   Lefebvre, *Space*, pp. 12–14, 27.
8   M. Cassidy-Welch, *Monastic Spaces and Their Meanings: Thirteenth-Century English Cistercian Monasteries*, Medieval Church Studies 1 (Turnhout, 2001); Cassidy-Welch, 'Space and Place'.

socio-political identities and subjectively influence the sense of 'self-location' within communities and the wider world.[9] Religious buildings themselves require, and define, a socially recognised 'sacredness'; equally, a collective belief in a 'higher power' informs the use and shape of the physical religious space. Roberta Gilchrist's analysis of Norwich Cathedral (in 2005) used archaeological, architectural and literary sources to identify a hierarchy within sacred spaces relating to degrees of sanctity.[10] Naturally, altars were sacred, and the high altars of cathedral priories embodied the most sacred spaces for whole dioceses. As a result, noted Gilchrist, these spaces became loci of holiness, and buildings as well as people were ranked in relation to their proximity to this divinity.[11] But, at what point does sacred space become 'profane space' (a terminological distinction championed by Mircea Eliade)?[12] Would the saints' shrines remain sacred areas when surrounded by lay visitors?

As Cassidy-Welch argued: 'we can no longer suppose that spatial boundaries around the sacred were immutable, or even thought to be so by medieval people'.[13] It is time to change, or re-define, the manner in which such topics are approached. What is now required is a consideration of 'monastic space' and, more importantly, the access lay cure-seekers were given to this space. What could cure-seekers, having journeyed to the monasteries with the hope of procuring the saints' assistance, expect from their hosts, and where within the monastic grounds might they visit? The fact that miracle stories identify the presence of lay cure-seekers within the church and the monastic precinct is proof of their presence within these spaces. The key issue is *how* lay presence within the monastery was balanced with ecclesiastical usage of key areas.

Guests of the Monastery, Visitors to the Shrine

There were numerous reasons why laypeople visited the monasteries; some came for business, others out of necessity. Not all visitors came with the same motivations, or expectations from their hosts. As many cure-seekers only made shorter journeys to the place of their cure, spending a night in the *hospitium* might not have been required. Indeed, as the cure-seekers were focused on their petitioning of the saints, it might be expected that they would remain

[9]   Cassidy-Welch, 'Space and Place', 3–4.
[10] R. Gilchrist, *Norwich Cathedral Close: The Evolution of the English Cathedral Land-scape*, Studies in the History of Medieval Religion (Woodbridge, 2005), p. 11.
[11] Ibid.
[12] M. Eliade, *The Sacred and Profane: The Nature of Religion*, trans. W. R. Trask (New York, 1987).
[13] Cassidy-Welch, 'Space and Place', 6.

resolutely at the tomb or shrine until they were either successful or lost hope, as Kerr also concludes.[14] No suggestion is made within the hagiographies that cure-seekers were constantly coming and going between shrine and *hospitium* over the course of their time within the precinct. This would hardly be the greatest show of devotion or a desire to be cured. Does this suggest there was a distinction between those who were cure-seekers and those who were guests of the monastery? The requirements of cure-seekers were potentially quite different from those of other visitors, so too were the ways in which they interacted with the monastery and monastic community. But can such a clear-cut separation be made between the two?

It is important to understand that from the twelfth century the term *peregrini* (pilgrims) was beginning to be used to distinguish a certain type of visitor, as separate from other *hospites* (guests).[15] Abbot Geoffrey distinguished between the two in *M. Moduenne*, recording that, during her life, Modwenna ensured that one-third of the monastery's revenues were to be used for the support of 'peregrinorum et hospitum' ('pilgrims and guests').[16] *Hospites* would have visited a monastery for various reasons, but the term could also indicate social standing. A noble, for example, might have been a guest of the monastery's superior even if they sought cure from the shrine, and it cannot be assumed that guests would not have visited the tomb or sought the saint's intercession. *Peregrini*, however, as Yarrow commented, implied an estrangement from the world.[17] Regarding their presence at cult centres, pilgrims were a very specific group of visitors who were focused on accessing specific areas of the monastery, namely the saints' shrines. Cure-seekers must be seen in the same light as other pilgrims, in that their focus was the shrine, the location where the sacred and temporal came together.[18] Contemporary churchmen, including Geoffrey of Burton, evidently distinguished between pilgrims (including the cure-seekers), and other guests. This distinction was similarly reflected in the necessity for monasteries to have varying officials to deal with different categories of visitor.[19] Lanfranc's *Decreta* instructs the guest-master to act as a tour guide by showing interested visitors around the

[14] Kerr, *Monastic Hospitality*, p. 9 n. 37.

[15] Ibid., p. 10.

[16] Geoffrey of Burton, *M. Moduenne* 15, ed. Bartlett, pp. 62–3.

[17] S. Yarrow, 'Pilgrimage', in *The Routledge History of Medieval Christianity 1050–1500*, ed. R. Swanson (London, 2015), pp. 159–71 (160).

[18] Rawcliffe, 'Curing Bodies and Healing Souls', p. 120.

[19] For detailed discussion of Benedictine hospitality, see Kerr, *Monastic Hospitality*, pp. 50–85, 92–3.

monastery's buildings if they desired to see them.[20] Presumably, this was hardly of primary importance to a cure-seeker but would have been of interest to a guest with the luxury of having time to spend in their surroundings. It follows, therefore, that regulations regarding hospitality primarily concerned themselves with general guests of the monastery. The striking consequence of this is that twelfth-century regulations regarding cure-seekers and pilgrims appear almost non-existent. After all, unless the saint's shrine happened to be in a location outside the main monastic church, there would be little need, or surely desire, for a cure-seeker to venture into other areas of the monastery. However, on occasion, the focus of devotion was not within the usual setting of the church.

Moving Shrines and Dual Locations

During the formative years of William of Norwich's cult, the boy-martyr's tomb underwent a series of translations. After an initial translation from Thorpe Wood to the monks' cemetery in 1144, the sarcophagus was moved into the chapter house in 1150. A year later it was translated into the cathedral itself where it was first placed to the south of the high altar, and then in the north transept's chapel of the holy martyrs in 1154.[21] Both the monks' cemetery and the chapter house might be presumed to be locations where lay presence was unwelcome, yet *M. Willelmi* presents them as having been accessible to both laymen and laywomen. During William's year in the chapter house, thirty curative miracles were recorded. Twenty of these cures occurred within the chapter house itself, with eight men and twelve women cured on-site.[22] Of the remaining healing miracles, twenty-seven occurred between 1151 and 1172 (the dates of the tomb's translation into the cathedral and *M. Willemi*'s last recorded miracle).[23]

The frequent coming and going of devotees to Norwich's chapter house in 1151, and the consequent translation of William's tomb into the church, is evidence of William's popularity and the growing perception of his sanctity. However, *M. Willelmi*, albeit subtly, reveals that the disruption caused by these lay devotees to the daily lives of the monks was becoming problematic and that this also influenced the decision to translate the tomb into the cathedral.[24]

---

[20] Lanfranc, *Decreta* 90, ed. Knowles and Brooke, pp. 130–3.

[21] Thomas of Monmouth, *M. Willelmi*, ed. Jessop and James, pp. lxxx, lxxxix–xc; Yarrow, *Saints and Their Communities*, p. 129.

[22] Thomas of Monmouth, *M. Willelmi* III.4–IV.13, ed. Jessop and James, pp. 128–83.

[23] For further discussion regarding the translation into Norwich Cathedral, see Yarrow, *Saints and Their Communities*, p. 140.

[24] Thomas of Monmouth, *M. Willelmi* V.1, ed. Jessop and James, p. 186.

At Norwich, while the laity had not been barred from accessing the chapter house, it was seen as beneficial that the tomb was translated to a more fitting location which would allow the lay and religious communities to use the space in parallel. Situating saints' shrines within the churches must be considered both a mark of reverence and also one with practical benefits.

Coldingham Priory appears to have taken a step further. While Æbbe's tomb had been translated to the priory church, it was the location of her own earlier monastery at Kirk Hill that developed as the primary focus for pilgrimage.[25] In 1188 the clifftop focus was marked by the building of an oratory, first by local layman Henry, and soon replaced by the priory with a more suitable building.[26] Miracles followed swiftly with thirty-three cures occurring at Kirk Hill: either at the oratory itself or at the associated springs. Only six of the miracle cures were at Æbbe's tomb, with one further cure occurring in the churchyard. In only two accounts is it unclear whether the cure-seeker was at the oratory or at the church.[27] The emphasis on Kirk Hill is striking and raises questions about possible earlier, local practices of devotion, and about the levels of interaction between the monks at Coldingham and the laity. On the surface it appears that this arrangement could have limited lay presence at the priory. The prominence of women among Æbbe's cure-seekers, and the prevailing attitudes towards women at their motherhouse, Durham Cathedral Priory, might suggest that the monks were keen to avoid unnecessary interaction with the laity.[28] Nevertheless, and regardless of the fact the two locations were approximately two miles apart, they were connected through Æbbe's perceived presence at both, and through the process of pilgrimage. Detailed analysis of *M. Æbbe* reveals that a key part of the successful cure-seeking process was returning from Kirk Hill to the priory to report the cure to the monastic community. A paralysed woman from Aycliffe spent three days fasting and in prayer before receiving her desired cure. During that time three Coldingham monks came to the oratory and 'eam uiderunt et illius miserie quam plurimum condoluerunt' ('saw her and sympathised deeply with her misery').[29] On the day following her cure she made her way to the priory and, after attending mass, reported the miracle to the officiating priest.

Æbbe's cult highlights an important element of 'sacred space' in relation to the saints. Æbbe's presence was seen to be most manifest at Kirk Hill,

25 *M. Æbbe* III, ed. Bartlett, 20–31.
26 Ibid., pp. 26–31.
27 Salter, 'Beyond the *Miracula*'.
28 For further discussion, see ibid.; Salter, 'Memory, Myth, and Creating the Cult of St Æbbe', 42–3.
29 *M. Æbbe* IV.38, ed. Bartlett, pp. 64–5.

connecting the pilgrims to the landscape which she had once also experi-enced.[30] But this did not mean that Coldingham's monks detached themselves from the cult and Æbbe's cure-seekers. Æbbe's powers were also manifest in the priory church where her tomb resided, and both the monks and the laity spent time at the oratory and the priory. True, there must have been benefits to the community in having an external locale as the focus of devotion, but the monks were not unaware of the lay visitors, nor were they unmoved by the plight of sufferers who sought Æbbe's aid. Just as at other monasteries, the monks of Coldingham took their duty of hospitality and charity seriously. Most notably, the monks allowed a Lothian musician to remain with them for four months while he recovered from the effects of a local famine, and ahead of being cured by Æbbe of his gout.[31] Where the musician was stationed during his recovery is not specified, but the Coldingham monks were evidently keen to oversee his return to health. That most of Æbbe's cure-seekers visited both Kirk Hill and the priory church also emphasises that the two locations both had an important role to play in the cult.

Access and Charity

The emphasis in the *Regula S. Benedicti* on the need for monastic hospitality towards guests is reflected in this being one of the longer chapters in the rules.[32] Pilgrims and the poor were represented as being especially worthy guests owing to their likeness to Christ whose depiction in the New Testa-ment led to an association with the 'outsider'.[33] Nevertheless, the *Regula S. Benedicti* stipulated that monks should not leave the confines of the monas-tery.[34] The First Lateran Council (1123) did not forbid lay presence within the monastery but was similarly conscientious in regulating interaction between monastic and lay communities; monks (including abbots) were not to leave their communities to tend to the sick or provide other public services.[35] The Third and Fourth Lateran Councils (1179 and 1215 respectively) pressed even further for monastic separation.[36] Ironically, limiting the monks in this way

[30] Powell, 'Pilgrimage, Performance and Miracle Cures', pp. 77–80.

[31] *M. Æbbe* IV.6, ed. Bartlett, pp. 38–41.

[32] *Regula S. Benedicti* 53, ed. McCann, pp. 118–23.

[33] Matthew 18.5, 25.41–5; *Regula S. Benedicti* 53, ed. McCann, pp. 118–23; Kerr, *Monastic Hospitality*, p. 26.

[34] *Regula S. Benedicti* 66, ed. McCann, pp. 152–3.

[35] *Concilium Lateranense I* 16, ed. Tanner, p. 193.

[36] P. Draper, *The Formation of English Gothic: Architecture and Identity* (New Haven, 2006), pp. 50, 125, 199, 206.

might have increased the necessity for lay people to come to the monks themselves, and these visitors, including the cure-seekers, might well have expected
a reasonably hospitable welcome.

In reality, the wealthy were often more warmly welcomed because of their
status and their potential patronage.[37] A concerned Abbot Hugh II (d. 1199)
recognised this imbalance as a growing problem at Reading, despite hospitality to all being emphasised in Henry I's foundation charter.[38] Hugh II's
solution was to construct a new *hospitium* outside the precinct, presumably
close to the main, west gate and not far from the earlier hospital of St John's
that was positioned just inside the west entrance.[39] This position might have
been a practical decision but the location of hospitals on the boundaries of
the monastic complex was also symbolic of the connection, and separation,
between the lay and religious communities.

Yet, as *M. Willelmi* illustrates, the laity were not necessarily barred from
the claustral buildings. Indeed, none of our seven *miracula* represent lay access
to the cloister as forbidden. Reading Abbey, as a royal foundation, was in fact
called upon for use as a meeting place for royal councils.[40] Nevertheless, such
access had potential to cause disruption and tension. Hence the decision to
translate William's tomb into the cathedral. The later visitation records of
Bishop Ralph of Walpole (d. 1302) show that he was concerned with lay
access and the Ely monks' engagement with the laity. He excluded women
from the cloister, refectory, dormitory, infirmary, and the choir, although on
certain occasions – consecrations, indulgences, principal feasts and funerals
– these restrictions were to be lifted.[41] Noblewomen were also to be exempt
as it was not possible to deny them if they had an honourable reason to be
present.[42] Walpole also ordered that a 'diversorium statim erigatur' ('partition
[was to] be immediately built') between Æthelthryth's altar and the vestry
to ensure that the contemplation of the monks was not hindered by laity at

[37] Burton, *Monastic and Religious Orders in Britain*, pp. 152–3.

[38] *Reading Abbey Cartularies*, 'Royal Acts 1', ed. Kemp, I, 33–5.

[39] Ibid., 'Abbatial Acts and Abbey Documents 224', I, 185–6.

[40] B. Kemp, *Reading Abbey: An Introduction to the History of the Abbey*, Reading Abbey
     2 (Reading, 1968), pp. 39–41; B. Kemp, 'Reading Abbey and the Medieval Town',
     in *The Growth of Reading*, ed. M. Petyt (Stroud, 1993), pp. 31–55 (37–41). It is also
     worth noting that in 1359 Reading Abbey hosted the marriage of John of Gaunt
     to Blanche, the daughter of Henry Duke of Lancaster.

[41] *The Statutes of Bishop Ralph of Walpole, 1300* 13, in *Ely Chapter Ordinances and Vis-
     itation Records, 1241–1515*, ed. S. Evans, Camden 3rd series 17 (London, 1940),
     pp. 6–23 (11).

[42] Ibid.

the shrine.[43] Importantly, Æthelthryth's shrine was to remain accessible to all laypersons, men and women, even if higher-status visitors were likely to receive a warmer welcome.

Access for the poor was rather different and connected with charitable activities. At Saint-Denis, near Paris, three selected poor men were taken into the chapter house every Wednesday, Friday and Saturday between Lent and the Kalends of November to have their hands and feet washed as part of the *mandatum* ritual.[44] At Peterborough, elderly and worthy poor men would assemble in the cloister on Palm Sunday to have their feet washed and dried by the abbot.[45] Treatment of this kind was in keeping with the *Regula S. Benedicti* and mirrored Christ's own treatment of the poor (and of his disciples).[46] Charitable care towards poor cure-seekers was also documented in the miracles; *M. Moduenne* recorded that a paralysed laywoman was supported by 'elemosina monachorum' ('the monks' charity') before being healed miraculously.[47]

As noted, monastic communities would not have treated all visitors in the same manner, nor would all visitors have the same requirements. Of course, there could be some cross-over between lay guests and cure-seekers, especially if the motivation for the visit was an important church feast. Nevertheless, if the purpose and focus of the individual's visit are taken into account it is possible to recognise cure-seekers as a very specific category of lay visitors within monastic spaces. References to immediate cure and to night vigils at the shrines, as discussed below, additionally emphasise that cure-seekers were unlikely to require the use of *hospitia*. Undoubtedly, the preferred location for all cure-seekers was the shrine itself, but was such access possible? Where were the cure-seekers at the point of their cure?

Locating the Healing Miracles

Both explicitly and implicitly the miracle accounts highlight that most cure-seekers recorded were located within the cult centre at the time of their cure. Cures that took place within 'lay-friendly' areas, such as the outer

---

[43] Ibid., p. 23.

[44] S. Von Daum Tholl, 'Life According to the Rule: A Monastic Modification of Mandatum Imagery in the Peterborough Psalter', *Gesta* 33 (1994), 151–8 (153). It is worth noting that 'mandatum' means 'commissioned', and is the origin of Maundy.

[45] Ibid., 154.

[46] John 13.1–17.

[47] Geoffrey of Burton, *M. Moduenne* 48, ed. Bartlett, pp. 198–9.

monastic precinct, the nave of the church, or the shrines, would have been less disruptive than if they had occurred within areas of more restricted access such as the cloister or claustral buildings. Attention, therefore, needs to be paid to identifying where within the monastery complex the saints provided cures. As mentioned above, not all cults followed the typical format of having the shrine located within the monastic church, at least not for the duration of the cult. It is important to bear this in mind when considering those cults that behaved atypically, such as William's at Norwich.

That pilgrims, including cure-seekers, saw the shrines as the focus of their intercessory powers is reflected in their unsurprising desire for closeness, as the miracles reflect (Table 6.1). Only a handful of cures occurred elsewhere within the monasteries, emphasising that cure-seekers' presence was focused on, and encouraged at, the shrines. This was a location in which lay devotion was expected and accepted and in which, for many cults, the presence of the laity would prove to be of minimal disruption.

Table 6.1. Locations of the cure-seekers at the time of their miraculous cure[*]

	M. Swithuni	M. Dunstani	L. Eliensis	M. Moduenne	M. Willelmi	M. Æbbe	M. Jacobi	Total
At the cult centre								
At the shrine	25	13	11	0	57	28	2	136
Within the church	10	0	4	12	1	6	9	42
Within another church building	1	1	0	0	0	0	0	2
Within the grounds	0	0	1	1	3	6	2	13
At an external location								
At home	4	3	3	0	18	0	5	33
Within another church	5	0	0	0	0	0	1	6
Other identifiable location	2	1	4	0	2	0	1	10
Unclear or unspecified location	3	3	3	0	3	2	4	18

* Regarding Æbbe's cure-seekers, 'at the shrine' is used to refer to the oratory at Kirk Hill; 'within the church' refers to the church at Coldingham Priory; and 'within the grounds' refers to external locations at both sites. For further, detailed analysis of the locations of Æbbe's cure-seekers see Salter, 'Beyond the *Miracula*', table 4.

The shrines also proved important to those who travelled to fulfil vows after their cure. Edward Haver was close to death from 'febris sinocha' ('a continuous fever').[48] After being cured through drinking the water of St James (water in which the relic had been immersed), Edward came to the abbey with his daughter, who had also recovered from the fever, and both presented votives at the shrine and offered their thanks to God and St James.[49] In accounts of young children too ill to leave home, it was the parents who visited the shrine on their behalf. When William Polcehart and his wife offered a candle the size of their son at William's shrine, their son was immediately cured.[50]

Proximity to the relics was recognised as an important aspect of the process of miraculous cure, as was prolonged proximity for those not cured immediately on arrival. The miracle reports contain records of devotees who spent extended periods of time in prayer at the shrine, including the aforementioned woman from Aycliffe.[51] As Emma Wells has discussed, devotion at the shrines was an extremely physical affair, with pilgrims not only spending extended periods of time at the shrines but also kissing and touching them.[52] The importance of prolonged and yet personal proximity to relics was such that shrines were increasingly designed with apertures and other aids to access. Surviving tombs, such as that of St Osmund at Salisbury Cathedral, include openings along their length that would have allowed for cure-seekers to reach into these saintly spaces. Matthew Paris's *Vita S. Eduardi, Regis et Confessoris* depicts pilgrims getting as close as possible to the relics of the canonised king in Westminster Abbey, with one devotee seemingly inside the tomb.[53] The patient crowd, illustrated to the right, wait for their turn and act as witnesses to the miracle granted to a kneeling male visitor.

York Minster's fifteenth-century stained glass at William of York's shrine similarly shows pilgrim engagement: one window depicts cure-seekers reaching to collect the holy oil that the tomb secreted, another shows a cure-seeker presenting a foot-shaped votive at the shrine.[54] With the presence of both

---

[48] M. Jacobi, fol. 172ra–b; Kemp, '*The Hand of St James*' V, 8. Kemp translates 'sinocha' as 'hectic' in his translation but 'continuous' is more faithful to the Latin.

[49] M. Jacobi, fol. 172rb; Kemp, '*The Hand of St James*' VI, 8.

[50] Thomas of Monmouth, M. Willelmi V.18, ed. Jessop and James, pp. 209–10.

[51] M. Æbbe IV.38, ed. Bartlett, pp. 64–5.

[52] E. J. Wells, 'Making "Sense" of the Pilgrimage Experience of the Medieval Church', *Peregrinations: Journal of Medieval Art and Architecture* 3 (2011), 122–46 (122, 135, 142).

[53] Matthew Paris, *Vita S. Eduardi, Regis et Confessoris*, Cambridge, CUL, MS Ee.3.59, fol. 33r.

[54] T. French, *York Minster: The St William Window*, Corpus vitrearum Medii Aevi (Great Britain) Summary Catalogue 5 (Oxford, 2000), plate 12. Also see T. French,

monks and laypeople at the shrine in mind, the miniature from Paris's *Vita S. Eduardi* is also noteworthy for its inclusion of a shrine-keeper.[55] This monk is not presented as actively policing the shrine or surrounding area but sits observing the pilgrims with hands raised to his face in awe. Seated in authority, but attentively watching the shrine with a manuscript open in front of him, the shrine-keeper is shown to have no qualms over the presence of the laity, both men and women, and their entry into the openings beneath Edward's tomb.

Women appear as welcome as men at most shrines promoted in these visual materials as well as the miracle accounts, and they were clearly as interested in securing physical closeness to the saints. Cuthbert's cult at Durham Cathedral however sits in contrast to this. Developing in the late eleventh century, but with justification reaching back to Cuthbert's dismay over *Coludi urbs*'s fall after Æbbe's death, Durham (under the guise of Cuthbert's wishes) banned women from entering the majority of the cathedral complex, including the church itself.[56] Such actions though were not the norm and many monasteries welcomed women as cure-seekers and as possible patrons. Lady Mabel de Bec was one such benefactor at Norwich. She was rewarded by being permitted to take part of William's tomb slab away with her in order that she and her family might benefit from its efficacy in times of poor health by mixing scrapings from the stone with holy water to produce a thaumaturgic drink.[57] The presence of women at shrines was clearly a generally established and accepted practice. The women recorded as having visited our case-study shrines appear to have enjoyed full and equal access to the saints with their male counterparts. But what could a visitor expect of these shrine spaces?

The Shrine Spaces

Screens such as the above-mentioned one Walpole ordered Ely to erect developed in the later Middle Ages. Nicola Coldstream has shown that earlier screens were much less invasive.[58] Over time, screens became more robust and minimised the visibility previously afforded to the laity. The laity of the earlier and high Middle Ages, including cure-seekers, would have been able

'The St William Window, York Minster', *British Academy Review* 3 (2000), 28, <https://www.thebritishacademy.ac.uk/documents/1586/ba-review03.pdf> [accessed October 2020].

55   Matthew Paris, *Vita S. Eduardi*, fol. 33r.

56   Symeon of Durham, *Libellus de exordio* II.7, ed. Rollason, pp. 104–8; V. Tudor, 'The Misogyny of Saint Cuthbert', *Archaeologia Aeliana*, 5th series 12 (1984), 157–67.

57   Thomas of Monmouth, *M. Willelmi* III.11, ed. Jessop and James, pp. 135–6.

58   N. Coldstream, *Medieval Architecture*, Oxford History of Art (Oxford, 2002), p. 139.

to see into the heart of the church, to the altar and choir, and to the monastic community's daily prayers, even if they could not physically enter these areas.

It is difficult to say for certain what the ambient environment of our seven shrines would have been like in the twelfth century. Later changes within these spaces (especially the destruction of shrines in the sixteenth century) have had an irreversible impact. There was no singular location for shrine placement, as noted in the cases of Æbbe and William, but there was a recognition that the east end of the church, in line with the orientation towards Jerusalem, was the more holy.[59] However, there are certain features that would have been common to a number of shrines, such as the presence of coverings on the altars or tomb-shrines, and the candles donated by those hopeful of engaging the saints, or thanking them for aid already provided. At wealthier institutions the furnishings were often of the highest quality.[60]

Medieval terminology rarely details the size of the shrine.[61] Nevertheless, the appearance of the shrine itself would have been dependent on whether this was a tomb-shrine or a smaller reliquary (in which perhaps only part of the saint was housed). Of our seven monasteries only one institution, Reading Abbey, did not claim to have the tomb of their cult saint. Nevertheless, as a royal donation and an apostolic saint, the shrine for St James was likely impressive. While M. Jacobi indicates that the relic was not accessible at the shrine, the account of Reading-local William's cure from paralysis records that there was an image of the saint on the altar.[62] Due to the poor survival of Reading Abbey the precise location of James's shrine within the abbey church cannot be known, yet Ronald Baxter has suggested it was possibly located in the inner south transept chapel.[63] Even at the cult centres that did house the saints' tombs, however, it was possible that smaller shrines might be established, Æbbe's oratory at Kirk Hill being a key example. Tomb-shrines, naturally, were less portable, often fixed, features that influenced not just the architecture of the churches but also the use of the space by the monastic community and visitors to the shrine.[64] Consequently, great thought had to be given to how to best balance the use of these spaces.

---

[59] Bartlett, *Why Can the Dead Do Such Great Things?*, p. 253. For further discussion of shrine location see B. Nilson, *Cathedral Shrines of Medieval England* (Woodbridge, 2001), pp. 63–81.

[60] Bartlett, *Why Can the Dead Do Such Great Things?*, p. 254.

[61] Ibid., p. 265.

[62] *M. Jacobi*, fols. 173rb; Kemp, 'The Hand of St James' XIII, 11.

[63] Baxter, *The Royal Abbey of Reading*, p. 209.

[64] Bartlett, *Why Can the Dead Do Such Great Things?*, p. 253.

Well-planned placement of shrines could filter cure-seekers and pilgrims around the important sites within the monastic church, and the development of ambulatories in Gothic pilgrim churches during the twelfth century benefited this.[65] Within English establishments, as elsewhere, shrines were rarely at, or in, the high altars.[66] Rather, shrines tended to be placed east of the high altar, often in special chapels, accessed via the ambulatories, and separated from the monks' choir by a screen. The initial development of these new architectural features was in France, first at Saint-Denis, but a number of institutions in England had also adopted ambulatories and retro-choirs by the close of the twelfth century.[67] The major religious sites like Canterbury Cathedral increasingly required a solution to balance their duties of hospitality and their liturgical requirements.[68]

The development of retro-choirs and ambulatories in the twelfth century undoubtedly benefited the lay visitors as well as the monks by streamlining access to the shrines while providing the monks with their required seclusion for the performance of their daily offices.[69] For the cure-seekers, and other visitors, this process of moving through the church to a clearly designated location connected to their would-be saintly intercessor must have added to the sense that they were entering the home of the saint, from which emanated God's divine power. But were the shrines as accessible as the miracle reports suggest?

Open to All and Open All Hours?

The miracles imply that there were few restrictions on visiting shrines, or even on entering monasteries at all. However, it is worth noting that the later, fifteenth-century customary for Becket's shrine stipulated that two *feretrars* (shrine custodians) were to guard the shrine day and night and, when locking up during dinner-time, were to ensure that no thieves (or mad dogs) had stowed away there.[70] These custodians were also to be on hand to open the shrine to visitors (signalled with the ringing of a bell), to recite the canonical

---

[65]   R. A. Scott, *The Gothic Enterprise: A Guide to Understanding the Medieval Cathedral* (Berkeley, 2011), pp. 128–9.

[66]   Nilson, *Cathedral Shrines*, p. 66.

[67]   L. Grant, *Abbot Suger of St-Denis: Church and State in Early Twelfth-Century France*, Medieval World (London, 1998), pp. 272–3.

[68]   Fergusson, *Canterbury Cathedral Priory*, p. 1.

[69]   Grant, *Abbot Suger*, pp. 30–1, 247; Bartlett, *Why Can the Dead Do Such Great Things?*, p. 253.

[70]   London, British Library, Add. MS 59616, fols. 1r–11v, cited in Bartlett, *Why Can the Dead Do Such Great Things?*, p. 259.

hours and to celebrate the Mass of St Thomas there.[71] Indication that access to the shrines was not necessarily a full-time reality, and that the gates would close at certain times, can also be found in *M. Moduenne*. Prior Jordan recounted that he went to the gates of the monastery one night to find a French penitent pilgrim who wished to access Modwenna's shrine, a request that he granted.[72] There is no mention of a porter at Burton Abbey's gate or any suggestion that the man might have been refused entry. Yet, as per the *Regula S. Benedicti*, there would have been an *ostiarius* (porter) at the gate at all times to receive visitors.[73]

A rare account to directly acknowledge that access could be restricted can be found in the *Miracula S. Margarite Scotorum Regine*, produced *c.* 1240–70.[74] An English woman suffering from a large tumour came to Dunfermline following a vision of St Margaret, and after visiting many other shrines across Europe.[75] Arriving late on Palm Sunday, the woman requested permission to remain at the shrine overnight from 'exterioris ecclesie custode cleric quodam, Scotico quidem genere et nimis proteruo' ('the guardian of the outer church, a certain clerk who was a Scot by birth and a very impudent man').[76] He responded violently and insisted she could not enter the 'sacris edibus' ('holy precincts') alone but only on 'noctibus semper singula sabbata precedentibus, in quibus maxima infirmancium multitudo uigilare solet' ('the ordained nights preceding each Saturday when a great crowd of sick people is accustomed to keep vigil').[77] Following the cleric's attempt to physically remove the woman, she prayed to God and Margaret for help before falling to the ground. After remaining like this for an hour, her health was restored.[78] No mention is made of what happened to the cleric or whether his refusal was an abbey policy or his own initiative. However, at Dunfermline, in the mid-thirteenth century, some officials were attempting to limit cure-seekers' access to the shrine. Similarly evident is that *M. Margarite*'s hagiographer thought little of this cleric; although whether this was due to his treatment of visitors or his nationality is

[71] Bartlett, *Why Can the Dead Do Such Great Things?*, p. 259.

[72] Geoffrey of Burton, *M. Moduenne* 51, ed. Bartlett, pp. 216–19. Also see above, pp. 134–5.

[73] *Regula S. Benedicti* 66, ed. McCann, pp. 152–3.

[74] *Miracula S. Margarite Scotorum Regine* (hereafter *M. Margarite*), in *M. Æbbe of Coldingham and Margaret of Scotland*, ed. R. Bartlett, OMT (Oxford, 2006), pp. 69–145.

[75] Ibid., 1, pp. 70–5.

[76] Ibid., pp. 74–5.

[77] Ibid.

[78] Ibid.

unclear. Importantly, Margaret's positive and welcoming response to the sick woman was promoted as triumphing over the cleric's officious enforcement.

If the above account is correct in stating that Dunfermline only granted overnight access to the laity on Friday evenings, there is another question to consider: how would a cure-seeker, especially one coming from some distance, know if admittance would be granted on their arrival? Considering this occurred on Palm Sunday, a major feast in the liturgical calendar, it is particularly surprising that a pilgrim would be turned away and it is possible that the woman had deliberately chosen this date owing to the likelihood of being granted access. This account thus raises questions of whether cure-seekers generally had to show patience and wait for an appropriate time to be admitted. The miracle accounts indicate that there were no uniform rules regarding the admittance of cure-seekers. Limiting access to cure-seekers, and other visitors, would have potentially impacted any financial benefits that might come to the monasteries.[79] Strikingly, *M. Margarite* records no further incidents of refused admittance; later in *M. Margarite* both a local blind woman and a woman with a stomach tumour partook in overnight prayers and vigils at the shrine.[80] Possibly the first account was a one-off example of an individual attempting to regulate access, or perhaps the resulting miracle revised attitudes at Dunfermline. Certainly, in the rest of *M. Margarite*, Dunfermline is shown to recognise the importance of lay visitors, and approves of their partaking in vigils, including nocturnal ones.

Within the seven case-study *miracula*, there is a single account that reflects a similar series of events to *M. Margarite*. A poor man from Northamptonshire who suffered from a long-term illness arrived at Ely at 'hora, qua cotidiana alimenta fratres et refectionem corporis percipere invitarentur' ('the hour when the brothers were invited to take their daily food and refreshment of the body').[81] At this point in the day, *L. Eliensis* notes, 'quando maxime introitus et exitus obserari solent et custodiri' ('the entrances and exits are customarily bolted and kept under guard').[82] The man thus found his entrance refused by a guard who even 'ei alapam dedit et abire precepit' ('gave him a slap and told him to go away').[83] The man continued pleading and requested that he be allowed to at least go to Æthelthryth's spring. The guard continued to

---

[79] Regarding the shrines as sources of revenue, see Nilson, *Cathedral Shrines*, pp. 134–43, 182–5.

[80] *M. Margarite* 3–4, ed. Bartlett, pp. 78–83.

[81] *L. Eliensis* III.116, ed. Blake, p. 366, trans. Fairweather, p. 451.

[82] Ibid.

[83] Ibid.

refuse but also began to fear that 'tamen quia peregrinum offenderat' ('he had behaved offensively to the pilgrim') and that the monks would be displeased if news reached them.[84] Eventually, despite the guard's actions, the man was able to drink from the spring and gained his desired cure. *L. Eliensis* here implies that this over-zealous guarding would not have been supported by the monastic community itself, suggesting this was not a general policy. The indication in *L. Eliensis* is that cure-seekers should be welcomed even when the gates were closed, and it has more in common with Jordan's admitting of the French penitent in *M. Moduenne*, than with the cleric in *M. Margarite*. The shrines appear to have been widely accessible, with conflict arising only if lay presence risked distracting the monks from their religious calling. Additionally, the miracles represent the shrines not just as open to anyone, but at any time, with many cure-seekers undertaking overnight vigils as part of the healing process. But was access really as unlimited as the miracles tend to represent?

Unlimited Access?

Saints did not always act immediately on the cure-seeker's request, and the miracle reports indicate that many cure-seekers spent hours at the shrine. A number even kept vigil overnight, occasionally staying longer still in their hope for a cure. Furthermore, hagiographers often indicated that this was no solitary undertaking, rather the shrines might be frequented by crowds of people. These assembled crowds bore witness to the miracle's occurrence. Their presence also alluded to the fact that the shrines were always open to all who wished to visit. In short, miracle accounts imply that monastic institutions took an extremely relaxed, open-door policy to when, and how many, laypeople could visit these sites.

The evidence implies that cure-seekers expected to spend time in prayer and vigil, and that overnight stays were not uncommon, leading to the necessity for overnight wardens.[85] But what was such an experience like, and how easy was it to obtain permission to remain in vigil throughout the night? Was permission even required, and if so, how willingly was it granted? As the accounts in *M. Margarite* and *L. Eliensis* illustrated, certain establishments, or at least certain officials, were less willing to welcome the laity at times, but generally

---

[84]   Ibid., pp. 451–2.

[85]   D. Knowles, *The Monastic Order in England: A History of Its Development from the Times of St Dunstan to the Fourth Lateran Council, 940–1216*, 2nd edn (Cambridge, 1963), p. 481.

the miracles remain silent on this.[86] Reading's preferential treatment of the nobility is recorded in *M. Jacobi*'s account of the woman from Collingbourne who was able to view the hand of St James only because her arrival coincided with that of William, second earl of Gloucester.[87] As noted, St James's relic was often not accessible to the public, nevertheless the shrine itself is shown to have been open.

Reading might have been cautious about permitting access to the relic, but James's shrine itself appears as open and accessible as any other shrine, with cure-seekers remaining overnight and visiting in crowds. The crowds recorded in many miraculous healings are relatively inactive and provide only a back-drop for the account. *L. Eliensis*, however, offers insight into the actions of such crowds of devotees in recounting the cure of a blind woman.[88] The woman from Cottenham had been blind for four years and spent the night in prayer, recovering her sight at dawn. Those who were nearby tested her regained eye-sight and 'proiecti sunt ei oboli et quadrantes diversi nummismatis, quorum caracteres ipsa certissime [. . .] distinguebat' ('half-pennies were thrown at her, and farthing-pieces of different mintings, the embossed designs of which she would distinguish between with complete certainty').[89] Her ability to identify the coins thrown by the crowds proved the cure and, following this, 'clerus et populus' ('the clergy and people') both sang in commendation.[90] Importantly, the crowd was proactive in verifying the miracle and celebrating the cure, with the latter uniting the laity and the clergy. The timing of this account is very precisely given as the night of Æthelthryth's feast, an important date in Ely's calendar and one on which lay presence was possibly less restricted than usual. The reference to the assembled crowd having half-pennies and farthings indicates that these were people ready with monetary donations for Æthelthryth's cult and church, while the various mintings of the coins could suggest that this event had drawn some cure-seekers and pilgrims from further afield.

A similar account, albeit replacing coins with apples, was recorded by Eadmer. A poor woman had brought her young, blind daughter to Dun-stan's shrine, and spent many days in vigil, pleading with the Christ Church monks to assist with their prayers.[91] After ten days, her daughter began to

---

86   *M. Margarite* 1, ed. Bartlett, pp. 70–5; *L. Eliensis* III.116, ed. Blake, pp. 365–6, trans. Fairweather, pp. 450–2.

87   *M. Jacobi*, fol. 173ra; Kemp, '*The Hand of St James*' XI, 10–11. Also see above, p. 136.

88   *L. Eliensis* III.57, ed. Blake, p. 305, trans. Fairweather, p. 373.

89   Ibid.

90   Ibid.

91   Eadmer of Canterbury, *M. Dunstani* 6, ed. Turner and Muir, pp. 164–5.

see, telling her mother that Dunstan had instructed her to look at all the beautiful things around her. News of the cure spread through the church, drawing a celebratory crowd. Some of the crowd threw apples on to the paving stones 'an ea more paruulorum directo gressu comprehendere posset' ('hoping to determine if the little girl could chase after them as children do').[92] The girl saw the apples and ran to collect them before returning to her mother, thus confirming the miracle.

The hagiographic depiction of cure-seekers spending the night in constant vigil at the tomb also accentuates the difference between them and other guests of the monasteries who might have required accommodation in the *hospitium* or the superior's lodgings. There would have been advantages and disadvantages to the monasteries in these instances. Although those desiring a cure focused their attention on the shrine, possibly forgoing the provision of sustenance or a bed for the night, especially during major festivities, these locations within the church might well become overcrowded with devotees, as in an instance recounted by Suger of Saint-Denis (d. 1151) that occurred prior to his enlargement of the abbey church.[93] Controlling these crowds was not without its difficulties, as Peter the Venerable discovered, complaining that Cluny's openness had resulted in the disruption of the monks' spiritual life and had caused the cloister to become akin to a public street.[94] While he acknowledged that the laity had the right to visit parts of Cluny, and attend some services, Peter resolved to return certain areas of the precinct to the sole use of the monks.[95]

As Benedictine establishments were primarily independent, the way our cult centres dealt with the presence of the laity would have been particular to not only the locations but the wishes of their superiors. A cure-seeker might spend no more than one night in prayer and vigil or, if the saint was less forthcoming with results, multiple days and nights might be spent at the tomb. One man spent three days at St Abb's Head before his eyesight was restored with

---

[92] Ibid.

[93] Suger of Saint-Denis, *On the Abbey Church of St Denis and Its Art Treasures*, ed. and trans. E. Panofsky, 2nd edn (Princeton, 1979), pp. 88–9. Also see Kerr, 'Health and Safety', 12–13.

[94] Peter the Venerable 'Statute 23', cited in G. Constable, 'The Monastic Policy of Peter the Venerable', in *Pierre Abélard – Pierre le Vénérable. Les courants philosophiques, littéraires et artistiques en Occident au milieu du XIIe siècle. Abbaye de Cluny, 2–9 julliet 1972*, Colloques internationaux du Centre national de la recherche scientifique 546 (Paris, 1975), pp. 119–38 (134).

[95] Ibid.

the curative waters of Æbbe's fountain.[96] *M. Dunstani* records the arrival of a man with lower body paralysis on Good Friday who was cured via a stretching of the sinews on Easter Sunday.[97] A local pensioner spent four days in prayer to Modwenna before being healed of his paralysis.[98]

Hagiographies were, understandably, keen to promote the openness of the shrines, and it is important that this is not forgotten when reading these materials. That the miracles, like that of the Cottenham woman cured at Ely, occurred during important feasts, when the policy towards lay presence might be more relaxed, is worth noting.[99] Similarly, in *M. Jacobi* a Reading boy named William was cured of paralysis when 'annua deuotione populus ad ecclesiam congregatur' ('the people had assembled in the church in their annual devotion') on Christmas Eve.[100] Nevertheless, the majority of the miracles do not refer to specific feasts, implying that cure-seekers were welcomed at any time of the year. After all, a hagiographer would be likely to mention a major liturgical event if a miracle coincided with its celebration. The miracle accounts, unsurprisingly, represent the overall approach at the shrine as cordial, regardless of the number of cure-seekers or pilgrims, and regardless of the time of day. This convivial approach is further emphasised by the fact that some members of the local lay community developed strong relationships with the monastic community, highlighting that monastic care went beyond the shrines.

Developing Relationships

Although not always explicitly stated in the miracles, some lay cure-seekers must have been known to the cult-centre communities owing to their persistent visits to the shrine, or because they were recipients of alms. The importance of pre-existing, long-term relationships should not be underestimated. Through observing afflicted persons at the shrines, as well as through their charitable acts, it is easy to see how the monks would have felt sympathy and compassion towards cure-seekers, and cure-seekers would have surely valued the care they received through monastic charity.

[96]   *M. Æbbe* IV.27, ed. Bartlett, pp. 58–9.
[97]   Eadmer of Canterbury, *M. Dunstani* 15, ed. Turner and Muir, pp. 176–7.
[98]   Geoffrey of Burton, *M. Moduenne* 45, ed. Bartlett, pp. 184–7. Also see pp. 115, 170.
[99]   *L. Eliensis* III.57, ed. Blake, p. 305, trans. Fairweather, p. 373; Eadmer of Canterbury, *M. Dunstani* 15, ed. Turner and Muir, pp. 176–7.
[100] *M. Jacobi*, fol. 173rb; Kemp, '*The Hand of St James*' XIII, 11.

That monastic communities responded sympathetically to cure-seekers has already been noted in the case of the woman from Aycliffe cured by Æbbe.[101] The Lothian musician who, before Æbbe cured his gout, had been taken in by the prior and had spent four months at Coldingham recovering from the effects of famine found the monks similarly supportive.[102] One poor woman, paralysed in her lower body, was well known to the Burton monks and was 'in cenobio sustentabatur' ('supported in the monastery').[103] A regular visitor to the abbey church, she often spent the night in prayer there in the hope of securing Modwenna's intercession. On the anniversary of Modwenna's translation she was finally cured and the miracle was celebrated by those present, causing Abbot Nigel to cry for joy when it was reported to him the next day.[104] Owing to this change in her circumstances, however, her clothes were now too short and, now able to stand, 'erat nudata pars interior corporis indecenti aspectu' ('the inner part of her body was laid bare in an indecent way').[105] This resulted in Nigel ordering new clothes for her. The celebrations of those present, and Abbot Nigel's continued charity to the woman after her cure, suggest an invested interest of both the monastic and local lay community in this woman's change of fortunes.

Accounts such as these emphasise the relationship that could develop between lay cure-seekers and the monastic communities. The monks are shown to have been concerned with the health of those who sought cure and prepared to engage with visitors. Indeed, the accounts of the Aycliffe and Burton women also reveal that male monastic communities charitably, and even affectionately, supported laywomen. This is worth keeping in mind when contrasted with the concerns shown in Walpole's later regulations for Ely regarding female presence within the priory.[106] Although it is worth emphasising that Walpole did not attempt to limit access to Æthelthryth's shrine, rather he did not wish for devotees from the shrine to traverse into the vestry or beyond into the cloister. Nevertheless, monastic communities were clearly observant of, and attentive to, the cure-seekers who came to the shrines and responded charitably and compassionately to their presence.

Occasionally the long-term compassion from, and care provided by, the monasteries could spread over several years. *M. Swithuni* provides a memorable

---

[101] *M. Æbbe* IV.38, ed. Bartlett, pp. 64–5.

[102] Ibid., IV.6, pp. 38–41.

[103] Geoffrey of Burton, *M. Moduenne* 48, ed. Bartlett, pp. 198–9.

[104] Ibid., pp. 200–1.

[105] Ibid.

[106] *The Statutes of Bishop Ralph of Walpole, 1300* 13, 39, ed. Evans, pp. 11, 23.

example of this in the eventual cure of a deaf and mute boy who, before being taken in by the cathedral priory's almoner, had had to support himself by begging in the city.[107] While little is disclosed of the boy's life preceding his admittance by the almoner to the 'domo pauperum' ('poor house'), the account implies that he had little or no family as he depended on the monks for some years prior to receiving his cure.[108] The boy, who could only communicate through signs and gestures, 'in domo et curia fratrum diu conuersatus et diuturna conuersatione probatus' ('lived for a long time in the house and courtyard of the monks and through his daily presence was accepted by them').[109] No explanation was provided for the boy's continued presence within the priory, but it is clear that the monks had no issue with his residing among them. Yet, *M. Swithuni* makes no suggestion that the boy officially joined the monastic community either. During this time, the boy must have developed strong relationships with at least some of the monks, such as the almoner. This account from *M. Swithuni*, as also those from *M. Æbbe* and *M. Moduenne*, is indicative of the hospitable reception cure-seekers could expect from their monastic hosts.

The Miraculous Cure

For the most part, cure-seekers appear to have been well-received in the cult centres, and welcome to remain for as long as necessary in order to secure their healing miracle. But what of the miracle itself? Accounts vary greatly in their reporting of the moment of cure. Some provide a clear sense that the cure-seeker perceived they were visited by the saint, in other instances they woke having been cured, while some even appear to be healed with little more than their prayers or vows. The saints might interact with the cure-seeker but the miracles also record accounts where healing is brought about without the saints directly engaging with them. As there was not one expected format in which miracle healing might be bestowed, it is worth returning to some of the cure-seekers recorded in the seven *miracula*, to consider their experiences of securing their desired remedy.

On their eventual arrival at Swithun's shrine, the three blind women from the Isle of Wight who had been abandoned on the mainland by their neighbours, and the deaf man who guided them to Winchester, found their cure 'sine omni dilatione' ('without any delay') on praying to the saintly bishop.[110]

[107] *M. Swithuni* 52, ed. Lapidge, pp. 684–7.

[108] Ibid., pp. 684–5.

[109] Ibid., pp. 686–7.

[110] Ibid., 6, pp. 654–5.

The son of Gurwan the tanner in Norwich, who had been ill for eighteen weeks, and to whom a woman from London had relayed William's message of recovery, experienced a 'festina [. . .] incolumitate' ('speedy restoration') of his health after his parents had delivered a candle to William's shrine.[111] Gurwan and his wife, who acted on behalf of their child, had also been instructed by the boy-martyr that they were to donate a candle to William's shrine every year for the prolonged health of their son. In both of these instances the act of prayer, and in the latter case the donation of a candle, was enough to result in the recovery of the cure-seeker. Gurwan's obligation to make an annual donation to William's shrine is an unusual addition that highlights that longer-term connections could arise between the cure-seeker and the saint.

Alditha, widow of Toke, had become isolated due to her increasing deafness, and feared other people's reactions to her impairment.[112] Having been cured of an illness through William's merits before, she turned her attention to the boy-martyr again and brought a candle to his tomb.[113] Having prayed at the tomb for some time, she was 'fidei tacta feruore aures utrasque quo sepulchrum tegebatur oppleuit pallio' ('stung by the fervour of faith, she stopped both her ears with the cloth that covered the tomb'); and Alditha instantly recovered her hearing.[114] Raven, a blind beggar from Tutbury, was drawn to Burton and Modwenna's shrine on hearing the big bell of the abbey.[115] Arriving with his guide, Raven prostrated himself in prayer requesting Modwenna to pity him. After some time, Raven 'raptus est subito tanquam in mentis excessum' ('was suddenly seized by a kind of trance'), and a beautiful nun appeared in front of him.[116] The nun, Modwenna, 'que manica uestis sue ambos oculos eius tetigit et confestim cecitatem' ('touched both his eyes with the sleeve of her garment, immediately wiping away his blindness').[117] Alditha and Raven were cured through different methods, both having engaged with the saint or their shrine. That some occasions resulted in direct interaction with the saint is intriguing, but there is also something poetic in the wiping away of blindness or, as in the previously mentioned case from *M. Dunstani*, the saint commanding the blind

---

[111] Thomas of Monmouth, *M. Willelmi* IV.2, ed. Jessop and James, p. 167. Also see above, p. 186.

[112] Ibid., V.23, pp. 217–18. Also see above, p. 116.

[113] Ibid., III.14, V.23, pp. 147, 218.

[114] Ibid., V.23, p. 218.

[115] Geoffrey of Burton, *M. Moduenne* 45, ed. Bartlett, pp. 186–9. Also see above, p. 80.

[116] Ibid., pp. 186–7.

[117] Ibid.

to see.[118] These interactions reflect the saints' Christ-like qualities of care and cure, as per the Gospels' description of Christ's healing miracles.[119]

Not all miracle cures were so peacefully obtained. The paralysed man from the Edinburgh area, who had applied fire and iron to his body to cure his impairment, came to Kirk Hill after having no luck at Canterbury or other shrines.[120] The two-mile journey from Coldingham to the oratory took him a day to complete because of his impairment and, owing to his tiredness, he fell asleep on arrival. Æbbe appeared and 'loca dolorum manibus explorans fortiter attrectauit' ('explored with her hands the places where he felt pain, touching them quite roughly').[121] This caused the man to cry and he later told the monks that he felt 'tantum inde paciebatur angustie acsi membrum aliquid auulsum fuisset e corpore' ('so much anguish as if a limb had been wrenched from his body').[122] The man spent the next day in vigil, waking from sleep the second night to find himself fully cured. No mention was made of Æbbe visiting him for a second time. This cure-seeker was not alone in receiving slightly rougher hands-on care from Æbbe. Her *miracula* also records mute cure-seekers whose tongues were touched or pulled by the saint to loosen them.[123] The discomfort felt by these cure-seekers, it should be noted, was fleeting and acted as a sign of transformation from the impaired to healthy body, and thus a marker of the saint's intercession.

Ysembela, the paralysed girl whom St James instructed to come to his shrine, had a similarly turbulent experience on her eventual arrival at Reading. James was not recorded as having directly engaged with her at the abbey, but 'est super eam manus domini et anxiatus est in ea spiritus eius' ('the Lord came upon her and his Spirit was troubled within her').[124] Ysembela 'pauimentum corruit et in uocem clamoremque acutissimum prorumpens usquequaque ingemuit' ('threw herself on the pavement and, letting out the most piercing cries, screamed in all directions').[125] For three hours, she shook her hair, and 'capud contudit corpus que suum ita absque sui respectu ad petram elisit'

---

[118] Eadmer of Canterbury, *M. Dunstani* 6, ed. Turner and Muir, pp. 164–5.

[119] Mark 8.22–6; Luke 4.38–9.

[120] *M. Æbbe* IV.5, ed. Bartlett, pp. 36–9. Also see above, pp. 85–5, 169.

[121] Ibid., pp. 38–9.

[122] Ibid.

[123] For example: *M. Æbbe* IV.10, ed. Bartlett, pp. 48–9. For further discussion see Salter, 'Beyond the *Miracula*'.

[124] *M. Jacobi*, fol. 174va; Kemp, 'The Hand of St James' XX, 15.

[125] Ibid.

('banged her head and dashed her body against the stone').[126] *M. Jacobi's* author recorded that it was as if 'se ipsam uelle conterere' ('she wished to destroy herself').[127] After this time, Ysembela recovered and was moved away from the shrine, presumably by the monks, and taken to the altar of Mary Magdalen. Tired from her struggles she slept, and on waking expelled a 'uirus sanguineus' ('bloody poison') and vomited blood until 'humor qui nocuerat' ('the humour which had harmed her') had been fully expelled.[128] As no mention of ingesting any poison was made in recording the cause of Ysembela's impairment – sleeping outside one summer's night – it is unclear how this bad *humor* was connected to her paralysis. But it is evident that this visceral reaction was taken as a visible sign of the conclusion to her suffering.

Alice, like Ysembela, had suffered from a partial paralysis when her arm had fused to her chest (she had additionally experienced temporary insanity).[129] Having had no luck at other shrines, Alice eventually came to Reading where she spent six days in prayer before, disheartened, she decided to return home. James appeared to Alice, forestalling her departure; she then bought a candle and returned to the church where she told the sacrist of her vision. After mass, William, the sub-prior, brought the reliquary containing James's hand to Alice and held it over her arm that 'aruerat' ('had withered'), while another monk, Nicholas, poured water over the relic and bathed her arm.[130] Immediately Alice began to recover and over the course of the next few hours her pain intensified until her arm was loosened. *M. Jacobi* comments that 'cutis a costis auulsa adhuc ex brachio dependebat' ('the skin had been torn from her ribs and was still hanging down from her arm'), and her arm 'plurimum fetebat et dolebat nimis que intumescebat' ('smelt and ached badly and became very swollen').[131] Eventually, Alice completely recovered and, grateful for James's aid, she took a position serving the abbey as a laundress.

There was not one single process through which miraculous healing was experienced. For some the process was sudden, for others it took more time and discomfort. What is important in these accounts, however, is that there was a perceived change in the body's health, and this change was noticed not just by the cure-seekers but by others who were present within these spaces. Those, like the Edinburgh man and Ysembela, whose cure resulted in physical

[126] Ibid.

[127] Ibid.

[128] Ibid. It should be noted that Kemp translated *humor* as fluid rather than humour.

[129] *M. Jacobi*, fol. 172rb–172vb; Kemp, '*The Hand of St James*' VIII, 9–10.

[130] Ibid.

[131] *M. Jacobi*, fol. 172vb; Kemp, '*The Hand of St James*' VIII, 9.

reactions undoubtedly drew the attention of others present who could attest to seeing saintly healing at work. What is more, these visible reactions to healing add a sensory and corporeal facet to the experiences of the shrines. These were not necessarily quiet places of contemplation; the shrines also became active sites of healing experienced not just by the cure-seeker but by any who witnessed the process.

When petitioning the saint, or after receiving their healing, many cure-seekers also left donations at the shrines. In some instances, as illustrated in the case of the Cottenham woman, these donations might be monetary, but more frequently they would have been offerings, like the candle brought by Gurwan and his wife. *M. Willelmi*, it should be noted, is particularly illustrative of such donations, with Thomas of Monmouth commenting that William had a particular love of candles because he was born on Candlemas.[132] Other cure-seekers left markers of their previous affliction including crutches that were no longer needed as mobility aids.[133] Canes and crutches are still to be found at shrines today, with St Winifred's Well, Oswestry, offering a British example of this continued practice.[134] Such donations would have been visible evidence of previous successful cures and must have instilled hope in subsequent cure-seekers that they too could obtain the healing they desired. That mementoes like these would have been left behind is a reminder of the multi-sensory nature of the shrines: the sounds of praying monks and pilgrims would have combined with the smell of the burning candles and incense, and visually, the decorated shrines, stained glass, and symbols of previous successes like the crutches would have added to the evocative nature of these spaces.[135]

What happened after the cure and when the cure-seeker returned home? Miracle accounts seldom provide an answer but it is worth considering the nature of the healing miracle and what this meant for the individual who believed they had benefited from the saint's assistance. Benedict of Peterborough's miracles for Thomas Becket are unusual for including seemingly less successful cure-seekers.[136] However, as Finucane asked, what would medieval

[132] Thomas of Monmouth, *M. Willelmi* III.12, ed. Jessop and James, p. 138.

[133] Ibid., VII.11, p. 271.

[134] 'Winifride (Wenefred, Gwenfrewi) (7th century)', in *ODS*, pp. 408–9.

[135] For further discussion of the shrines as multi-sensory spaces, see Wells, 'Making "Sense" of the Pilgrimage Experience', 122–46.

[136] For examples, see Benedict of Peterborough, *Miracula Sancti Thomae Cantuariensis* II.17, IV.3, in *Materials for the History of Thomas Becket, Archbishop of Canterbury*, ed. J. C. Robertson, 7 vols (London, 1875–85), II (1876), 21–281 (67–8, 182–3). Also see Koopmans, *Wonderful to Relate*, pp. 165–6.

cure-seekers consider to have been 'a cure'?[137] Would this have been a full
return to good health, the partial remission of the former complaint, or an
easing of any accompanying discomfort? Cures did not have to be a complete
return to health, nor did they necessarily have to be permanent.[138] Relapses of
the complaint could occur, but when such occurrences appear in the miracles
they are explained away as being due to a reliance on secular medicine, or the
failure to fulfil a vow to come to the shrine.[139] *M. Dunstani* even includes an
account of a previously-paralysed priest who, having been healed by Dunstan,
suffered a fatal return of his complaint after claiming Dunstan had had no
part in his cure.[140] Retrospectively, we might be tempted to argue that this
priest was never actually cured; however, such an approach does not aid us
in understanding medieval experiences nor does it take into account the perceived religious aspect of such cures (or punishments).[141] When considering
the experiences of our cure-seekers, it is worth acknowledging that they would
have perceived themselves to have been the recipients of a healing miracle.

*   *   *

The hagiographies imply that, in the twelfth century, shrines were always open
and welcoming to those in search of saintly assistance. Cure-seekers coming to
Norwich Cathedral were even able to access William's shrine during the year
his tomb was in the chapter house. Finding regulation of lay access within hagiographical sources would be unusual, but would such 'openness' be expected
either? Whilst the shrines are depicted in the miracles as accessible for lay
devotion and prayers, the lack of references to strict monastic guardianship of
the shrines goes further than anticipated in showcasing the accessibility which
could be attained. Surviving visual resources support the 'lay-friendly' attitude
of the shrines in most institutions.

Analysis of where the laity sought and found cures further supports this by
revealing that cure-seekers not only wished to, but were predominantly able to,
petition the saint in as close a proximity to their shrines and earthly remains
as possible. A number of cure-seekers were only cured following a night of

---

[137] R. C. Finucane, 'The Use and Abuse of Medieval Miracles', *History* 60 (1975), 1–10
(8).

[138] Ibid.

[139] Thomas of Monmouth, *M. Willelmi* IV.9, ed. Jessop and James, pp. 174–7; *M. Jacobi*, fol. 174vb–175ra; Kemp, *'The Hand of St James'* XXII, 16.

[140] Eadmer of Canterbury, *M. Dunstani* 4, ed. Turner and Muir, pp. 162–3.

[141] McCleery, '"Christ More Powerful Than Galen?"', p. 143.

vigil, or even longer, suggesting an allowance and acceptance of their extended presence by monastic communities. Evidence of ecclesiastical intervention is rare within miracle reports, and images of the tombs, such as that in the *Vita S. Eduardi*, illustrate a relatively relaxed, and accepting, ecclesiastical approach to lay presence.

More important still is to recognise that, in references to apprehensions regarding lay access, the primary concern is not the presence of the laity but the disruption or deviation that this could cause for the monastic community. Nowhere is there the sense that lay presence would affect the sanctity of the shrine or monastery. Even Walpole's visitations do not suggest that all lay presence to the cloisters should be disallowed, and women might be permitted depending on occasion and social rank. Nor, when ordering the erection of a screen to the vestry, did Walpole prevent lay access to Æthelthryth's shrine. Here, as in the earlier *Regula S. Benedicti* and the regulations of the First Lateran Council, it is evident that concern rests upon the impact that lay presence, at a more pressing and practical level, might have on the brothers' monastic resolve.

When monks were witnesses to the petitions of cure-seekers, it is clear that they were compassionate and sympathetic to those who sought saintly intercession. The monastic communities were certainly not inattentive to the suffering of the laity, as the miracles confirm. The young deaf and mute boy remained for some time with Winchester's monastic community, and charity was shown at Burton to the cured woman who no longer fitted into her clothes. Whilst charity and hospitality were written into the *Regula S. Benedicti*, so was the idea that the monastic community should avoid excessive interaction with the temporal world. Yet the hagiographies suggest communities were not above providing help to those who needed assistance within the monasteries themselves. With such mixed messages of seclusion and inclusion it is perhaps no wonder that sources appear vague or conflicted on the issue of lay presence within monastic institutions. Finding a balance between welcoming hospitality and spiritual retreat within one space was no easy task.

What then of Æbbe's cult, with its dual locations two miles apart? It is easy to suggest that the development of the Kirk Hill oratory presented the Coldingham monks with an ideal solution to this issue of lay intrusion. However, while Æbbe's oratory was the prominent location for healing miracles, *M. Æbbe* reveals that both locations had a role to play in the pilgrimage process. Reporting the miracle at Coldingham Priory was the concluding feature of many accounts. The monks also visited the oratory and provided hospitality for cure-seekers in Coldingham itself, with the Lothian musician being cared for over a period of four months.

Guests to the monastery might also be cure-seekers, but for most cure-seekers it must be understood that the shrine was paramount. In finding a cure it was important for sufferers to make an association between themselves and the saint both through prayer and, where possible, through physical proximity, the importance of which was clearly recognised by monks and lay visitors. There was an innate sense of tangibility to the shrines, spaces where the temporal and divine coincided, and cure-seekers wished for contact not just in their supplications but in their cures; Alditha used the cloth that covered William's tomb to cure her deafness, and Edward Haver was cured (albeit before arriving at the shrine) after drinking water that had washed James's hand.

Although questions remain over the exact level of 'openness' allowed to the laity, these monastic communities found a balance between their duties of devotion and charity. This cannot have proved easy. This willingness to welcome cure-seekers suggests a recognition by the monks not just of cure-seekers' desires but also an understanding of the need to find cures for ill health, and the place of saintly intercession within the broader remit of high-medieval healthcare.

Conclusion

With the cure-seekers having arrived at the end of their journey for miraculous healing so this book comes to its conclusion. The journey taken by both the cure-seekers and this work began with the initial health complaint, the impairment or illness that drew these individuals to seek out saintly intercession. The journey then moved on, identifying who these cure-seekers were and what their experience of the road to recovery was like, before arriving at the shrines and the desired remedy. In taking this journey, this work set out to answer the questions of how cure-seekers experienced the miraculous cure-seeking process they undertook, and how the hagiographical materials presented healthcare.

Throughout this book consideration has been given to understanding the place of healing miracles within the broad spectrum of medieval healthcare that was on offer, and to investigating the experiences of those who sought remedy through the saints' intercession. The miracle accounts recorded in *miracula* provide an insight into these experiences of affliction and recovery that few other contemporary sources can. In using these materials, the research presented here has stood on the shoulders of giants in this field, including Finucane whose pivotal work also demonstrated the benefits of analysing posthumous hagiographies from a statistical standpoint.[1] Here, this methodology was combined with a focused case-study approach, as has also been taken by Yarrow and Trenery.[2] Concentrating on seven select texts, relating to what might best be termed localised saints' cults (in terms of their predominant popular appeal), has allowed for close engagement with a select group of cure-seekers whose quests for holy healing were recorded in these twelfth-century miracle accounts. This close analysis has additionally offered the opportunity to consider what the hagiographers (and the monastic communities more broadly) knew of ill health and healing, and the dynamic between the various avenues of healthcare.

To place miraculous healing within both its healthcare context, and the saints' cults within their monastic setting, Chapter 1 addressed the medical knowledge and remedial practices that were present within England. What

---

[1] Finucane, *Miracles and Pilgrims*; Finucane, *The Rescue of the Innocents*.
[2] Yarrow, *Saints and Their Communities*; Trenery, *Madness, Medicine and Miracle*.

were the alternative therapeutic avenues on offer, and where did healing mir-acles sit within this wider spectrum of healthcare? The surviving evidence of monastic book collections and library catalogues, especially with regard to the seven case-study cult centres, was a valuable line of enquiry. Although only a handful of these once-great high medieval book collections and book lists survive, one thing was striking: even when both medical manuscript and library catalogues (such as the 1190s catalogue from Reading Abbey) survive, the catalogues rarely list the medical works. Naturally, medical manuscripts – including the herbals, bestiaries, and lapidaries – would not have been suitable for the *lectio divina* (the daily spiritual reading undertaken by the monks), rather these were specialist texts. Only those whose duties might require recourse to this knowledge, such as the infirmarer, or those who were in a prominent enough position to have private collections, markedly the monastic superiors, would have had access to such volumes.

Not every monk, and thus not every hagiographer, would therefore have had access to, and knowledge of, scholastic medicine. However, monks would have received regular treatments, including phlebotomy, that would have brought them into contact with the practical applications of medical practice. For many twelfth-century monks then, observation and personal experience of healthcare were as, if not more, important in shaping ideas of ill health and healing as the texts on learned medicine that were housed within the monasteries. Similar experiences must have influenced the decisions of many cure-seekers, lay or religious, although recourse to learned medicine would have proved very difficult for the less affluent. In such instances cure-seekers might have first turned to herbal remedies, charms or other avenues of healing, but the hagiographers rarely mention such attempts; rather the miracles stress the superiority of the power of divine healing over the temporal efforts of the *medici*, the alternative that appears to have been recognised as the shrines' greatest competition.

Although the miracles champion the miraculous powers of God, brought about through the saints, theories and concepts of learned medicine also inter-twined with theological understandings of the connection between sickness and sin. Within the monastic communities, as the letters of Bernard of Clair-vaux and Herbert of Losinga exemplified, care of the soul was stressed over that of the body. This biblical precedent also influenced the way in which the saints were understood in their role as intercessors, especially as providers of healing. Following the precedent laid down by Christ, as recorded within the Gospels, the saints were seen as intermediaries of God whose divine powers were able to work through them. The cults of the saints were thus a pivotal fea-ture of the medieval church, with the saints acting as intercessors between the temporal and celestial worlds. In terms of where this placed healing miracles with regard to contemporary healthcare, it is important to note the sense of due process that can be seen within the miracle accounts; many cure-seekers first sought earthly remedies before turning to the saints. Of course, the miracles do not include accounts in which these medicines proved effective but this does suggest an understanding of an inherent hierarchy; the saints, as agents of the divine, were only to be turned to once other options had failed or when the affliction was deemed incurable.

This attitude was not only reflected in the miracle stories' critical recording of medical attempts to provide healing but in the notably high proportions of healing miracles that involved curing the untreatable, namely the loss of sight or mobility and serious illnesses. Blindness and paralysis could prove to be disabling impairments, while illness could prove fatal and required a swift solution. All three proved challenging, if not impossible, for temporal medicine to remedy and, like Christ before them, the saints were able to offer a thaumaturgic option that worldly medicines could not compete with. In following on from this, attention turned to the miracles themselves, and to the cure-seekers. Of importance here was to ask what brought these individuals into contact with the saints. What types of affliction were the saints recorded as having healed, and what do the miracle accounts reveal about cure-seeking and medical awareness, inside and outside the monastery?

While the miraculous cure of blindness, paralysis and illness proved prominent in the miracles, other health complaints featured less often – these included complaints of other sensory impairments. That these were recorded less frequently is suggestive that such impairments were often seen to be less disabling. Blindness could be congenital but could also be the result of numerous other health complaints, including poor diet, meaning complaints such as blindness had a range of potential causes. Paralysis, likewise, could be inherent from birth or could result from lifestyle or occupational complications. Cases of difficult labour were also notably rare (with only two accounts of this within the seven *miracula*). Nevertheless, *M. Jacobi*'s record of Aquilina's miraculous remedy provided a fascinating reference to the use of precious stones to ease labour. Although the stones were not named in *M. Jacobi*, it was important to note that lapidaries supported the use of particular precious stones during labour including jasper and sard. A similar investigation was also made into the possible herbal remedies which Abbot Osbert of Notley, also in *M. Jacobi*, might have applied to his eye and which only worsened his complaint. Osbert's case was important for its reference to a specific form of treatment, even if this medical knowledge was seemingly misplaced in Osbert's case.

In considering the medicinal aspects of the healing miracles and the miracle reports, it was important to determine the language used in recording the afflictions. Eye afflictions (predominantly cases of blindness), paralysis and tumours (including swellings and growths) highlighted that the Latin was usually generic. This was particularly the case in accounts of blindness; however, there was evidence of semantic medicalisation in some of the accounts connected to swellings.

References to medical practitioners were also found within the miracles. In these instances, physicians were, unsurprisingly, criticised for their costs and unsuccessful or exacerbating treatments. What came as a surprise was the instance of 'self-burning' found in *M. Æbbe*. While this was unique among our seven case-studies, another *miracula*, Reginald of Durham's hagiography for Cuthbert, included a reference to cautery. While the latter account implied this was undertaken by a practitioner, it was intriguing that these two hagiographies, both with a connection to Durham Cathedral Priory, included cases with treatments of a similar nature. That Durham Cathedral held at least one manuscript relating to cautery – and including miniatures illustrating cautery points – highlights an awareness of medical practices at Durham and its daughter-house, making the two references even more fascinating. This indicates potential medical knowledge on the part of *M. Æbbe*'s hagiographer. The account of the Edinburgh man also demonstrates that some were willing to undergo invasive methods of treatment for even seemingly incurable complaints, and these might be attempted prior to petitioning the saints. As noted, this implied that the saints were not the first remedial resort for many cure-seekers. This hinted at an unspoken etiquette to cure-seeking practices which would have ensured that saintly assistance was not requested without due respect and reverence.

So, who were the cure-seekers who turned to these seven saints? The laity were prominent in all seven *miracula*, with *M. Æbbe* and *M. Moduenne* both only recording the healing of lay cure-seekers. With the *miracula* dating from across the twelfth century it was evident that the recording of such instances was both a pattern and a reflection on the importance of saintly intercession for lay cure-seekers; the seven case-study cults thus fitted within broader patterns of cure-seeking, as both Finucane and Sigal had previously shown.

If the high presence of the laity was a predictable pattern across these sources, what was unexpected was the prominence of pre-adult cure-seekers, especially in the later twelfth-century *miracula*. The recording of these young cure-seekers offers a great insight into the cults and into the levels of parental care and concern over the well-being of their offspring. Linguistic study also highlighted the clear identification among these younger cure-seekers of a range of ages spanning from newborns to those on the cusp of adulthood. Conversely, the miracle accounts were less likely to identify more senior cure-seekers, and here language had just as much of a part to play. Elderly women were more likely to be identifiable through use of terms such as *matrona*, but as social and sexual status for male cure-seekers did not change, identifying which male cure-seekers were more senior required attention to the context of the account, as was the case with the recording of the pensioner in *M. Moduenne*. The presence of a wide age range among the cure-seekers recorded in the miracles reflects the desire to represent the saints and their cults as being welcoming to all, and must surely also indicate wider contemporary understandings of these holy figures and their roles as patrons and protectors, especially in matters of ill health and healing.

One other social group that, while accounting for less than a tenth of cure-seekers, was a notable presence was the churchmen (the monks and clerics). The inclusion of religious men, both from the cult centre's own community and from other religious institutions, revealed that these men were not averse to turning to saintly assistance. However, the prominence of the laity, as represented within the miracles, did suggest that churchmen potentially had access to better medical care. Moreover, as evidenced by Bernard of Clairvaux's letter to the monks of St Anastasius, monks were expected to bear bodily suffering because care for the health of their soul was of greater concern. What this made clear was that further investigation into not only the levels of medical knowledge, but also the experiences of ill health and healing within the monasteries, would prove rewarding. Attention to the religious recorded in the miracle reports also revealed another striking feature: nowhere within the seven sources were nuns included among the cure-seekers. Although it was expected that their presence would be limited, the complete absence of religious women was surprising. Where were the nuns? *L. Gilberti* highlighted that nuns were likely to experience miraculous occurrences within their own communities. Thus, miracle accounts suggest that stricter rules of enclosure were already imposed upon nuns in the twelfth century. These same levels of enclosure were not evident in the accounts of the churchmen, a third of whom were not members of the cult centre's community. Clearly the monastic communities recognised that the saints were able to provide holy healing, but the laity were evidently the prominent demographic among those who came to the shrines.

The prominence of the laity highlighted a crucial point: travel to the saints' shrines would have been a key part of the process for many cure-seekers. While some attention has been paid to the origin-sites of pilgrims, previous studies (such as those of Finucane and Yarrow) have tended to look outward from the shrines to consider the spread of the cult. Here, that concept was reversed to approach distances travelled from the perspective of the cure-seekers themselves. Moreover, the practicalities of undertaking journeys to the shrines have been little discussed despite being an essential element of the cure-seeking process. The following two chapters sought to remedy this with an in-depth analysis of the distances covered by the cure-seekers and consideration of the nature of travel in twelfth-century England.

In looking at the distances travelled by cure-seekers from origin-site to the cult centre, it emerged that the greatest numbers of our recorded cure-seekers were healed by their local saint. *M. Moduenne* represented Modwenna's cult to be an especially localised affair. That cure-seeking should first be undertaken close to home made a great deal of sense in terms of devotion to local patron saints and practical considerations. Many of our cure-seekers found that their local cure-seeking resulted in successful recovery, and this in itself is reflective of how firm the belief in the connection between patron saint and local community was. Local cure-seeking was the generally expected and accepted method for securing healing miracles. That numbers of cure-seekers should have declined as the distance between origin-site and shrine increased was to be anticipated, but it left open for debate those accounts that made no mention of origin-site. Although no distance could be estimated for these accounts, it can be assumed that a number of individuals who fell into this category would have lived relatively locally, and that the distance they covered was not seen to be noteworthy.

The miracles also revealed that most cure-seekers made the journey to the shrine themselves prior to receiving their desired healing. A small, but significant number were recorded as having been successful in securing their cure through the making of a vow and were thus able to complete the journey and fulfil their vow having already been healed. Fewer cure-seekers still made no journey to the shrine themselves. For young children, parents might take on the role of petitioning the saint. For others, such as the London *matrona*, cured at home through contact with Dunstan's chasuble held at Westminster Abbey, and for whom there is no mention of a visit to the shrine, it was likely that news of the miracle passed through monastic channels of communication. That the miracles do record varying methods for obtaining miracle cures highlights that there was not a singular process, but that there was an understanding and a desire to make an appeal to the saints at the site of their shrines where possible. What then when a cure-seeker had to seek cure further afield? Here the comments made to St James by the young, paralysed Ysembela – that she had not heard of Reading so did not know the way, that she had no money, and was worn out by her affliction – provide a rare and fascinating insight into the practical concerns many cure-seekers likely had about seeking holy healing further afield.

Taking these practicalities into account was the aim of the following chapter. Cure-seekers, like any other pilgrims, would primarily make physical journeys to the shrine and would thus experience time on the road. It is essential that this is considered when understanding how the process of cure-seeking was experienced, especially as so many cure-seekers made this journey while in poor health. In order to understand the experiences of the cure-seekers, this chapter cast a wider net to establish what the road network in twelfth-century England was like, and what travellers more generally might encounter on the roads. As well as considering the evidence for the network of roads and trackways, it was important to recognise the potential dangers faced during travel. Law codes, such as *L. Henrici*, indicated that royal protection was limited to certain key roads, and that there were a range of penalties for attacks on the road. But such punishment would have been consequential to the crime itself. More pro-active were the attempts made by figures such as Abbot Leofstan who endeavoured to make the roads through the wooded parts of the east Chilterns less advantageous for both animal and criminal attacks. While later evidence revealed that this was not a wholly successful undertaking, it was clear that there was a recognition of the potential dangers that might face any traveller, including pilgrims and cure-seekers.

This chapter also considered the ways in which cure-seekers made their journeys to the shrine. If roads could prove problematic, would cure-seekers look to England's waterways? Analysis of the miracle accounts revealed that specific references to water travel were only made in instances where this was a necessity. The roads, while potentially slower, were at least free, and many cure-seekers (including Ysembela) had little in the way of finances to support their journey. In part this reflected the financial reality for many cure-seekers but it also reflected broader ideals of pilgrimage. Quinciana, recorded in *M. Æbbe*, was one clear example of a cure-seeker who purposefully left worldly possessions behind when she turned her attention to seeking out miraculous healing. Of course, those who were successful closer to home would have spent less time on the road to recovery, but one thing that united the cure-seekers (with the exception of the few who did not travel) was the end result: reaching the saint's shrine to either petition the saint or to fulfil the vow for the miracle healing already provided. These longer, and more arduous, journeys were also reflective of the underlying spiritual element of undertaking the trip. There was surely a sense for some, if not all, cure-seekers that travelling to the shrines was part of the overall process and that challenges faced on the road were tests of faith.

Arrival at the shrine brought the cure-seekers to the end of their cure-seeking process and brought this book to its final chapter. The shrines were a central point, an anchor for the saints who were able to manoeuvre between the temporal and celestial worlds. As the majority of recorded cure-seekers were laypeople, this meant permitting lay access to, and allowing lay presence within, these areas. However, these shrines were also located within religious spaces in which monastic communities lived and worshipped. How then were these purposes, with their potentially conflicting needs, balanced? This raised the issue of 'sacred space' and the fact that it is not identifying these spaces but considering how they were used and experienced that is key to understanding them in the context of cure-seeking and miracle healing. Important here then was to question the reasons why the laity might have visited the monasteries, and whether cure-seekers would have fallen into the category of guests. While it cannot be denied that guests of the monasteries might also petition the saints, the majority of cure-seekers embodied a very specific type of visitor: one who came with a particular purpose and whose focus was on a specific part of the monastic complex. Cure-seekers were not likely to wish for a tour of the monastic buildings, as Lanfranc's *Decreta* permitted for guests. Like other *peregrini*, their attention was principally focused on the church where the shrines of the saints tended to be located.

Two of the seven cults, however, did not follow this structure. William of Norwich's shrine was translated numerous times during the twelfth century, with his year in the chapter house seeming a particularly productive one. Æbbe, in contrast, was firmly rooted within the landscape with attention drawn to the oratory at Kirk Hill – the site of her own seventh-century monastery – rather than at her translated tomb within Coldingham Priory's church. Both cults provided worthy studies for shrines that do not fit the broader norms. Despite their differences, the evidence from Coldingham and Norwich revealed that, regardless of the shrine's location, there was interaction between the laity and the monks within these spaces. Indeed, there was generally a sense within the miracle reports that the laity, including cure-seekers, were to be welcomed at the shrine no matter the time of day.

On the rare occasions when the miracle accounts record challenges to this, the actions of officious individuals who barred access are depicted as having been at fault, and the subsequent miraculous cure was seen to be further evidence for the saints' willingness to help anyone at any time. This level of care and concern was also reflected by the monastic communities themselves in the charity and compassion shown to the cure-seekers. Not only was this in keeping with the model of Christ, and the *Regula S. Benedicti*, but it became evident that some cure-seekers developed more personal relationships with the monastic communities. This was notably reflected in the experiences of one poor woman cured by Modwenna; the Burton community provided for her for many years prior to her cure, and even after her paralysis was miraculously healed the abbot ensured that she had clothing that suitably covered her. This level of care and observance mirrors the awareness that monastic communities had towards ill health, healthcare, and healing within their own communities. Witnessing suffering due to illness and impairment was not limited to the cloister, and the monks along with other lay visitors present at the shrine would also celebrate the miraculous recovery, be that an immediate recovery or one that took longer to achieve and might require direct contact with the saint or, as *M. Æbbe* and *M. Jacobi* recorded, a prolonged and even painful process.

As with any topic, there will always be more that awaits to be explored. This book has asked, and answered, certain key questions relating to cure-seekers and the place of healing miracles within the broader remit of medieval healthcare. The saints and their cults were central to medieval Christianity and medieval Christian society, and these smaller cults, with their predominantly localised cure-seeking clientele, provide a fascinating insight into the processes and experiences of miraculous healing in high medieval England. Ever-present and universally accessible, the saints, via their cults, extended their power and influence through all levels of society.

Appendix 1:
A List of the Named Cure-Seekers
Within the Seven *Miracula**

	Laymen	Laywomen	Monks and clerics
M. Swithuni	Æthelsige		
M. Dunstani	Ælfweard		Æthelweard
	Lambert		Lanfranc (*Archbishop of Canterbury*)
L. Eliensis	Ælred	Reinburgis	Ælfhelm
	Baldwin		Edwin
	Leofmær		John
	Richard		Ralph of Dunwich
	Robert de Alta Ripa		Thomas
	Ulf		
	Wihtgar		
M. Moduenne	Godric		
	Raven		
M. Willelmi	Adam (*son of John*)	Ada	Edmund
	Adam (*nephew of Edward of Yarmouth*)	Agnes (*wife of Reginald*)	Peter Peverell
	Baldwin	Agnes [Hoc]	Thomas
	Blythburgh	Alditha	Walter
	Ebrard Fisher	Bothilda (*wife of Girard*)	William
	Gaufrid (*from Canterbury*)	Botilda (*wife of Toke*)	
	Gaufridus (*clerk of William de Cheyney*)	Clarica	
	Godric	Emma de Wighton	
	Herbert	Gillilda	

	Laymen	Laywomen	Monks and clerics
M. Willelmi (*continued*)	Hildebrand	Gilliva	
	Kobert	Goda	
	Lewin	Goldeburga	
	Ralph (*the moneyer*)	Hathewis	
	Ralph [de Hadeston]	Huelina	
	Reimbert	Ida	
	Robert (*a knight*)	Leva	
	Robert (*son of Herveus*)	Matilda (*daughter of Rathe*)	
	Robert [de Crachesford]	Matildis (*from Langham*)	
	Robert (*from Norwich*)	Muriel	
	Schet	Ravenilda	
	Sieldeware	Wimarc	
	Thomas		
M. Æbbe		Quinciana	
M. Jacobi	Edward Haver	Alice	John
	Gilbert	Aquilina	Osbert (*abbot of Notley*)
	John	Goda	Roger Hosatus
	Mauger Malcuvenant	Ysembela (*wife of Sewel*)	Thomas
	Peter [de Leuns]	Ysembela (*daughter of John*)	
	Ralph Gibuin		
	Robert of Stanford		
	William		

* Parentheses are used where the *miracula* contains more than one person of the same name. Square brackets provide a surname or moniker recorded in association with a family member, such as a father or husband.

Appendix 2:
A List of the Occupations Recorded for Laypersons Within the Seven *Miracula*

	Laymen	**Laywomen**
M. Swithuni	Servant (*to a priest on the Isle of Wight*)	
	Servant (*to a man named Richard*)	
M. Dunstani	Servant (*to Archbishop Anselm*)	
L. Eliensis		Servant (*to a priest*)
		Servant (*to Ralph, son of Colsuein*)
M. Moduenne	Carpenter	
	Cleric	
	Workman	
M. Willelmi	Clerk (*Adam, nephew of Edward of Yarmouth*)	
	Clerk (*Robert, son of William de Crachesford*)	
	Clerk (*to William de Cheyney, sheriff*)	
	Moneyer (*of Norwich*)	
	Money-changer (*of Norwich*)	
	Miller (*of the seneschal [below]*)	
	Seneschal (*Reimbert, for the abbot of Battle*)	
	Workman (*for the moneyers of Norwich*)	
M. Æbbe	Needle-seller	
	Musician	
	Smith	
M. Jacobi	Clerk (*John, from Barking*)	
	Hound-keeper (*Gilbert, from the north of England*)	

Appendix 3:
A List of the Place Names Recorded Within
Thomas of Monmouth's *M. Willelmi*

	Place name	Additional comments
5 miles or under		
	Grimeston	Now known as Grimston
	Markshall	
	Norwich	
	Postwick	
6–20 miles		
	Bedingeham	Now known as Bedingham.
	Belaugh	
	Flordon	
	Hadeston, Bunwell	
	Loddon	
	Needham	
	Ormesbury	Neighbouring villages Ormesbury St Margaret and Ormesbury St Micheal are nineteen miles from Norwich.
	Repps	
	Swafield	
	Taverham	
	'The Wells' near Ely	Upwell, Outwell and Welney are neighbouring villages. Upwell and Outwell are a mile apart and Welney just over seven miles to the south. All three are fifty miles from Norwich.
	Tivetshall	Neighbouring villages Tivetshall St Margaret and Tivetshall St Mary are sixteen miles from Norwich.
	Tuttington	

	Place name	Additional comments
21–50 miles		
	Bury St Edmunds	
	Dunwich	
	Great Yarmouth	
	Hasketon	
	Haughley	
	Langham	
	Lindsey	
	Lothingland	
	Mildenhall	
	North Creake	
	St Edmund, North Lynn	
	Setchy	
	Thornage	
	Tudenham	
	Wighton	
	Wormegay	
	Wortham	
51–100 miles		
	Bardney	
	Lincoln	
101 miles or over		
	Battle	
	Canterbury	
	London	
	York	

Place name	Additional comments
Unidentifiable	
Hempstead	There are two places with this name in Norfolk, one near North Walsham, the other near Holt. Only Hempstead near Holt is identifiable on a modern map. North Walsham is fifteen miles, and Holt is twenty-two miles from Norwich.
Rochesburch	There is no place identifiable with this name. Jessop and James suggested that it could refer to either Roxham or Rockland. Roxham is forty-two miles west of Norwich; Rockland All Saints and Rockland St Peter are neighbouring villages eighteen miles west of Norwich; and Rockland St Mary is six and a half miles south-east of Norwich.
Tudenham	This could refer to either Tudenham near Bury St Edmunds or Tudenham near Ipswich, both of which are approximately forty-two miles from Norwich. However, this could also refer to North Tuddenham which is only twelve miles from Norwich. It is the latter that Jessop and James favoured in their edition of *M. Willelmi.*

Bibliography

Primary Sources

Selected Manuscripts

Aberdeen, Aberdeen University Library, MS 24.
Cambridge, Cambridge University Library, MS Ee.3.59.
Durham, Durham Cathedral Library, MS. Hunter 100.
Gloucester, Gloucester Cathedral Library, MS 1.
Imola, Biblioteca Comunale di Imola, MS III.
Oxford, Bodleian, MS Bodley 130.
Oxford, Corpus Christi College, MS 157.

Printed Sources

Aimery Picaud, *The Pilgrim's Guide to Santiago de Compostela*, ed. and trans. W. Melczer (New York, 1993).
The Alphabet of Galen: Pharmacy from Antiquity to the Middle Ages: A Critical Edition of the Latin Text with English Translation and Commentary, ed. and trans. N. Everett (Toronto, 2012).
Ancient Christian Writers 52: Cassiodorus. Volume 2: Explanation of the Psalms, trans. P. G. Walsh (New York, 1990).
An Anglo-Norman Medical Compendium (Cambridge, Trinity College MS 0.2.5 (1109)), ed. T. Hunt, Anglo-Norman Text Society Plain Text Series 18 (Oxford, 2014).
An Anglo-Norman Medical Compendium (Oxford, Bodleian Library MS Bodley 761), ed. T. Hunt, Anglo-Norman Text Society Plain Text Series 19 (Oxford, 2017).
Anglo-Norman Medicine. Volume I: Roger Frugard's Chirurgia and The Practica Brevis of Platearius, ed. T. Hunt (Cambridge, 1994).
Anglo-Norman Medicine. Volume II: Shorter Treatises, ed. T. Hunt (Cambridge, 1997).
Augustine of Hippo, *Sancti Aurelii Augustini, Hipponensis Episcopi. Opera Omnia*, ed. J.-P. Migne, *Patrologiae cursus completus, series latina* 32–47, 12 vols (Paris, 1844–65).
Bede, *Historia Ecclesiastica Gentis Anglorum*, ed. and trans. B. Colgrave and R. A. B. Mynors, OMT (Oxford, 1991).
———, *The Reckoning of Time*, trans. F. Wallis, Translated Texts for Historians 29 (Liverpool, 1999).
———, *Vita Sancti Cuthberti auctore Beda*, in *Two Lives of Saint Cuthbert: A Life by an Anonymous Monk of Lindisfarne and Bede's Prose Life*, trans. B. Colgrave (Cambridge, 1940), pp. 141–307.
Benedict of Peterborough, *Miracula Sancti Thomae Cantuariensis*, in *Materials for the History of Thomas Becket, Archbishop of Canterbury*, ed. J. C. Robertson, 7 vols (London, 1875–85), II (1876), 21–281.

Bernard of Clairvaux, *The Letters of St Bernard of Clairvaux*, ed. B. S. James (Stroud, 1998).

Boniface, *The Letters of St Boniface: Translated with an Introduction*, trans. E. Emerton, Records of Civilization Sources and Studies 31 (New York, 1940).

The Book of St Gilbert, ed. and trans. R. Foreville and G. Keir, OMT (Oxford, 1987).

Charters of the Medieval Hospitals of Bury St Edmunds, ed. C. Harper-Bill, Suffolk Charters 14 (Woodbridge, 1994).

Chaucer, Geoffrey, *A Variorum Edition of the Works of Geoffrey Chaucer, 2. The Canterbury Tales: The General Prologue*, ed. M. Andrew et al., 1 vol. in 2 parts (Norman, OK, 1993).

Chronicon Monasterii de Abingdon, ed. J. Stevenson, 2 vols, RS 2 (London, 1858).

Conchubranus, *Vita S. Monenna*, in 'The *Life of St Monenna* by Conchubranus, Part I', ed. and trans. Ulster Society for Medieval Latin Studies, Seanchas Ardmhacha 9 (1979), 250–73.

———, *Vita S. Monenna*, in 'The *Life of St Monenna* by Conchubranus, Part II', ed. and trans. Ulster Society for Medieval Latin Studies, Seanchas Ardmhacha 10 (1980), 117–41.

———, *Vita S. Monenna*, in 'The *Life of St Monenna* by Conchubranus. Part III', ed. and trans. Ulster Society for Medieval Latin Studies, Seanchas Ardmhacha 10 (1982), 426–54.

Daniel, Walter, *The Life of Ailred of Rievaulx by Walter Daniel*, trans. F. M. Powicke, Medieval Classics (London, 1950).

Decrees of the Ecumenical Councils, ed. and trans. N. Tanner, 2 vols (London, 1990), I, *Nicaea I – Lateran V*.

Douay-Rheims Bible, <http://www.drbo.org/> [accessed 10 October 2020].

Eadmer of Canterbury, *Miracula S. Dunstani*, in Eadmer of Canterbury, *Lives and Miracles of Saints Oda, Dunstan and Oswald*, ed. and trans. A. Turner and B. Muir, OMT (Oxford, 2006), pp. 160–211.

———, *Miracula S. Oswaldi*, in Eadmer of Canterbury, *Lives and Miracles of Saints Oda, Dunstan and Oswald*, ed. and trans. A. Turner and B. Muir, OMT (Oxford, 2006), pp. 290–323.

———, *Life of St Anselm: Archbishop of Canterbury, by Eadmer*, ed. and trans. R. W. Southern, OMT (Oxford, 1972).

Ely Chapter Ordinances and Visitation Records, 1241–1515, ed. S. Evans, Camden 3rd series 17 (London, 1940).

Geoffrey of Burton, *Life and Miracles of St Modwenna*, ed. and trans. R. Bartlett, OMT (Oxford, 2002).

Gerald of Wales, *Itinerarium Kambriae et Descriptio Kambriae*, ed. J. F. Dimock, RS 6 (London, 1868).

———, *The Journey through Wales and The Description of Wales*, trans. L. Thorpe (London, 1978).

Gervase of Canterbury, *Instructio nouiciorum*, in *The Monastic Constitutions of Lanfranc*, ed. and trans. D. Knowles and C. Brooke, OMT (Oxford, 2002), pp. 197–221.

Henry of Huntingdon, *Anglicanus Ortus: A Verse Herbal of the Twelfth Century*, ed. and trans. W. Black, Studies and Texts 180 (Oxford, 2012).

————, *Historia Anglorum: The History of the English People*, ed. and trans. D. Greenway, OMT (Oxford, 1996).

Herman the Archdeacon, *Miracula S. Edmundi*, in *Herman the Archdeacon and Goscelin of St-Bertin: Miracles of St Edmund*, ed. and trans. T. Licence, OMT (Oxford, 2014), pp. 1–125.

Hildegard von Bingen's Physica: The Complete English Translation of Her Classical Work on Health and Healing, trans. P. Throop (Rochester, 1998).

Hippocrates, Heracleitus, *Nature of Man. Regimen in Health. Humours. Aphorisms. Regimen 1–3. Dreams. Heracleitus: On the Universe*, trans. W. H. S. Jones, Loeb Classical Library 150 (Cambridge, MA, 1931).

'Il Salterio inglese (MS 111)', Biblioteca Comunale di Imola, <http://www.bim.comune.imola.bo.it/content.php?current=8628#top> [accessed 27 June 2020].

John of Salisbury, *Metalogicon*, ed. J. B. Hall and K. S. B. Keats-Rohan, *Corpus Christianorum Continuatio Mediaevalis* 98 (Turnhout, 1991).

Kemp, B., '*The Miracles of the Hand of St James*: Translated with an Introduction', *Berkshire Archaeological Journal* 65 (1970), 1–19.

Lanfranc, *Decreta Lanfranci Monachis Canturiensibus Transmissa*, in *The Monastic Constitutions of Lanfranc*, ed. and trans. D. Knowles and C. Brooke, OMT (Oxford, 2002), pp. 2–195.

Leechdoms, Wortcunning and Starcraft of Early England. Being a Collection of Documents, for the most part never before printed, illustrating the History of Science in the Country before the Norman Conquest, ed. and trans. O. Cockayne, 3 vols, RS 35 (London, 1864–66).

Leges Edwardi Confessori, in B. O'Brien, *God's Peace and King's Peace: The Laws of Edward the Confessor*, The Middle Ages Series (Philadelphia, 1999), pp. 158–203.

Leges Henrici Primi, ed. and trans. L. Downer (Oxford, 1972).

Letters and Papers, Foreign and Domestic, Henry VIII, Volume 13 Part 2, August–December 1538, ed. J. Gairdner (London, 1893).

Liber Eliensis, ed. E. Blake, Camden 3rd series 92 (London, 1962).

Liber Eliensis: A History of the Isle of Ely, from the Seventh Century to the Twelfth, trans. J. Fairweather (Woodbridge, 2005).

The Life, Letters and Sermons of Bishop Herbert de Losinga and Sermons of Bishop Herbert de Losinga, ed. E. M. Goulburn and H. Symonds, 2 vols (Oxford, 1878).

Miracula S. Margarite Scotorum Regine, in *Æbbe of Coldingham and Margaret of Scotland*, ed. Bartlett, OMT (Oxford, 2006), pp. 69–145.

Miracula S. Swithuni, in *The Anglo-Saxon Minsters of Winchester: The Cult of St Swithun*, ed. and trans. M. Lapidge, Winchester Studies 4.ii (Oxford, 2003), pp. 641–97.

The Old English Herbarium, in A. Van Ardsall, *Medieval Herbal Remedies: The Old English Herbarium and Anglo-Saxon Medicine* (New York, 2002), pp. 119–230.

Omnia opera Ysaac, ed. A. Turinus, 2 vols (Lyons, 1515), via the Bibliothèque Interuniversitaire de Santé, <http://www.biusante.parisdescartes.fr/histoire/medica/resultats/index.php?cote=00122&do=livre> [accessed 10 September 2020].

Reading Abbey Cartularies. British Library Manuscripts: Egerton 3031, Harley 1708 and Cotton Vespasian E xxv, ed. B. Kemp, Camden 4th series 31, 33, 2 vols (London, 1986–87).

Reginald of Durham, *Libellus de Admirandis Beati Cuthberti Virtutibus quae novellis Patratæ sunt Temporibus*, ed. J. Raine, Surtees Society 1 (London, 1835).

Regularis Concordia: Anglicae Nationis Monachorum Sanctimonialiumque. The Monastic Agreement of the Monks and Nuns of the English Nations, ed. and trans. T. Symons, Medieval Classics (London, 1953).

Rolls of the Justices in Eyre being the Rolls of Pleas and Assizes for Lincolnshire 1218–19 and Worcestershire 1221, ed. and trans. D. Stenton, Seldon Society 53 (London, 1934).

The Rule of St Benedict: In Latin with an English Translation, ed. and trans. J. McCann (Tunbridge Wells, 1969).

Suger of Saint-Denis, *On the Abbey Church of St Denis and Its Art Treasures*, ed. and trans. E. Panofsky, 2nd edn (Princeton, 1979).

Symeon of Durham, *Libellus de exordio atque procursu istius, hoc est Dunhelmensis, ecclesie. Tract on the Origins and Progress of this the Church of Durham*, ed. and trans. D. Rollason, OMT (Oxford, 2000).

The 'Things of Greater Importance': Bernard of Clairvaux's Apologia and the Medieval Attitude toward Art, ed. and trans. C. Rudolph (Philadelphia, 1990).

Thomas of Monmouth, *The Life and Miracles of St William of Norwich*, ed. and trans. A. Jessop and M. R. James (Cambridge, 1896).

——, *The Life and Passion of St William of Norwich*, trans. M. Rubin (London, 2014).

The Trotula: An English Translation of the Medieval Compendium of Women's Medicine, ed. and trans. M. H. Green (Philadelphia, 2002).

Vita et Miracula S. Æbbe Virginis, in *Æbbe of Coldingham and Margaret of Scotland*, ed. R. Bartlett, OMT (Oxford, 2006), pp. 1–67.

Vita S. Swithuni Episcopi et Confessoris, in *The Anglo-Saxon Minsters of Winchester: The Cult of St Swithun*, ed. and trans. M. Lapidge, Winchester Studies 4.ii (Oxford, 2003), pp. 611–39.

Walsingham, Thomas, *Gesta abbatum monasterii Sancta Albani a Thoma Walsingham, regnante Ricardo Secundo, ejusdem ecclesiae praecentro, compilata*, ed. H. Riley, 3 vols, RS 28 (London, 1867).

William of Canterbury, *Miracula Sancti Thomae Cantuariensis*, in *Materials for the History of Thomas Becket, Archbishop of Canterbury*, ed. J. C. Robertson, 7 vols (London, 1875–85), I (1875), 137–546.

William of Malmesbury, *Gesta Pontificum Anglorum*, ed. R. M. Thomson and M. Winterbottom, 2 vols, OMT (Oxford, 2007).

William of St Thierry et al., *Vita Prima Sancti Bernardi Claraevallis Abbatis: Liber Primus*, ed. P. Verdeyen and C. Vande Veire, *Corpus Christianorum Continuatio Mediaevalis* 89B (Turnhout, 2011).

Secondary Literature

Arbesmann, R., 'The Concept of '*Christus Medicus*' in St Augustine', *Traditio* 10 (1954), 1–54.

Arias-Santiago, S., et al., 'Phytophotodermatitis due to *Ruta graveolens* prescribed for fibromyalgia', *Rheumatology* 48 (2009), 1401.

Ariès, P., *Centuries of Childhood*, trans. R. Baldick (London, 1996).

Arrizabalaga, J., 'Problematising Retrospective Diagnosis in the History of Disease', *Asclepio* 54 (2002), 51–70.

Bailey, A. E., 'Flights of Distance, Time and Fancy: Women Pilgrims and Their Journeys in English Medieval Miracle Narratives', *Gender and History* 24 (2012), 292–309.

——, 'Representations of English Women and Their Pilgrimages in Twelfth-Century Miracle Collections', *Assuming Gender* 3 (2013), 59–90.

——, 'Wives, Mothers and Widows on Pilgrimage: Categories of "Woman" Recorded at English Healing Shrines in the High Middle Ages', *Journal of Medieval History* 39 (2013), 197–219.

——, 'The Rich and the Poor, the Lesser and the Great', *Cultural and Social History* 11 (2014), 9–29.

——, 'Women Pilgrims and Their Travelling Companions in Twelfth-Century England', *Viator* 46 (2015), 115–34.

——, 'Miracle Children: Medieval Hagiography and Childhood Imperfection', *Journal of Interdisciplinary History* 47 (2016), 267–85.

——, 'Miracles and Madness: Dispelling Demons in Twelfth-Century Hagiography', in *Demons and Illness: Theory and Practice from Antiquity to the Early Modern Period*, ed. S. Bhayro and C. Rider (Leiden, 2016), pp. 235–55.

——, 'Reconsidering the Medieval Experience at the Shrine in High-Medieval England', *Journal of Medieval History* 47.2 (2021), 203–29.

Banham, D., *Food and Drink in Anglo-Saxon England* (Stroud, 2004).

——, 'Medicine at Bury in the Time of Abbot Baldwin', in *Bury St Edmunds and the Norman Conquest*, ed. T. Licence (Woodbridge, 2014), pp. 226–46.

Bartlett, R., *Why Can The Dead Do Such Great Things? Saints and Worshippers from the Martyrs to the Reformation* (Princeton, 2013).

——, 'Medieval Miracle Accounts as Stories', *Irish Theological Quarterly* 82 (2017), 113–27.

Basford, V., 'Medieval Resource Assessment for the Isle of Wight', Oxford Archaeology (2006), 1–23, <https://oxfordarchaeology.com/images/pdfs/Solent_Thames/County_resource_assessments/Late_Medieval_IOW.pdf > [accessed 18 July 2020].

Baxter, R., *The Royal Abbey of Reading*, Boydell Studies in Medieval Art and Architecture (Woodbridge, 2016).

Bennett, G., 'William of Norwich and the Expulsion of the Jews', *Folklore* 116 (2005), 311–14.

Bishop, L. M., *Words, Stones and Herbs: The Healing Word in Medieval and Early Modern England* (Syracuse, 2007).

Black, W., 'Henry of Huntingdon's Lapidary Rediscovered and His *Anglicanus ortus* Reassembled', *Medieval Studies* 68 (2006), 43–87.

Bouquet, D., and Nagy, P., *Medieval Sensibilities: A History of Emotions in the Middle Ages*, trans. R. Shaw (Cambridge, 2018).

Brand, P., 'The Travails of Travel: The Difficulties of Getting to Court in Later Medieval England', in *Freedom of Movement in the Middle Ages: Proceedings of the 2003 Harlaxton Symposium*, ed. P. Horden (Donington, 2007), pp. 215–28.

Brenner, E., *Leprosy and Charity in Medieval Rouen*, Royal Historical Society Studies in History, New Series (Woodbridge, 2015).

————, 'The Transmission of Medical Culture in the Norman Worlds, c.1050–c.1250', in *People, Texts and Artefacts: Cultural Transmission in the Norman Worlds of the Eleventh and Twelfth Centuries*, ed. D. Bates, E. D'Angelo and E. van Houts, IHR Conference Series (London, 2017), pp. 47–64.

————, 'The Medical Role of Monasteries in the Latin West, c. 1050–1300', in *The Cambridge History of Medieval Monasticism in the Latin West. Volume 2: The High and Late Middle Ages*, ed. A. I. Beach and I. Cochelin (Cambridge, 2020), pp. 865–81.

Brown, P., *The Cult of Saints: Its Rise and Function in Latin Christianity*, 2nd edn (Chicago, 2015).

Bullough, V. L., *Universities, Medicine and Science in the Medieval West*, Variorum Collected Studies 781 (Aldershot, 2004).

Burnett, C., *The Introduction of Arabic Learning into England*, Panizzi Lectures 1996 (London, 1997).

————, 'The Twelfth-Century Renaissance', in *The Cambridge History of Science. Volume 2: Medieval Science*, ed. D. C. Lindberg and M. H. Shank (Cambridge, 2013), pp. 365–84.

Burrow, J. A., *The Ages of Man: A Study in Medieval Writing and Thought* (Oxford, 1986).

Burton, J., *Monastic and Religious Orders in Britain, 1000–1300*, Cambridge Medieval Textbooks (Cambridge, 1994).

The Cambridge Dictionary of English Place-Names: Based on the Collections of the English Place-Name Society, ed. V. Watts (Cambridge, 2004).

Cameron, M., *Anglo-Saxon Medicine*, Cambridge Studies in Anglo-Saxon England 7 (Cambridge, 2006).

Cassidy-Welch, M. *Monastic Spaces and Their Meanings: Thirteenth-Century English Cistercian Monasteries*, Medieval Church Studies 1 (Turnhout, 2001).

————, 'Space and Place in Medieval Contexts', *Parergon* 27 (2010), 1–12.

Catalogi Veteres Librorum Ecclesiæ Cathedralis Dunelm: Catalogues of the Library of Durham Cathedral at Various Periods, from the Conquest to the Dissolution including Catalogues of the Library of the Abbey of Hulne and the MSS. Preserved in the Library of Bishop Cosin, at Durham, ed. B. Botfield, Surtees Society 7 (London, 1838).

Childs, W. R., 'Moving Around', in *A Social History of England, 1200–1500*, ed. R. Horrox and W. M. Ormrod (Cambridge, 2006), pp. 260–75.

Clark, J. G., *The Benedictines in the Middle Ages*, Monastic Orders (Woodbridge, 2011).

Clifton-Taylor, A., *The Cathedrals of England* (London, 1967).

Coates, A., *English Medieval Books: The Reading Abbey Collections from Foundation to Dispersal*, Oxford Historical Monographs (Oxford, 1999).

Coldstream, N., *Medieval Architecture*, Oxford History of Art (Oxford, 2002).

Constable, G., 'The Monastic Policy of Peter the Venerable', in *Pierre Abélard – Pierre le Vénérable. Les courants philosophiques, littéraries et artistiques en Occident au milieu du XIIe siècle. Abbaye de Cluny, 2–9 julliet 1972*, Colloques internationaux du Centre national de la recherche scientifique 546 (Paris, 1975), pp. 119–38.

————, *The Reformation of the Twelfth Century*, Trevelyan Lectures 1985 (Cambridge, 1996).

Cooper, A., 'The King's Four Highways: Legal Fiction Meets Fictional Law', *Journal of Medieval History* 27 (2000), 351–70.

————, 'The Rise and Fall of the Anglo-Saxon Law of the Highway', *The Haskins Society Journal: Studies in Medieval History* 12 (2002), 46–9.

Craig, L.-A., *Wandering Women and Holy Matrons: Women as Pilgrims in the Later Middle Ages*, Studies in Medieval and Reformation Studies 138 (Leiden, 2009).

Crook, J., *English Medieval Shrines*, Boydell Studies in Art and Architecture (Woodbridge, 2011).

Cunningham, A., 'Identifying Disease in the Past: Cutting the Gordian Knot', *Asclepio* 54 (2002), 13–34.

Daniell, C., *Atlas of Medieval Britain* (London, 2011).

Darby, H. C., *The Draining of the Fens*, 2nd edn, Cambridge Studies in Economic History (Cambridge, 1956).

Davies, H. E. H., 'Designing Roman Roads', *Britannia* 29 (1998), 1–16.

Demaitre, L., *Medieval Medicine: The Art of Healing from Head to Toe*, Praeger Series on the Middle Ages (Santa Barbara, 2013).

Draper, P., *The Formation of English Gothic: Architecture and Identity* (New Haven, 2006).

Duffy, E., *The Stripping of the Altars: Traditional Religion in England, c.1400–c.1580*, 2nd edn (New Haven, 2005).

Dyas, D., *Pilgrimage in Medieval English Literature, 700–1500* (Cambridge, 2001).

Eliade, M., *The Sacred and Profane: The Nature of Religion*, trans. W. R. Trask (New York, 1987).

English Benedictine Libraries: The Shorter Catalogues, ed. R. Sharpe et al., Corpus of British Medieval Library Catalogues 4 (London, 1996).

Fergusson, P., *Canterbury Cathedral Priory in the Age of Becket* (New Haven, 2011).

Finucane, R. C., 'The Use and Abuse of Medieval Miracles', *History* 60 (1975), 1–10.

————, 'Pilgrimage in Daily Life: Aspects of Medieval Communication Reflected in the Newly-Established Cult of Thomas de Cantilupe (d. 1282), Its Dissemination and Effects upon Outlying Herefordshire Villagers', in *Walfahrt und Alltag in Mittelalter und früher Neuzeit. Internationales Round-Table-Gespräch, Krems an der Donau, 8. Oktober 1990*, ed. G. Jaritz and B. Schuh (Vienna, 1992), pp. 165–218.

————, *Miracles and Pilgrims: Popular Beliefs in Medieval England* (London, 1995).

————, *Rescue of the Innocents: Endangered Children in Medieval Miracles* (New York, 1997).

Frampton, M., *Embodiments of Will: Anatomical and Physiological Theories of Voluntary Animal Motion from Greek Antiquity to the Latin Middle Ages* (Saarbrücken, 2008).

French, T., *York Minster: The St William Window, Corpus vitrearum Medii Aevi* (Great Britain) Summary Catalogue 5 (Oxford, 2000).

————, 'The St William Window, York Minster', *British Academy Review* 3 (2000), 28, <https://www.thebritishacademy.ac.uk/documents/1586/ba-review03.pdf> [accessed October 2020].

Gameson, R., *The Earliest Books of Canterbury Cathedral: Manuscripts and Fragments to c.1200*, Canterbury Sources 4 (London, 2008).

Gilchrist, R., *Contemplation and Action: The Other Monasticism* (London, 1995).

————, *Norwich Cathedral Close: The Evolution of the English Cathedral Landscape*, Studies in the History of Medieval Religion (Woodbridge, 2005).

————, *Medieval Life: Archaeology and the Life Course* (Woodbridge, 2012).

Gilchrist, R., and Sloane, B., *Requiem: The Medieval Monastic Cemetery in Britain* (London, 2005).

Glaze, F. E., 'Salerno's Lombard Prince: Johannes 'Abbas de Curte' as Medical Practitioner', *Early Science and Medicine* 23 (2018), 177–216.

Goodrich, M., *Worcester Nunneries: The Nuns of the Medieval Diocese* (Chichester, 2008).

Google Maps, <https://www.google.co.uk/maps/> [accessed 15 July 2020].

Gordon, E. C., 'Child Health in the Middle Ages as Seen in the Miracles of Five English Saints, A.D. 1150–1220', *Bulletin of the History of Medicine* 60 (1986), 502–22.

Grant, L., *Abbot Suger of St-Denis: Church and State in Early Twelfth-Century France*, Medieval World (London, 1998).

Green, M. H., 'The Re-Creation of Pantegni, Practica, Book VIII', in *Constantine the African and 'Ali ibn al-'Abbas al-Magusi: The 'Pantegni' and Related Texts*, ed. C. Burnett and D. Jacquart, Studies in Ancient Medicine 10 (Leiden, 1994), pp. 121–6.

———, 'Gendering the History of Women's Healthcare', *Gender and History* 20 (2008), 487–518.

———, *Making Women's Medicine Masculine: The Rise of Male Authority in Pre-Modern Gynaecology* (Oxford, 2008).

———, 'Salerno on the Thames: The Genesis of Anglo-Norman Medical Literature', in *Language and Culture in Medieval Britain: The French of England, c.1100–c. 1500*, ed. J. Wogan-Browne et al. (York, 2009), pp. 220–32.

———, 'Medical Books', in *The European Book in the Twelfth Century*, ed. E. Kwakkel and R. Thomson, Cambridge Studies in Medieval Literature 101 (Cambridge, 2018), pp. 277–92.

———, '"But of the Practica of the Pantegni he translated only three books, for it had been destroyed by the water": The Puzzle of the Practica', *Constantinus Africanus* (22 March 2018), <https://constantinusafricanus.com/2018/03/22/but-of-the-practica-of-the-pantegni-he-translated-only-three-books-for-it-had-been-destroyed-by-the-water-the-puzzle-of-the-practica/> [accessed 10 September 2020].

Gullick, M., 'An Eleventh-Century Bury Medical Manuscript', in *Bury St Edmunds and the Norman Conquest*, ed. T. Licence (Woodbridge, 2014), pp. 190–225.

Hagen, A., *Anglo-Saxon Food and Drink* (Little Downham, 2010).

Harrison, D. F., *The Bridges of Medieval England: Transport and Society, 400–1800*, Oxford Historical Monographs (Oxford, 2004).

Harvey, B., *Living and Dying in England, 1100–1540: The Monastic Experience* (Oxford, 1993).

Haskins, C. H., *The Renaissance of the Twelfth Century* (Cambridge, MA, 1927).

Hawkes, J. W., and Fasham, P. J., *Excavations on Reading Waterfront Sites, 1979–1988*, Wessex Archaeology Report 5 (Salisbury, 1997).

Hayward, P. A., 'Saints and Cults', in *A Social History of England, 900–1200*, ed. J. Crick and E. Van Houts (Cambridge, 2011), pp. 309–20.

Hindle, B. P., 'The Road Network of Medieval England and Wales', *Journal of Historical Geography* 2 (1976), 207–21.

———, 'Seasonal Variations in Travel in Medieval England', *The Journal of Transport History* 4 (1978), 170–8.

———, *Medieval Roads*, Shire Archaeology 26 (Princes Risborough, 1982).

———, *Roads, Tracks and Their Interpretation*, Know the Landscape (London, 1993).

A History of the County of Berkshire: Volume 2, ed. P. H. Ditchfield and W. Page, VCH (London, 1907).

A History of the County of Hampshire: Volume 2, ed. H. A. Doubleday and W. Page, VCH (London, 1903).

A History of the County of Staffordshire: Volume 3, ed. M. W. Greenslade and R. B. Pugh, VCH (London, 1970).

A History of the County of Staffordshire: Volume 9, Burton-on-Trent, ed. N. J. Tringham, VCH (London, 2003).

A History of the County of Suffolk: Volume 2, ed. W. Page, VCH (London, 1975).

A History of the County of Wiltshire: Volume 3, ed. R. B. Pugh and E. Crittall, VCH (London, 1956).

Horden, P., 'A Non-Natural Environment: Medicine without Doctors and the Medieval European Hospital', in *The Medieval Hospital and Medical Practice*, ed. B. S. Bowers, AVISTA Studies in the History of Medieval Technology, Science and Art 3 (Aldershot, 2007), pp. 133–46.

——, *Hospitals and Healing from Antiquity to the Later Middle Ages*, Variorum Collected Studies (Aldershot, 2008).

——, 'Medieval Medicine', in *The Oxford Handbook of the History of Medicine*, ed. M. Jackson (Oxford, 2011), pp. 40–59.

——, 'Sickness and Healing', in *The Oxford Handbook of Christian Monasticism*, ed. B. M. Kaczynski (Oxford, 2020), pp. 403–17.

Hunt, T., 'The Medical Recipes in MS. Royal 5 E. vi', *Notes and Queries* 33 (1986), 6–9.

——, 'The Anglo-Norman Book', in *The Cambridge History of the Book in Britain. Volume 2*, ed. N. J. Morgan and R. M. Thomson (Cambridge, 2008), pp. 367–80.

James, M. R., *A Descriptive Catalogue of the Manuscripts in the Library of Jesus College, Cambridge* (London, 1895).

Kealey, E. J., *Medieval Medicus: A Social History of Anglo-Norman Medicine* (Baltimore, 1981).

Kemp, B., *Reading Abbey: An Introduction to the History of the Abbey*, Reading Abbey 2 (Reading, 1968).

——, 'Reading Abbey and the Medieval Town', in *The Growth of Reading*, ed. M. Petyt (Stroud, 1993), pp. 31–55.

Ker, N. R., *Medieval Libraries of Great Britain; A List of Surviving Books*, 2nd edn (London, 1964).

Kerr, J., *Monastic Hospitality: The Benedictines in England, c. 1070–c. 1250*, Studies in the History of Medieval Religion 32 (Woodbridge, 2007).

——, 'Health and Safety in the Medieval Monasteries of Britain', *History* 93 (2008), 3–19.

——, *Life in the Medieval Cloister* (London, 2009).

Kinder, T. N., *Cistercian Europe: Architecture of Contemplation* (Grand Rapids, 2002).

Kitson, P., 'Lapidary Traditions in Anglo-Saxon England: Part 1, the Background; the Old English Lapidary', *Anglo-Saxon England* 7 (1978), 9–60.

Knowles, D., *The Monastic Order in England: A History of Its Development from the Times of St Dunstan to the Fourth Lateran Council, 940–1216*, 2nd edn (Cambridge, 1963).

Knowles, D., and Hadcock, R. N., *Medieval Religious Houses: England and Wales*, 2nd edn (London, 1971).

Koopmans, R., *Wonderful to Relate: Miracle Stories and Miracle Collecting in High Medieval England*, The Middle Ages Series (Philadelphia, 2011).

———, 'Thomas Becket and the Royal Abbey of Reading', *English Historical Review* 131 (2016), 1–30.

Kuuliala, J., *Childhood Disability and Social Integration in the Middle Ages. Constructions of Impairments in Thirteenth- and Fourteenth-Century Canonization Processes*, Studies in the History of Daily Life 4 (Turnhout, 2016).

Langmuir, G. I., 'Thomas of Monmouth: Detector of Ritual Murder', *Speculum* 39 (1984), 820–46.

Lawrence, A., 'The Artistic Influence of Durham Manuscripts', in *Anglo-Norman Durham, 1093–1193*, ed. D. Rollason, M. Harvey and M. Prestwich (Woodbridge, 1998), pp. 451–70.

Lawrence-Mathers, A., 'John of Worcester and the Science of History', *Journal of Medieval History* 39 (2013), 1–20.

Lawrence-Mathers, A., and Escobar-Vargas, C., *Magic and Medieval Society*, Seminar Studies in History (London, 2014).

Lefebvre, H., *The Production of Space*, trans. D. Nicholson-Smith (Oxford, 1991).

Lett, D., *L'Enfant des miracles: Enfances et familles au Moyen Âge (XIIe–XIIIe siècles)* (Paris, 1997).

Leyser, H., *Medieval Women: A Social History of Women in England, 450–1500* (London, 1996).

Leyser, K., 'Frederick Barbarossa, Henry II and the Hand of St James', *English Historical Review* 90 (1975), 481–506.

Linguistic Geographies: The Gough Map of Great Britain, <http://www.goughmap.org/> [accessed 24 June 2020].

Lipman, V. D., *The Jews of Medieval Norwich* (London, 1967).

Locker, M., *Landscapes of Pilgrimage in Medieval Britain* (Oxford, 2015).

Mahood, H., 'The Liminality of Care: Caring for the Sick and Needy on the Boundaries of Monasteries', *The Maladies, Miracles and Medicine of the Middle Ages: Selected Papers from the Postgraduate and Early-Career Researcher Conference, March 2014. The Reading Medievalist: A Postgraduate Journal* 2 (2015), 50–70, <http://blogs.reading.ac.uk/trm/2015/04/01/proceedings-of-the-gcms-postgraduate-conference-2015-the-maladies-miracles-and-medicine-of-the-middle-ages/> [accessed 17 July 2020].

McCall, A., *The Medieval Underworld* (New York, 1979).

McCleery, I., '"Christ More Powerful Than Galen?" The Relationship between Medicine and Miracles', in *Contextualising Miracles in the Christian West, 1100–1500: New Historical Approaches*, ed. M. M. Mesley and L. E. Wilson, Medium Ævum Monographs 32 (Oxford, 2014), pp. 127–54.

McCulloch, J. M., 'Jewish Ritual Murder: William of Norwich, Thomas of Monmouth, and the Early Dissemination of the Myth', *Speculum* 72 (1997), 698–740.

Metzler, I., *Disability in Medieval Europe: Thinking about Physical Impairment during the High Middle Ages, c. 1100–1400*, Routledge Studies in Medieval Religion and Culture 5 (London, 2006).

————, *A Social History of Disability in the Middle Ages: Cultural Considerations of Physical Impairment*, Routledge Studies in Cultural History 20 (London, 2013).

Meyvaert, P., 'The Medieval Monastic Claustrum', *Gesta* 12 (1973), 53–9.

Millea, N., *The Gough Map: The Earliest Road Map of Great Britain?*, Treasures from the Bodleian Library (Oxford, 2008).

Morrison, S. S., *Women Pilgrims in Late Medieval England: Private Piety and Public Performance*, Routledge Research in Medieval Studies 3 (London, 2000).

Moseman, C. P., and Shelton, S., 'Permanent Blindness as a Complication of Pregnancy Induced Hypertension', *Obstetrics and Gynecology* 100 (2002), 943–5.

Mynors, R. A. B., *Durham Cathedral Manuscripts to the End of the Twelfth Century* (Oxford, 1939).

Newton, H., *The Sick Child in Early Modern England, 1580–1720* (Oxford, 2014).

Nilson, B., *Cathedral Shrines of Medieval England* (Woodbridge, 2001).

Ohler, N. *The Medieval Traveller*, trans. C. Hillier (Woodbridge, 2010).

Oldfield, P., *Sanctity and Pilgrimage in Southern Italy, 1000–1200* (Cambridge, 2014).

Ordnance Survey Historical Map: Roman Britain, 6th edn (Southampton, 2010).

Orme, N., *Medieval Children* (New Haven, 2001).

Orme, N., and Webster, M., *The English Hospital, 1070–1570* (New Haven, 1995).

Oxford Dictionary of National Biography (Oxford, 2004), <https://www.oxforddnb.com/> [accessed 24 July 2020].

The Oxford Dictionary of Saints, ed. D. H. Farmer (Oxford, 1978).

Pandemic Disease in the Medieval World: Rethinking the Black Death, ed. M. H. Green, The Medieval Globe 1 (Amsterdam, 2015).

Patrick, P., *The 'Obese Medieval Monk': A Multidisciplinary Study of a Stereotype*, BAR British Series 590 (Oxford, 2014).

Paxton, F. S., '*Signa mortifera*: Death and Prognostication in Early Medieval Monastic Medicine', *Bulletin of the History of Medicine* 67 (1993), 631–50.

Phillips, K. M., *Medieval Maidens: Young Women and Gender in England, 1270–1540*, Manchester Medieval Studies (Manchester, 2003).

Pluskowski, A., *Wolves and the Wilderness in the Middle Ages* (Woodbridge, 2006).

————, 'The Wolf', in *Extinctions and Invasions: A Social History of British Fauna*, ed. T. O'Connor and N. Sykes (Oxford, 2010), pp. 68–74.

Powell, H., '"Once upon a time there was a saint. . .": Re-evaluating Folklore in Anglo-Latin Hagiography', *Folklore* 121 (2010), 171–89.

————, 'The "Miracle of Childbirth": The Portrayal of Parturient Women in Medieval Miracle Narratives', *Social History of Medicine* 25 (2012), 795–811.

————, 'Following in the Footsteps of Christ: Text and Context in the *Vita S. Mildrethae*', *Medium Aevum* 82 (2013), 23–43.

————, 'Pilgrimage, Performance and Miracle Cures in the Twelfth-Century *Miracula* of St Æbbe', in *Medicine, Healing and Performance*, ed. E. Gemi-Iordanou et al. (Oxford, 2014), pp. 71–85.

————, 'Saints, Pilgrimage and Landscape in Early Medieval Kent *c.* 800–1220', in *Early Medieval Kent, 800–1220*, ed. S. Sweetinburgh, Kent History Project 10 (Woodbridge, 2016), 133–53.

Rawcliffe, C., *The Hospitals of Medieval Norwich*, Studies in East Anglian History 2 (Norwich, 1995).

————, '"On the Threshold of Eternity": Care for the Sick in East Anglian Monasteries', in *East Anglia's History: Studies in Honour of Norman Scarfe*, ed. C. Harper-Bill, C. Rawcliffe and R. G. Wilson (Woodbridge, 2002), pp. 41–72.

————, 'Curing Bodies and Healing Souls: Pilgrimage and the Sick in Medieval East Anglia', in *Pilgrimage: The English Experience from Becket to Bunyan*, ed. C. Morris and P. Roberts (Cambridge, 2002), pp. 108–40.

————, 'Sickness and Health', in *Medieval Norwich*, ed. C. Rawcliffe and R. Wilson (London, 2004), pp. 301–26.

————, *Leprosy in Medieval England* (Woodbridge, 2006).

————, 'Health and Disease', in *A Social History of England, 900–1200*, ed. J. Crick and E. Van Houts (Cambridge, 2011), pp. 66–75.

————, 'Medical Practice and Theory', in *A Social History of England, 900–1200*, ed. J. Crick and E. Van Houts (Cambridge, 2011), pp. 391–401.

————, *Urban Bodies: Communal Health in Late Medieval English Towns and Cities* (Woodbridge, 2013).

Reaney, P. H., *The Place-Names of Cambridgeshire and the Isle of Ely*, English Place-Name Society 19 (Cambridge, 1943).

Riddle, J. M., 'Pseudo-Dioscorides' *Ex herbis feminis* and Early Medieval Botany', *Journal of the History of Biology* 14 (1981), 43–81.

Risse, G. B., *Mending Bodies, Saving Souls: A History of Hospitals* (Oxford, 1999).

Rose, E. M., *The Murder of William of Norwich: The Origins of the Blood Libel in Medieval Europe* (Oxford, 2015).

Rosenthal, J. T., *Old Age in Late Medieval England*, The Middle Ages Series (Philadelphia, 1996).

Roth, C., *A History of the Jews in England*, 3rd edn (Oxford, 1964).

Rubenstein, J., 'Liturgy against History: The Competing Visions of Lanfranc and Eadmer of Canterbury', *Speculum* 74 (1999), 279–309.

Rubin, M., 'Making a Martyr: William of Norwich and the Jews', *History Today* 60 (2010), 48–54.

Salter, R. J., 'Memory, Myth, and Creating the Cult of St Æbbe of Coldingham', *Journal of Medieval Monastic Studies* 9 (2020), 31–49.

————, 'Minors and the Miraculous: The Cure-Seeking Experiences of Children in Twelfth-Century English Hagiography', in *Kids Those Days: Children in Medieval Culture*, ed. L. Preston-Matto and M. A. Valante (Leiden, 2021), 67–94.

————, 'Beyond the *Miracula*: Practices and Experiences of Lay Devotion at the Cult of St Æbbe, Coldingham', in *Northern Lights. New Directions in Late Medieval Insular Sanctity*, ed. C. Whitehead et al. (Turnhout, forthcoming).

Savage-Smith, E., 'Were the Four Humours Fundamental to Medieval Islamic Medical Practice?', in *The Body in Balance: Humoral Medicines in Practice*, ed. P. Horden and E. Hsu, Epistemologies of Healing 13 (New York, 2013), pp. 89–106.

Scott, R. A., *The Gothic Enterprise: A Guide to Understanding the Medieval Cathedral* (Berkeley, 2011).

Sears, E., *The Ages of Man: Medieval Interpretations of the Life Cycle* (Princeton, 1986).

Shahar, S., *Childhood in the Middle Ages* (London, 1990).

————, *Growing Old in the Middle Ages: 'Winter clothes us in shadow and pain'*, trans. Y. Lota (London, 1997).

Sigal, P.-A., *L'Homme et le miracle dans la France médiévale (XIe–XIIe siècle)* (Paris, 1985).

Siraisi, N., *Medieval and Early Renaissance Medicine: An Introduction to Knowledge and Practice* (Chicago, 1990).

Skinner, P., *Health and Medicine in Early Medieval Southern Italy*, The Medieval Mediterranean 11 (Leiden, 1997).

Stenton, F., 'The Road System of Medieval England', *The Economic History Review* 7 (1936), 1–21.

Sumption, J., *Pilgrimage* (London, 2002).

———, *The Age of Pilgrimage: The Medieval Journey to God* (Mahwah, NJ, 2003).

Sweetinburgh, S., *The Role of the Hospital in Medieval England: Gift-Giving and the Spiritual Economy* (Dublin, 2004).

Talbot, C., *Medicine in Medieval England*, Oldbourne History of Science Library (London, 1967).

Taylor, B., 'The Hand of St James', *Berkshire Archaeological Journal* 75 (1994–97), 97–102.

Theilmann, J., and Cate, F., 'A Plague of Plagues: The Problem of Plague Diagnosis in Medieval England', *Journal of Interdisciplinary History* 37 (2007), 371–93.

Thomson, R. M., *A Descriptive Catalogue of the Medieval Manuscripts in Worcester Cathedral Library* (Cambridge, 2001).

Thouroude, V., 'Medicine after Baldwin: The Evidence of BL, Royal 12. C. xxiv', in *Bury St Edmunds and the Norman Conquest*, ed. T. Licence (Woodbridge, 2014), pp. 247–57.

———, 'Sickness, Disability, and Miracle Cures: Hagiography in England, c.700–c.1200' (unpublished doctoral thesis, University of Oxford, 2015).

Tomalin, D., 'St Catherine's Oratory', *Archaeological Journal* 163 (2006), 51.

Touati, F.-O., 'How Is a University Born? Montpellier before Montpellier', *CIAN-Revista de Historia de las Universidades* 21 (2018), 41–78.

Trenery, C., *Madness, Medicine and Miracle in Twelfth-Century England* (Abingdon, 2019).

Tudor, V., 'Reginald of Durham and St Godric of Finchale: A Study of a Twelfth-Century Hagiographer and His Major Subject' (unpublished doctoral thesis, University of Reading, 1979).

———, 'The Misogyny of Saint Cuthbert', *Archaeologia Aeliana*, 5th series 12 (1984), 157–67.

Turner, P., 'Places of Worship in Britain and Ireland 1150–1350: An Introduction', in *Places of Worship in Britain and Ireland 1150–1350*, ed. P. S. Barnwell, Rewley House Studies in the Historic Environment 7 (Donington, 2018), pp. 1–9.

Van Ardsall, A., *Medieval Herbal Remedies: The Old English Herbarium and Anglo-Saxon Medicine* (New York, 2002).

Vauchez, A., *Sainthood in the Later Middle Ages*, trans. J. Birrell (Cambridge, 1997).

Voigts, L. E., 'A New Look at a Manuscript Containing the Old English Translation of the *Herbarium Apulei*', *Manuscripta* 20 (1976), 40–60.

Voigts, L. E., and McVaugh, M. R., *A Latin Technical Phlebotomy and Its Middle English Translation*, Transactions of the American Philosophical Society 74.2 (Philadelphia, 1984).

Von Daum Tholl, S., 'Life according to the Rule: A Monastic Modification of Mandatum Imagery in the Peterborough Psalter', *Gesta* 33 (1994), 151–8.

Waldron, T., 'Nutrition and the Skeleton', in *Food in Medieval England: Diet and Nutrition*, ed. C. M. Woolgar, D. Serjeantson and T. Waldron, Medieval History and Archaeology (Oxford, 2006), pp. 254–66.

Waller, R., 'Archaeological Resource Assessment of the Isle of Wight: Early Medieval Period', Oxford Archaeology (2006), 1–8, <https://oxfordarchaeology.com/images/pdfs/Solent_Thames/County_resource_assessments/Early_Medieval_IOW.pdf> [accessed 18 July 2020].

Ward, B., *Miracles and the Medieval Mind: Theory, Record and Event, 1000–1215* (Philadelphia, 1987).

Watson, S., 'The Origins of the English Hospital', *Transactions of the Royal Historical Society* 16 (2006), 75–94.

———, *On Hospitals: Welfare, Law, and Christianity in Western Europe, 400–1320*, Oxford Studies in Medieval European History (Oxford, 2020).

Webb, D., 'Women Pilgrims of the Middle Ages', *History Today* 48 (1998), 20–6.

———, *Pilgrimage in Medieval England* (London, 2000).

———, *Medieval European Pilgrimage*, European Culture and Society (Basingstoke, 2002).

Webster, P., *King John and Religion*, Studies in the History of Medieval Religion 43 (Woodbridge, 2015).

Wells, E. J., 'Making "Sense" of the Pilgrimage Experience of the Medieval Church', *Peregrinations: Journal of Medieval Art and Architecture* 3 (2011), 122–46.

Whatley, G., '*Vita Erkenwaldi*: An Anglo-Norman's Life of an Anglo-Saxon Saint', *Manuscripta* 27 (1983), 67–81.

———, 'Heathens and Saints: St Erkenwald in Its Legendary Context', *Speculum* 61 (1986), 330–63.

Wheatley, E., *Stumbling Blocks before the Blind: Medieval Constructions of Disability*, Corporealities: Discourses of Disability (Ann Arbor, 2010).

Whitehead, C., 'A Scottish or English Saint? The Shifting Sanctity of St Aebbe of Coldingham', in *New Medieval Literatures 19*, ed. P. Knox et al. (Cambridge, 2019), pp. 1–42.

Williams, J., *Mappa Mundi and the Chained Library: Treasures of Hereford Cathedral*, 2nd edn (Norwich, 2005).

Williams, S., *The Gregorian Epoch: Reformations, Revolutions, Reaction?*, Problems in European Civilization (Boston, 1964).

Wilson, D. M., *The Bayeux Tapestry: The Complete Tapestry in Colour: With Introduction, Description and Commentary* (London, 1985).

Wilson, L. E., 'Conceptions of the Miraculous: Natural Philosophy and Medical Knowledge in the Thirteenth-Century *Miracula* of St Edmund of Abingdon', in *Contextualising Miracles in the Christian West, 1100–1500: New Historical Approaches*, ed. M. M. Mesley and L. E. Wilson, Medium Ævum Monographs 32 (Oxford, 2014), pp. 99–125.

Woolgar, C. M., 'Meat and Dairy Products in Late Medieval England', in *Food in Medieval England: Diet and Nutrition*, ed. C. M. Woolgar, D. Serjeantson and T. Waldron, Medieval History and Archaeology (Oxford, 2006), pp. 88–101.

Yarrow, S., *Saints and Their Communities: Miracle Stories in Twelfth-Century England*, Oxford Historical Monographs (Oxford, 2006).

——, 'Narrative, Audience and the Negotiation of Community in Twelfth-Century English Miracle Collections', in *Elite and Popular Religion*, ed. K. Cooper and J. Gregory, Studies in Church History 42 (Woodbridge, 2006), pp. 65–77.

——, 'Pilgrimage', in *The Routledge History of Medieval Christianity 1050–1500*, ed. R. Swanson (London, 2015), pp. 159–71.

Ziegler, J., *Medicine and Religion c.1300: The Case of Arnau de Vilanova*, Oxford Historical Monographs (Oxford, 1998).

Index

Personal names of individuals recorded within accounts of miraculous healing are followed with the name of the hagiographic source in squared brackets.

complexions, the   31–2, 47, 86, 87 *see also* humours, the
Conchubranus   8, 9
Constantine the African   28, 29, 39, 44, 51, 74, 75, 82
Cottenham   193, 195, 201
Cowes   165
Cranwich   167
cure-seekers
    ailments of *see* individual health complaints
    children and youths as   14–15, 16, 21, 24, 63, 67, 76, 79, 80, 82, 93, 100, 102, 103, 105, 111, 112–15, 117, 118, 123, 128, 133, 137, 140, 141, 142, 143, 208, 210
    companions and supporters of   100, 113, 116, 117, 128, 144, 159, 160, 162, 166, 168, 170, 171, 172, 173, 174, 175, 184, 196, 197
    elderly cure-seekers   23, 100, 106–7, 108, 111, 112, 115–17, 167, 170, 195, 209, 210
    gender of   2, 69–73, 92, 93–6, 111, 117, 119, 160, 180, 184, 187, 209
    monks and clerics as   54, 55, 74–5, 82, 92, 103–11, 140–1, 118, 119, 131 145, 169, 207, 209
    names of   95, 96, 101–3 *see also* individually named cure-seekers
    occupations of (laity)   67, 96, 101–3, 118, 134, 160, 182, 196, 200, 203, 207
    patterns of cure-seeking   15, 62, 64, 68, 88, 89, 91, 93, 102, 103, 105–6, 118, 123, 126, 131, 134, 136, 203
    and pilgrimage *see peregrini* (pilgrims)
    social-status of   2, 47, 77, 91, 92, 93, 95, 96–101, 102, 115 119, 133, 138, 142, 143, 165, 179, 183–4, 187, 191, 193, 196, 197, 209, 213
    travel *see* travel
Cuthbert of Canterbury (archbishop)   159
Cuthbert of Northumbria (bishop, saint)   4, 50, 85, 93, 187, 208

Damigeron   46

deafness (and other ear afflictions)   24, 100, 101, 116, 117, 139, 197, 198, 203, 204
deafness and muteness (ear and speech impediments)   197, 203
Demaitre, Luke   66
difficult labour   16, 47, 68–9, 77–9, 95, 139, 140, 207
disability studies   18, 20
Dioscorides   39, 45
Dissolution of the Monasteries, the   37
Dover   148, 150, 164, 174
dropsy   82, 124
Duffy, Eamon   1, 14, 33
Dunfermline Abbey   190–1
Dunstan (archbishop, saint)   5, 6–7, 108, 110, 113, 122, 124, 130, 142, 193, 194, 202, 210
Durham Cathedral Priory   4, 9, 10, 37, 38, 39, 40, 43, 46, 85, 86, 87, 93, 137, 138, 181, 187, 208

Eadmer of Canterbury   6, 7, 38, 41, 78, 80, 116, 127, 128, 162, 193
Earconwald (saint)   4
Earley   124
East Lothian   137
Ecgfrith of Northumbria (king)   7, 8
Edgar of Scotland (king)   10
Edinburgh   84, 137, 138, 148, 169, 199, 200, 208
Edmund of Abingdon (archbishop, saint)   87
Edmund of Bury (king, saint)   129, 131, 141, 155, 168
Edward Haver [*M. Jacobi*]   139, 186, 204
    daughter of   139, 186
Edward the Confessor (king, saint)   48, 187
Eliade, Mircea   178
Ely   7–8, 123–4, 129, 148, 150, 153, 154, 163, 177
Ely Cathedral Priory   7–8, 42, 53, 55, 82, 98, 99, 104, 123–4, 129, 133, 140, 141, 147, 150, 154, 155, 163, 183, 187, 191, 193, 195, 196